LABORATORY
INSTRUMENTATION

Edited by

M. Robert Hicks, B.S., M.S., M.T. (ASCP)
Assistant Professor of Pathology and Microbiology
Assistant Professor, Division of Medical Technology, School of Allied
    Health Professions
University of Nebraska Medical Center;
Clinical Chemist, University Hospital
Omaha, Nebraska

Mary C. Haven, B.S., M.S.
Assistant Professor of Pathology and Microbiology
Assistant Professor, Division of Medical Technology, School of Allied
    Health Professions
University of Nebraska Medical Center;
Clinical Chemist, University Hospital
Omaha, Nebraska

Jerald R. Schenken, B.S., M.D.
Clinical Professor of Pathology and Microbiology
University of Nebraska Medical Center;
Director of Pathology
Nebraska Methodist Hospital and Children's Memorial Hospital
Omaha, Nebraska

C. A. McWhorter, M.D.
Professor of Pathology and Microbiology
University of Nebraska Medical Center
Omaha, Nebraska

With 26 Contributors

LABORATORY INSTRUMENTATION

Third Edition

J. B. LIPPINCOTT COMPANY

Philadelphia

London   St. Louis

Mexico City   São Paulo

New York   Sydney

Acquisitions Editor: Lisa Biello
Sponsoring Editor: Delois Patterson
Manuscript Editor: Margaret E. Maxwell
Indexer: Ann Cassar
Design Director: Tracy Baldwin
Design Coordinator: Anne O'Donnell
Production Supervisor: J. Corey Gray
Production Coordinator: Kathleen R. Diamond
Compositor: General Graphic Services
Printer/Binder: R. R. Donnelley & Sons Company
Cover Printer: Algen Press Corp.

Third Edition

6   5   4   3   2

Library of Congress Cataloging-in-Publication Data

Main entry under title:

Laboratory instrumentation.

   Includes bibliographies and index.
   1. Medical laboratories—Equipment and supplies.
2. Diagnosis, Laboratory—Instruments. I. Hicks,
M. Robert, DATE [DNLM: 1. Laboratories.
2. Technology, Medical—instrumentation.
QV 26 L123]
RB36.2.L33   1986   616.07'5'028   86-28
ISBN 0-397-50777-1

The authors and publisher have exerted every effort to
ensure that drug selection and dosage set forth in this text
are in accord with current recommendations and practice
at the time of publication. However, in view of ongoing
research, changes in government regulations, and the
constant flow of information relating to drug therapy and
drug reactions, the reader is urged to check the package
insert for each drug for any changes in indications and
dosage and for added warnings and precautions. This is
particularly important when the recommended agent is a
new or infrequently employed drug.

CONTRIBUTORS

Gene d'Allemand, B.S., M.S., M.T. (ASCP)
Assistant Chief Technologist, Pathology Center, Nebraska Methodist Hospital, Omaha, Nebraska
Chapter 3

John H. Eckfeldt, M.D., Ph.D.
Associate Professor of Laboratory Medicine and Pathology, University of Minnesota
    Medical School;
Director, Clinical Chemistry, Department of Laboratory Medicine and Pathology, University of
    Minnesota, Minneapolis, Minnesota
Chapter 20

Steven M. Faynor, B.A., Ph.D.
Director of Clinical Chemistry and Toxicology, International Clinical Laboratory,
    Nashville, Tennessee
Chapter 9

Ronald D. Feld, B.S., Ph.D.
Associate Professor of Pathology, University of Iowa College of Medicine; Director of Core
    Chemistry, University of Iowa Hospital and Clinics, Iowa City, Iowa
Chapter 21

Dale B. Haack, B.S., M.E., M.S.E.E.
Consulting Engineer, Granger, Indiana
Chapter 1

Guy T. Haven, B.S., M.D., Ph.D.
Medical Director, Louisiana Reference Laboratories, Baton Rouge, Louisiana
Chapter 15

Mary C. Haven, B.S., M.S.
Assistant Professor of Pathology and Microbiology,
Assistant Professor, Division of Medical Technology, School of Allied Health Professions,
    University of Nebraska Medical Center;
Clinical Chemist, University Hospital and Clinics, Omaha, Nebraska
Chapters 7, 15

Marietta M. Henry, A.B., M.S., M.D.
Clinical Assistant Professor of Pathology and Microbiology,
University of Nebraska Medical Center;
Pathologist, Bishop Clarkson Memorial Hospital, Omaha, Nebraska
Chapter 22

Marilyn K. Hiatt, B.A., M.T. (ASCP)
Clinical Project Manager, System Associates, Inc., Naperville, Illinois
Chapter 14

M. Robert Hicks, B.S., M.S., M.T. (ASCP)
Assistant Professor of Pathology and Microbiology,
Assistant Professor, Division of Medical Technology, School of Allied Health Professions,
University of Nebraska Medical Center;
Clinical Chemist, University Hospital and Clinics, Omaha, Nebraska
Chapters 4, 5

Jeffrey A. Huth, B.S., Ph.D.
Assistant Professor of Pathology and Microbiology, University of Nebraska Medical Center;
Clinical Chemist, University Hospital and Clinics, Omaha, Nebraska
Chapter 8

Carl R. Jolliff, B.S., SMAAM, CLSp (NCA)
Director, Clinical Laboratories Section, Lincoln Clinic, Lincoln, Nebraska
Chapter 12

Richard D. Juel, B.S., M.D.
Pathology Consultants, El Paso, Texas
Chapter 11

Ernest J. Kiser, B.S., M.S., Ph.D.
Director, Research and Development, Baker Instruments Corp., Allentown, Pennsylvania
Chapter 14

Arden E. Larsen, B.S., M.S., Ph.D., M.T. (ASCP)
Associate Professor of Pathology and Microbiology,
Associate Professor, Division of Medical Technology, School of Allied Health Professions,
University of Nebraska Medical Center, Omaha, Nebraska
Chapter 13

Arthur L. Larsen, B.A., M.D.
Professor Emeritus of Pathology and Microbiology, University of Nebraska Medical Center,
Omaha, Nebraska
Chapter 13

Catherine Leiendecker–Foster, B.S., M.S., CLS (NCA)
Instructor, Department of Laboratory Medicine and Pathology,
University of Minnesota Medical School;
Supervisor, Clinical Chemistry and Toxicology, Veterans Administration Medical Center,
Minneapolis, Minnesota
Chapter 20

Martin R. Lohff, B.S., M.D.
Clinical Assistant Professor of Pathology and Microbiology,
University of Nebraska Medical Center;
Associate Pathologist, Nebraska Methodist Hospital, Omaha, Nebraska
Chapter 6

Joan F. Mares, B.S., M.T. (ASCP), SH
Instructor, Division of Medical Technology, School of Allied Health Professions,
University of Nebraska Medical Center;
Supervisor, Hematology Section, Clinical Laboratories, University of Nebraska Hospital and
Clinics, Omaha, Nebraska
Chapter 16

Jim Noffsinger, B.S., M.S., Ph.D.
Clinical Assistant Professor, Division of Medical Technology, School of Allied Health Professions,
University of Nebraska Medical Center;
Clinical Chemist, Bishop Clarkson Memorial Hospital, Omaha, Nebraska
Chapters 13, 21

John D. Olson, B.S., B.A., M.D., Ph.D.
Associate Professor of Pathology, University of Iowa College of Medicine;
Director of Laboratories, University of Iowa Hospital and Clinics, Iowa City, Iowa
Chapter 17

Mary Ann Steinrauf, B.S., M.T. (ASCP)
Clinical Assistant Instructor, Division of Medical Technology, School of Allied Health Professions,
University of Nebraska Medical Center;
Clinical Chemist, Bishop Clarkson Memorial Hospital, Omaha, Nebraska
Chapters 10, 11

Wesley K. Tanaka, B.A., Ph.D.
Associate Professor, Chemistry Department and Allied Health Professions, University of
Wisconsin—Eau Claire, Eau Claire, Wisconsin
Chapter 19

Judith Thompson, B.S., M.S., M.T. (ASCP)
Product Manager, Laboratory Filtration Products, Amicon Division, W. R. Grace,
Danvers, Massachusetts
Chapter 2

Thomas L. Williams, B.S., M.D.
Clinical Assistant Professor of Pathology and Microbiology,
University of Nebraska Medical Center;
Associate Pathologist, Nebraska Methodist Hospital and Children's Memorial Hospital,
Omaha, Nebraska
Chapter 18

David L. Witte, B.A., M.D., Ph.D.
Laboratory Director, Laboratory Control, Limited, Ottumwa, Iowa
Chapter 19

PREFACE

The need for a book on laboratory instrumentation is as great today as it was at the time of the first two editions of *Laboratory Instrumentation*. The field of laboratory medicine is still expanding at a rapid pace. When I visited the technical exhibits at the fall meeting of the ASCP–CAP in Las Vegas in 1985, I was again greatly impressed with the number and variety of new instruments. It is indeed challenging, but difficult, to stay current with all of these new scientific and technical advancements. We have attempted to meet the challenge of this ever-changing and increasing knowledge and instrumentation as best we can.

The content and references of all chapters of *Laboratory Instrumentation, Third Edition* have been updated. Many chapters have been completely revised. We have added new chapters on automated chemistry, hematology, coagulation, and microbiology instruments.

The purposes of this book are the same as those originally set forward in the two previous editions.

1. To attempt to bridge the gaps that exist between the various textbooks on theory and the instrument manuals, provided in most cases by the manufacturers.
2. To attempt to explain the functions of the instrument's components to the student.

The great variation in the complexity of instrumentation makes understanding instrument operation difficult. It is hoped that teaching the basic principles of instrument operation will result in an improved ability to read and understand instrument manuals. This should be particularly helpful in introducing new instruments into the laboratory. The sections on operation, calibration, application, operational checks systems, and definitions make this an excellent text for a lecture course in instrumentation for medical technology students. Much of the information here will be invaluable to pathologists, pathology residents, and clinical chemists as well as to analytical chemists, biochemists, and college students in the physical sciences.

It should be clearly understood at the outset that reference in this book to any specific instrument is not an endorsement of that instrument, and that the failure to mention any specific instrument is in no way an indication of inferiority or unacceptability.

C. A. McWhorter, M.D.

PREFACE TO
FIRST EDITION

No field of medicine is expanding as rapidly as laboratory medicine. This expansion is primarily the result of the development of new procedures and the practical application of research to actual practice in the laboratory. It has also been stimulated by the development of refined instrumentation in other fields and the application of these to clinical pathology.

A combined medical technology program was developed through the recent affiliation of the Schools of Medical Technology at the Bishop Clarkson Memorial Hospital and the Nebraska Methodist Hospital with the University of Nebraska at Omaha and the University of Nebraska College of Medicine. With this enlarged faculty and revised curriculum, it became apparent that an instructional book on instrumentation would be a necessity in the education of medical technologists.

The purposes of *Laboratory Instrumentation* are the following:

1. To attempt to bridge the gaps that exist between the various textbooks on theory and the instrument manuals, provided in most cases by the manufacturers.
2. To attempt to explain the functions of the instrument's components to the student.

The great variation in the complexity of instrumentation makes understanding instrument operation difficult. It is hoped that teaching the basic principles of instrument operation will result in improved ability to read and understand instrument manuals. This should be particularly helpful in introducing new instruments into the laboratory. The sections on operation, calibration, application, operational checks systems, and definitions make this an excellent text for a lecture course in instrumentation for medical technology students. Much of the information here should be invaluable to pathologists, pathology residents, and clinical chemists as well as analytical chemists, biochemists, and college students in the physical sciences.

It should be clearly understood at the outset that reference in this manual to any specific instrument is not an endorsement of such instrument, and that the failure to mention any specific instrument is in no way an indication of inferiority or unacceptability.

I wish to express my sincere gratitude both to those who have contributed as authors and to those who have revised and edited this book.

C. A. McWhorter, M.D.

ACKNOWLEDGMENTS

We, the editors of *Laboratory Instrumentation, Third Edition*, wish to express our appreciation to our families and friends for their help, understanding, encouragement, and tolerance of our preoccupation during the preparation of this manuscript. We also wish to thank the authors for their advice and willing contributions in the composition and arrangement of this book.

M. Robert Hicks
Mary C. Haven
Jerald R. Schenken
C. A. McWhorter

CONTENTS

GLOSSARY OF ABBREVIATIONS

Word/Phrase Abbreviations

A	absorbance
ac	alternating current
A/D	analog to digital
alb	albumin
alk phos	alkaline phosphatase
bp	boiling point
BUN	blood urea nitrogen
CSF	cerebrospinal fluid
dc	direct current
DVM	digital voltmeter
e^-	electron
E	energy*
E	sensitivity*
EDTA	ethylenediaminetetraacetate
emf	electromotive force
Eq	equivalent
GLC	gas liquid chromatography
glu	glucose
Hct	hematocrit
Hgb	hemoglobin
I	current
ICU	intensive care unit
LC	liquid chromatography
ln	natural logarithm, $\log_e$
m	mass
MCH	mean corpuscular hemoglobin
MCHC	mean corpuscular hemoglobin concentration
MCT	mean cell threshold
MCV	mean cell volume*
MCV	mean corpuscular volume*
mp	melting point
pCO_2	partial pressure of carbon dioxide
pH	negative log of hydrogen-ion concentration
pO_2	partial pressure of oxygen
PCV	packed cell volume
R	resistance
RBC	red blood cell (erythrocyte)
RCF	relative centrifugal force
SD	standard deviation
SRM	standard reference materials
$\%T$	percent transmittance
T. bili	total bilirubin
TLC	thin layer chromatography
TP	total protein
TS	total solids
UV	ultraviolet
W	weight
WBC	white blood cell (leukocyte)

*Even though the same abbreviation represents two different terms, the context in which the abbreviation is used will make its meaning clear.

xvii

Unit Abbreviations

A	ampere	mEq/liter	milliequivalents per liter
Å	angstrom	MeV	million electron volts
C	coulomb	mg	milligram
°C	degree centigrade	ml	milliliter
cpm	counts per minute	mm	millimeter
cps	cycles per second	mm Hg	millimeters of mercury
dpm	disintegrations per minute	mOsm	milliosmolar
eV	electron volt	mV	millivolt
F	faraday	μ	micron
ft	foot	N	normal
g	gram	nm	nanometer
g	gravity	nsec	nanosecond
hr	hour	Ω	ohm
Hz	Hertz (cycles per second)	Osm	osmolar
in²	square inches	psi	pounds per square inch
J	joule	rpm	revolutions per minute
°K	degree Kelvin	sec	second
λ	wavelength	u	unified atomic units
lb	pound	V	volt
mμ	millimicron	W	watt
M	molar		

Prefixes for Decimal Factors

10^3	kilo	10^{-6}	micro
10^{-1}	deci	10^{-9}	nano
10^{-2}	centi	10^{-12}	pico
10^{-3}	milli		

Common Elements

Al	Aluminum	Cr	Chromium	Mg	Magnesium	Rn	Radon
Ar	Argon	Co	Cobalt	Hg	Mercury	Se	Selenium
Ba	Barium	Cu	Copper	Mo	Molybdenum	Si	Silicon
Be	Beryllium	F	Fluorine	Ne	Neon	Ag	Silver
Bi	Bismuth	Au	Gold	Ni	Nickel	Na	Sodium
B	Boron	He	Helium	N	Nitrogen	S	Sulfur
Br	Bromine	H	Hydrogen	O	Oxygen	Sn	Tin
Cd	Cadmium	I	Iodine	Pd	Palladium	W	Tungsten
Ca	Calcium	Fe	Iron	P	Phosphorus	U	Uranium
C	Carbon	La	Lanthanum	Pt	Platinum	Xe	Xenon
Cs	Cesium	Pb	Lead	K	Potassium	Zn	Zinc
Cl	Chlorine	Li	Lithium	Ra	Radium		

LABORATORY INSTRUMENTATION

1

PRINCIPLES
OF ELECTRICITY

Dale B. Haack

Definitions

Alternating Current: A current that is periodically changing direction and value.

Battery: A device constructed from solid and/or liquid chemicals that, through chemical action, will cause electrons (current) to flow from the negative to the positive battery terminals.

Capacitor: An electronic circuit component that utilizes the phenomenon of the attraction of opposite charges. This makes the capacitor capable of storing electrical energy. Capacitor values are expressed in farads.

Circuit: The total sum of all the components and hardware that comprise the electrical portion of the instrument being considered.

Current: An actual flow of electrons in an electrical conductor. The amount of current flow is quantitatively expressed in units of amperes.

D'Arsonval Galvanometer: An electromechanical device for measuring direct current. It consists of a current-carrying coil that is suspended between the poles of a permanent magnet. The deflection of this coil is indicated by a pointer-needle, and the amount of deflection is proportional to the current in the coil.

Direct Current: This current is always flowing in the same direction at some fixed voltage level.

Electric Field: That space surrounding an object that is electrically charged. An additional electrical charge will have a force exerted on it if it is brought into the vicinity of an electric field.

Magnetic Field: The field of electric activity surrounding any current-carrying conductor. The magnetic field intensity can be of sufficient strength to attract nonmagnetic soft ferrous materials.

Meter Movement: That part of an instrument used to measure an electrical activity that will mechanically display the quantitative value.

Ohm's Law: The quantitative relationship between volts, amperes, and resistance is expressed by $E = IR$ and is referred to as Ohm's Law.

Photocell: A device that will cause a flow of current when activated by a light source.

Potentiometer: A variable resistor used in a circuit to allow selection of a voltage value to meet circuit requirements.

Resistance: The impedance offered to the flow of electrons by a given conductive material is expressed in units of ohms of resistance.

Resistor: A precision-made device, usually of compacted carbon, used in electronic circuits to control and regulate the flow of current. Resistor values are expressed in ohms.

Rheostat: A resistor whose value can be easily changed by means of a knob or screwdriver to meet changing circuit requirements.

Scintillation Phosphors: Materials that, when ionized by the passage of high-speed electrons or γ rays, emit a very small amount of light, generally in the ultraviolet or blue part of the spectrum.

Thermocouple: A device that will develop a voltage potential when heat is applied to its bimetal thermojunction.

Voltage: That force that makes electrons flow in a wire, transistor, or any electrically conductive material.

Wheatstone Bridge: Circuit used to measure an unknown resistance.

Introduction

An understanding of the basic principles of electricity and electronics will help foster an operational knowledge of the electronic apparatus found in the hospital laboratory. It is not the intent here to enable the laboratorian to attempt any equipment repairs because the sophistication of modern equipment requires a qualified expert in electronics. Because lethal voltages are present, neither removal of covers and inspection plates nor disassembly for repair purposes should ever be attempted by the uninformed.

Electrical Analogy

An analogy of the flow of electricity can be made with the common everyday occurrence of water flow. Everyone is familiar with the ability of a water faucet to regulate the amount of water that flows from it. This simple illustration will be

Figure 1-1. Water and electrical system comparison.

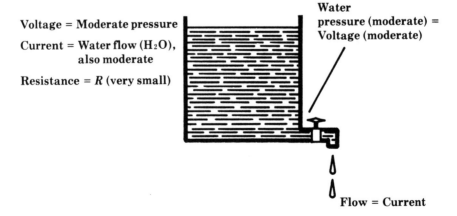

Voltage = Moderate pressure

Current = Water flow (H_2O), also moderate

Resistance = R (very small)

Water pressure (moderate) = Voltage (moderate)

Flow = Current

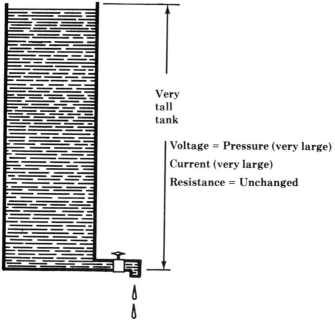

Figure 1-2.   Water height compared to large voltage potential.

developed to show how electricity can be regulated as it flows through a wire. Resistance performs this regulatory function. Several commonly used electronic components and their current applications are discussed.

Consider a large tank full of water with a small pipe at the bottom equipped with a faucet (Fig. 1-1). Assume that a pail is also under the faucet to catch the water when the faucet is opened. Compare the pressure of the water at the base of the tank (where the pipe is) to voltage. Similarly, compare the amount of water collected in the pail and measured out per unit time to a given quantity of current flow. Also, the volume of water flowing from the faucet will depend on the resistance of the outlet pipe on the bottom of the tank. This resistance to the flow of the water is the same as the resistance (R) that an electrical wire presents to the flow of an electrical current. Extreme cases to demonstrate the effects of varying any of the parameters are shown in Figures 1-2 and 1-3.

Types of Voltage and Current

The two types of current associated with voltage are direct current (dc) and alternating current (ac). We can say that the current and voltage will be of the same type in any single circuit. Because they do not function in the same manner, an ac voltage and current circuit cannot be substituted for a dc circuit. In fact, disastrous results may follow. Household voltage is an example of a common source of ac voltage. It is produced by generators that are usually driven by steam turbines or water power.

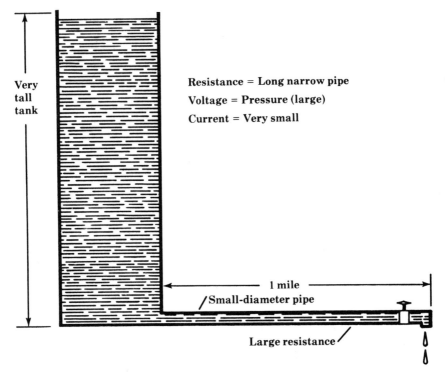

Very
tall
tank

Resistance = Long narrow pipe

Voltage = Pressure (large)

Current = Very small

1 mile

Small-diameter pipe

Large resistance

Figure 1-3.   Resistance effects on current.

A dc voltage is most easily and commonly produced by a battery. Other sources might be generators and rectifiers, which we shall treat in the electronics circuits portion of this chapter.

An ac voltage, as displayed on an oscilloscope, would appear as a wave form (Fig. 1-4). Several examples of a dc voltage on the screen of an oscilloscope are shown in Figure 1-5. The important feature of a dc voltage is the constant value it maintains. The most common application for a dc voltage is with transistor

Figure 1-4.   Waveshape of ac voltage; 60 cycles/second = frequency.

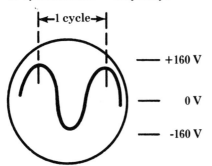

|←1 cycle→|

— +160 V

— 0 V

— -160 V

Figure 1-5.   Waveshape of dc voltage.

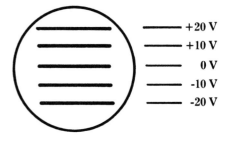

— +20 V

— +10 V

— 0 V

— -10 V

— -20 V

circuits and other electronic amplifiers. Voltage values can range from a few volts to several thousand volts.

Electricity from Chemical Action

There are primarily two sources of electrical energy for laboratory instrumentation. An electronic power supply is used when considerable amounts of current are required to power an instrument. A less expensive power source, when a simple reference voltage is required and when the current requirements are small, is a battery. Two types of batteries are discussed in this text. These batteries represent only a small part of the many power cells available for instrumental application.

PRIMARY CELL

A primary cell (dry cell) is made of a carbon rod, elemental metal case, and inorganic acids or salts (Fig. 1-6). These elements form the positive and negative poles and the electrolyte, respectively.

The primary cell is a common source of direct current for items that run the gamut from simple household flashlights to complicated laboratory instruments. A distinguishing feature of the primary cell is that the material of the cell is part of the chemical reaction that produces electricity. When exhausted, these cells cannot be recharged. The discharge reaction of the cell is irreversible because the case and electrolyte are chemically depleted during the discharge cycle.

Figure 1-6.   Cutaway section of a primary cell showing typical construction features.

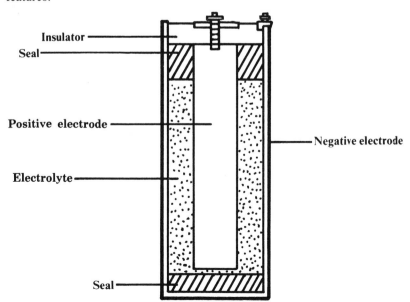

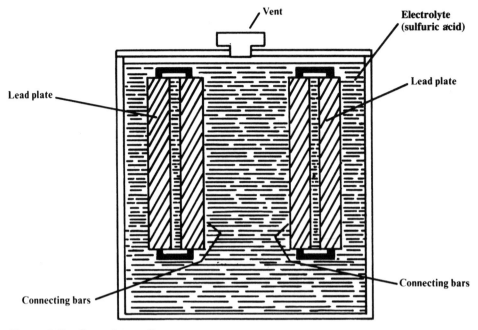

Figure 1-7. Secondary cell.

SECONDARY CELL

The secondary cell type of battery is most easily identified as the type of battery used in automobiles to start the engine, light the headlights, and run the radio and other car accessories (Fig. 1-7). It can produce large amounts of current when the power requirements are high, such as in the starter motor of an automobile. The electrolyte in the secondary cell is usually sulfuric acid. In the case of a rapid-charging cycle in which heat is likely to be produced, some of the water tends to evaporate from the electrolyte and water needs to be added. Allowing the electrolyte level to drop below the level of the plates can cause permanent

Figure 1-8. Quartz crystal showing voltage output.

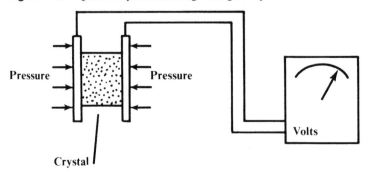

Thermocouple

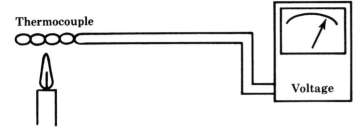

Figure 1-9. Thermocouple showing voltage output.

damage. For this reason, maintenance of proper electrolyte levels is important. During the cell discharge, the positive and negative plates change to lead peroxide. Batteries that are of the secondary cell type can be recharged to restore the battery to a fully charged condition.

Voltage Sources for Instrumentation

QUARTZ CRYSTAL

Crystals of certain materials, such as quartz, will develop an electrical charge if mechanical pressure is applied to them. Pressure applied to a quartz crystal placed between two plates results in a voltage (Fig. 1-8).

Although the actual use of pressure as a source to produce electricity is limited to a very low-power application, pressure is used in many types of equipment. Crystal microphones, headphones, phonograph pickups, and sonar equipment may use a crystal in this manner.

THERMOCOUPLE

Dissimilar metals twisted together to form a junction produce an electrical charge when heated (Fig. 1-9). This is referred to as a thermocouple. Although a thermocouple cannot generate a charge sufficient for a power source, it is useful as a temperature-indicating device. Thermocouple sensing devices are used as

Figure 1-10. Photocell where the dc voltage level varies with the intensity of light striking the selenium surface.

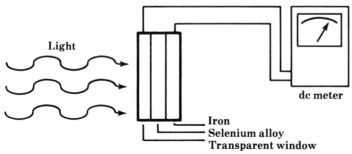

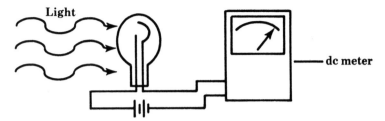

Figure 1-11. Photocell and meter circuit showing electron potential.

primary indicators in chromatography and osmometry. They are also used for temperature control in incubators and ovens.

PHOTOCELL

A photocell is constructed as shown in Figure 1-10. When light is transmitted through the transparent window and onto the selenium, an electrical charge develops across the two outside layers (selenium and iron) and can be measured with a dc voltmeter (Fig. 1-11). A light meter, such as the one commonly used in photography for determining the amount of light present, is an example of an application of this principle.

Automobile headlight dimmers and some automatic door openers use a photoelectric cell that requires a battery to furnish the electrical voltage needed for the detection of light. Photocells are used in spectrophotometers and many other laboratory instruments. In certain equipment in intensive care units, the photocell is used to activate alarm systems when a patient's heart rate, blood pressure, or respiration rate exceeds preset limits. The heart may be monitored as shown in Figure 1-12.

Electrical Controls

VARIABLE RESISTOR

Circuits often require resistors that are easily varied (as compared to the fixed-value resistor) to allow for calibration of an instrument or perhaps to allow for the speed control on a centrifuge motor. A variable resistor can be made of carbon

Figure 1-12. Heart rate monitor (side view).

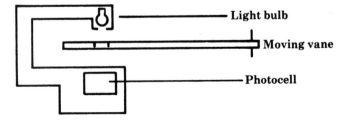

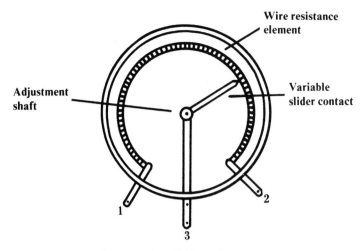

Figure 1-13.   Wire-wound variable resistor.

or wire wound on a porcelain or bakelite circular form. On this form, a contact wiper follows as the rotating shaft of the resistor is turned (Figs. 1-13 and 1-14). The material for the resistor depends on the current requirements of the system. Carbon is used for small currents and the wound wire is used for large currents.

RHEOSTAT

Variable resistors may have two or three terminals. Those with only two terminals can be used as rheostats only (Fig. 1-15).

Figure 1-14.   Carbon variable resistor.

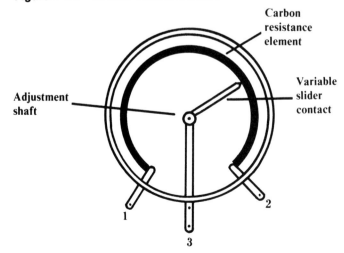

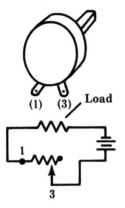

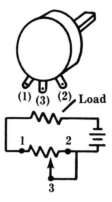

Figure 1-15. Rheostat-type two-terminal variable resistor circuit.

Figure 1-16. Three-terminal potentiometer-type circuit.

POTENTIOMETER

If three terminals of a variable resistor each connect to different parts of a circuit, the resistor is called a potentiometer. A potentiometer does not vary the total resistance between the end terminals, (*1*) and (*2*), but rather the resistance between each end, (*1*) and (*2*), and the center contact, (*3*); see Figure 1-16.

Physical Properties of Electricity

MAGNETIC FIELD

A current flowing in a wire always produces a magnetic field around it. A natural magnet does not depend on current flow from an external voltage source

Figure 1-17. The normal distribution of flux fields surrounding a magnet.

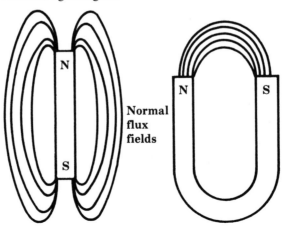

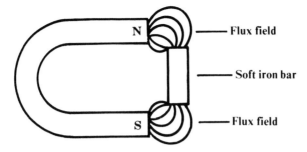

Figure 1-18. The concentration and displacement of the flux field by the action of a soft iron bar.

to produce a magnetic field. It possesses its own magnetic field due to a permanent distribution and alignment of its molecular structure (Fig. 1-17).

An interesting property of any magnetic field is that the invisible lines of force leaving one end of the magnet (north pole) and entering the other end (south pole) may be routed through a soft iron bar (Fig. 1-18). The explanation for this phenomenon is that the soft iron bar offers a path of lower resistance than the surrounding air for the flux field. With the use of a soft iron bar the lines of flux may be concentrated. The amount of concentration is limited, however, and the iron core becomes "saturated." The amount of saturation becomes a part of the characteristics of the material being used. Because some materials are stronger magnetics, they have a stronger flux field.

It can be assumed, therefore, that a current always has an associated magnetic field. The assumption can then be made that an existing magnetic field can be used to produce a voltage and cause current to flow in a conductor. A magnet can be used to generate a voltage by moving it past a wire (Fig. 1-19). A voltmeter will register a voltage in the wire. The amount of voltage generated depends on the strength of the magnet, the speed at which it is moved, and the number of turns of wire.

The flow of electrons is called current. Electrons participating in current flow

Figure 1-19. Generating a voltage by moving a magnet through a coil of wire.

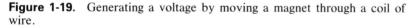

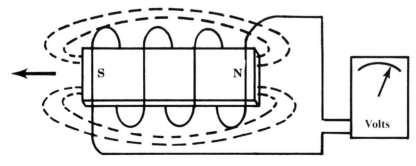

are always those in the so-called outer ring of the normal atom. The availability of the electrons varies greatly in different materials. Silver, copper, and aluminum have a very weak attractive force between the nucleus and the outer electrons and consequently are good conductors. Glass, plastics, and wood have a strong attractive force between the outer electrons and the nucleus. Hence, these materials are good insulators.

RESISTANCE

In the discussion of current, we mentioned that it is very difficult to find "free" electrons in some materials, owing to the strong force attracting them to the nucleus. These materials have, then, a high resistance. Factors other than the nature of the material that affect resistance are (1) length, (2) cross-sectional area, and (3) temperature.

1. A long conductor presents a greater resistance than a short one.
2. Resistance varies inversely with the cross-sectional area. Increasing the area reduces the resistance.
3. Increased temperature will increase wire resistance. The increased temperature will cause the atoms to hold onto the outer electrons more tightly.

Some materials, such as carbon and electrolyte solutions, lower their resistance as temperature increases. The effect of temperature on the resistance of materials such as copper and aluminum is very slight.

Measuring the Physical Properties

From the water-tank analogy we recall that voltage was compared to water pressure. In this case consider voltage to be an electron pressure that will respond something like water under certain conditions of varied pressure and resistance. The question may be asked: "How is voltage actually measured in a circuit?" Answer: "A voltmeter."

Figure 1-20.   A pivoted bar magnet showing the repulsion of like poles.

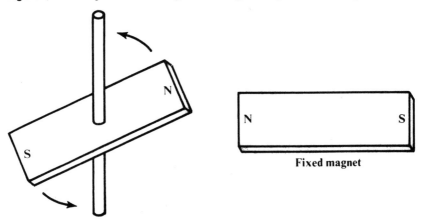

Fixed magnet

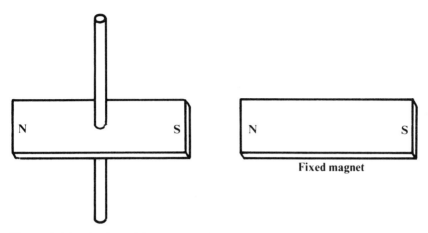

Figure 1-21. A pivoted bar magnet showing the attraction of unlike poles.

A voltmeter's construction is developed in Figures 1-20 through 1-23. A pivoted bar magnet and a fixed magnet are brought into close proximity with like-pole faces aligned as shown in Figure 1-20. The two north poles will repel each other and the pivoted bar magnet will turn until opposite poles are aligned as shown in Figure 1-21. Because opposite poles attract each other, the magnets will remain permanently in this position. The pivoted permanent magnet can now be replaced with an electromagnet (Fig. 1-22) and a voltage source. The resulting current flow in the coil of the electromagnet will magnetize the soft iron core on which the coil is wound. The direction of this current will determine the polarity

Figure 1-22. An electromagnetic circuit showing the action of electron flow.

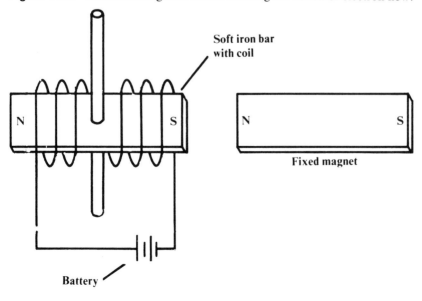

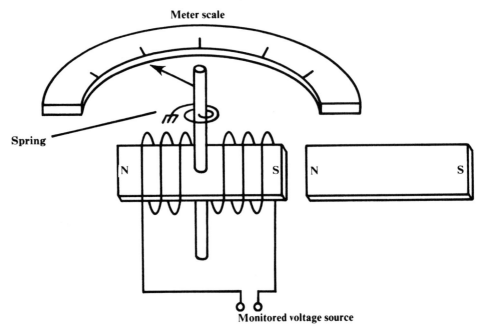

Figure 1-23.   Typical meter movement.

of the electromagnet. The pivoted electromagnet will align itself with the fixed bar magnet.

The addition of a pointer and a return spring to the shaft of the pivoted bar magnet will complete our voltmeter (Fig. 1-23). The voltage source to be measured now furnishes the current for the electromagnet portion of our voltmeter. The magnitude of the deflection of the pointer will be proportional to the voltage being measured. A meter scale, shown in Figure 1-23, is calibrated to read directly in units of voltage or any other parameter that the instrument may be measuring. The voltmeter may be incorporated into an instrument to measure parameters such as density, resistance, illuminescence, pressure, or light intensity.

The construction of an ammeter closely parallels that of a voltmeter, with one important difference. A shunt resistor is placed across the coil of the meter movement to bypass approximately 99% of the current around the coil (Fig. 1-24). This gives a very sensitive meter movement that will produce a full-scale deflection of the pointer with 0.05 mA.

VOLTAGE AND CURRENT

A voltmeter measures voltage differences across a selected portion of a circuit that is being investigated. It is not necessary to disturb the circuit in any way to make a voltage measurement (Fig. 1-25). In the case of a current measurement, the circuit being investigated is opened up and the current meter is inserted in

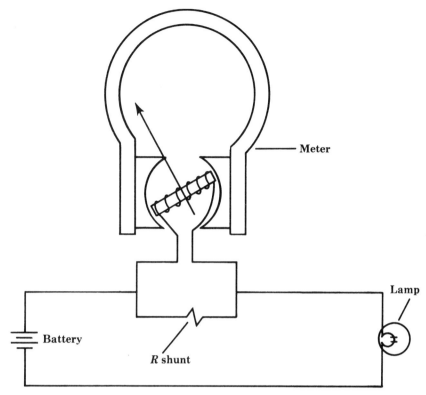

Figure 1-24. An ammeter circuit showing a shunt resistor.

series with the circuit (Fig. 1-26). It is sometimes physically impossible to make a current measurement directly; other means must be used to determine current values. This current value may be calculated using Ohm's Law if the voltage and resistance values are known.

PHOTOMULTIPLIER TUBE

The photomultiplier tube may be used alone to detect and quantify the intensity of light, or it may be used with scintillation phosphors to detect and measure β and γ rays. The amount of light generated within the phosphor is roughly proportional to the energy lost by the ray in the phosphor. It is possible, then, not only to detect a ray but also to measure the amount of its energy. These phosphor characteristics would make the scintillation detector ideal were it not for the fact that the amount of light generated by a single ray is indeed small, so small that it cannot be detected by an ordinary light detector such as a photocell. A much more sensitive device called a photomultiplier tube must be used to measure these small light flashes.

The photomultiplier has a photocathode surface that emits electrons when struck by light (Fig. 1-27). Because the total number of electrons emitted from

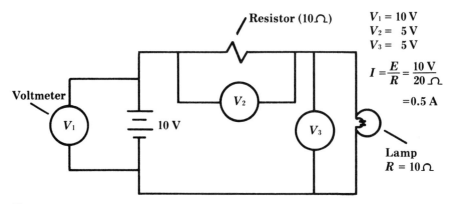

Figure 1-25.   Voltmeter placement in circuit.

the photocathode is very small, a number of multiplier stages (usually 10), called dynodes, are employed in the tube to amplify the "light signal." Each dynode is an anode at a slightly higher positive voltage than the one before so as to attract the electrons emitted from the preceding dynode stage and to accelerate them so that large numbers of electrons are emitted at each succeeding stage. Therefore, it is possible with a 10-stage photomultiplier tube to have, for each electron emitted from the photocathode, between 100,000 and 1,000,000 electrons at the output of the photomultiplier tube. The actual number of electrons at the final stage depends on parameters such as the voltage on the dynodes of the photomultiplier tube. The photomultiplier tube is used in precision spectrophotometric devices such as spectrophotometers, flame photometers, and atomic absorption spectrophotometers.

WHEATSTONE BRIDGE

For various reasons, it is often necessary to measure the value of an unknown resistance. The Wheatstone bridge is a device to measure such unknown resist-

Figure 1-26.   Ammeter placement in circuit.

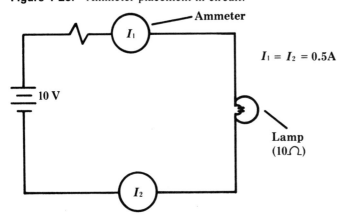

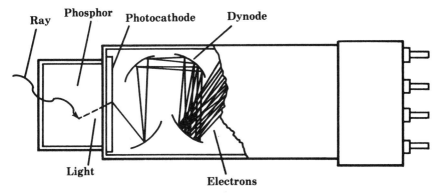

Figure 1-27. Photomultiplier tube.

ances. It finds many applications in the medical laboratory, where it is incorporated with other circuits in an instrument such as the osmometer or gas chromatograph.

The resistors R_A and R_B (Fig. 1-28) are known constant-value resistors; R is a variable resistor used as a rheostat and R_U is the unknown resistance being measured. When R_U is equal to R, the circuit is balanced and there will be no voltage difference between the terminals T_1 and T_2. At this time, the null detector will read zero volts (nulled). When the circuit is balanced or nulled, the following conditions exist.

$R_A = R_B$
I_1 is current through R_A and R_U
I_2 is current through R_B and R
$I_1 = I_2$

Figure 1-28. Wheatstone bridge.

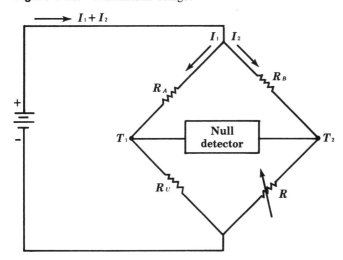

Then

$$I_1 R_A = I_2 R_B$$
$$(T_1 \text{ voltage} = T_2 \text{ voltage})$$
$$I_1 R_U = I_2 R$$

By proportion, then,

$$R_A/R_U = R_B/R \text{ therefore } R_U = (R_A/R_B)R$$
$$R_U = R \text{ because } R_A/R_B = 1$$

The value of R is read on a calibrated dial on the Wheatstone bridge and this equals R_U. The Wheatstone bridge can accommodate a wide range of R_Us by changing the R_A/R_B ratio, and this becomes simply a multiplier of R to obtain the R_U value.

By proper calibration, R_U can be a meaningful value for the medical instrument being used. This device, as was pointed out in the beginning of this section, may be any one of a great variety of laboratory measuring systems.

Electrical Safety

The modern hospital laboratory is equipped with a wide variety of instrumentation for processing physiological fluids and, in addition, often uses liquid chemical reagents. Because of this combination of electrical apparatus and electrically conductive fluids, special precautions must be taken to ensure the safety of laboratory personnel. All electrical instrumentation and apparatus must be designed and constructed so that electrical hazards do not exist. Careful design, component selection, and good quality manufacturing standards are all necessary to render electrical safety. The user, however, must be aware of the potential dangers any electronic instrument presents if proper operating procedures are not followed. Some of the most common electrical hazards arise from spilled liquids that come in contact with circuit boards inside the instrument, broken or damaged parts, faulty cords and plugs, or improper repairs.

The electrical power to all laboratory equipment must come from a three-wire distribution system. One wire is white (neutral wire), one is black (hot wire), and the third is green (ground wire). In addition, isolation transformers, ground-fault interrupters, and line isolation monitors may be used to provide greater electrical safety and improved operational stability. The three-wire electrical power distribution system is common to all instruments; it is imperative never to tamper with it. There are other important rules that must be followed to minimize electrical hazards. These rules are as follows:

1. Restrict the use of extension cords.
2. Ban the use of adapter plugs.
3. Immediately repair faulty cords and broken connectors.

All instrumentation used in the hospital laboratory must be inspected at periodic intervals for cleaning, calibration, electrical safety, and preventive maintenance. The electrical power receptacles in the laboratory must also be inspected for broken parts, blade tension, and polarity. The voltage and current requirements of the laboratory must be determined prior to installation of any new equipment and checked routinely at regular intervals. The responsibility for the periodic inspection of equipment and the maintenance of the facilities is usually given to the appropriate department whose staff has received training in those areas.

Suggested Reading

Beam RE (ed): Allied Dictionary of Electronic Terms, 6th ed. Chicago, Allied Radio Corp, 1962

Cooke NM (ed): Allied Electronics Data Handbook, 3rd ed. Chicago, Allied Radio Corp, 1963

Dictionary of Instrumentation Terminology. Compiled by engineers at Brush Instrument Div., Clevite Corp. Cleveland, Penton, 1967

Glossary of Electronics Terminology, 2nd ed. A glossary prepared by IRC, Philadelphia, 1967

Swaminathan M: Electronics: Circuits and Systems. Indianapolis, Howard W. Sams & Co, Inc, 1985

2

ANALYTICAL BALANCE

Judith Thompson

Definitions

Accuracy: The agreement between the measured weight and the calibrated weight of an object. It is dependent upon the calibration of the weight and the scale divisions of the balance. For equal-arm balances, accuracy is also dependent upon the lever arm error and variation of sensitivity due to load placed on the pan.

Balance: A mechanical instrument for the comparison of weights.

Capacity: The largest load that can be weighed on a balance. The capacity of most analytical balances is 200 g.

Mass: A measure of the quantity of matter in an object; a constant, independent of gravitational force.

Precision: The degree of agreement between repeated weighings of the same mass, expressed as one standard deviation in mass units.

Readability: The smallest fraction of the scale division that can be read. The validity of this reading depends upon the precision of the instrument.

Sensitivity: The ratio of the change in scale divisions to a specific weight change, expressed as scale-division deflection per mass unit. It is dependent upon the deflection of the beam and the optical magnification of this deflection.

Weight: The force with which a mass is attracted by earth. It is dependent upon gravity, which varies with location and time. The relationship is expressed as weight = mass × gravity.

Weighing: The comparison of an unknown mass to a calibrated one.

Weights: Objects of known mass, made from corrosion-resistant material (brass, gold, platinum, stainless-steel). The National Bureau of Standards has established classes of weights, setting acceptable tolerance limits and specifications for material and construction. In the clinical laboratory, Class S weights are used for routine calibration and accuracy checking of the analytical balance.

Introduction

The analytical balance is one of the most basic and accurate instruments in the clinical laboratory. It is used for the preparation of standard solutions and whenever accuracy of 1 mg or less is required. Most analytical balances have a capacity of 200 g. Semimicrobalances are capable of weighing up to 100 g, and microbalances have a capacity of 20 to 50 g. There are a variety of analytical balances available. Substitution balances have been standard equipment in the clinical laboratory, but electronic balances are now becoming more widely used.

Principles and Component Parts

MECHANICAL BALANCES

Mechanical balances are based on the principle of a first-class lever. The central moving part is the beam, which rests on the knife edge, acting as the fulcrum. This system allows for the direct comparison of masses rather than weights, so that correction for the effect of gravity is not necessary. There are two types of mechanical balances used for analytical work: the equal-arm balance and the single-pan substitution balance.

The equal-arm balance consists of a knife edge supporting the exact center of the beam (Fig. 2-1) so that the lengths of the two lever arms, L_1 and L_2, are

Figure 2-1. Equal-arm balance.

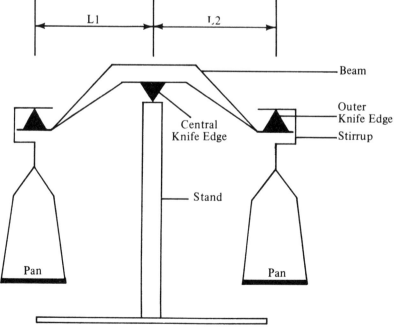

equal. The pans are linked to the ends of the beams by stirrups, which rest on two outer knife edges. The three knife edges lie in the same plane about which motion occurs. The lengths of the two lever arms are equal; therefore, the mass supported by each arm must be equal for the system to be in equilibrium. If an unknown mass, m_x, is added to one side, the beam is deflected. The deflection is offset by adding standard weights, m_s, until the beam returns to the horizontal position so that $m_x L_1$ equals $m_s L_2$. If L_1 equals L_2, then m_x equals m_s.

The beam of the single-pan substitution balance is situated unsymmetrically on the central knife edge (Fig. 2-2). The pan is supported by a stirrup placed on the outer knife edge. Again, both knife edges are in the same plane. A series of calibrated weights are supported from the same end of the beam from which the pan is suspended. A fixed-constant counterweight on the opposite end of the beam keeps the balance in equilibrium. The lengths of the lever arms, L_1 and L_2, are not equal; therefore, for the beam to remain in a horizontal position, the masses at either end of the lever arm are not equal. When an unknown weight is placed on the weighing pan, the beam deflects in the direction of the heavier side. To return the system to equilibrium, the corresponding mass of calibrated weights is removed from the front of the beam. The mass on the front of the beam is equalized by this substitution process, and the beam is restored to equilibrium. This is called weighing by substitution.

The condition of the knife edges is critical to the performance of the balance. The edges are made from an extremely hard material such as sapphire and must

Figure 2-2. Substitution balance.

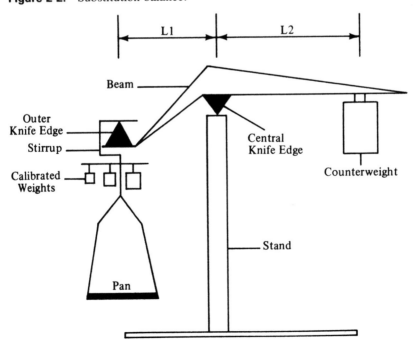

be precision ground to minimize the area of contact and reduce friction. There is considerable stress at the point of contact with the beam, and mechanical shock can easily damage these parts. To protect the knife edge, the beam support lifts the beam slightly from the knife edge. The pan arrests help control the movement of the pans. Both arrests should be engaged when the balance is not in use or when the pans are being loaded or unloaded.

Analytical balances are also equipped with dampers, which oppose the movement of the beam, allowing it to come to equilibrium rapidly. Magnetic dampers are commonly used with equal-arm balances and consist of a metal plate fixed to the beam and positioned between the poles of a magnet. When the beam is set in motion, the plate moves through the magnetic field that opposes the oscillations. The air damper is used on the substitution balance. It consists of a piston attached to the beam and a cylinder mounted on the balance case. When the beam is set in motion, the air within the cylinder expands and contracts, opposing the movement of the beam.

Most manufacturers use the substitution principle because the substitution balance has several advantages compared to the equal-arm balance. The weighing procedure using an equal-arm balance is time-consuming and demands considerable skill. With an equal-arm balance, the sensitivity is dependent upon the load placed on the balance. With increased loading there is increased friction due to mechanical imperfections in the knife edges and slight displacement of the terminal knife edges from the same plane as the central knife edge. The load is always constant on the substitution balance and, therefore, the sensitivity is constant. Lever-arm error is eliminated because comparison of the known mass with an unknown mass takes place on the same lever arm. Two knife edges instead of three reduces friction.

ELECTRONIC BALANCES

Electronic balances commonly used in the clinical laboratory consist of three basic component systems: a null detector, a feedback loop to control the balancing force, and a readout device.

The null detector senses the position of the balance beam and is used to determine the balance point at which the system is in equilibrium. The magnitude of the electrical current from the null detector is proportional to the sample weight.

To return the system to equilibrium, electromagnetic restoring forces are used in place of standard weights. The signal from the null detector is applied directly to control a current through an electromagnet to return the balance to equilibrium. When the null meter reads zero, the compensating force required to bring the balance to equilibrium is proportional to the weight on the pan. The current required to produce the compensating force is converted to a digital display of the weight.

Electronic balances have several advantages compared to mechanical balances. The precision is greatly increased with a digital display, replacing visual interpretation of a scale. Hand dialing to apply built-in weights is eliminated. In addition, electronic balances have automatic tare correction, which automatically subtracts the weight of the container. Therefore, the time required to make a weighing is substantially decreased.

Performance and Operation

The performance of an analytical balance should be judged by sensitivity, precision, accuracy, and readability. The sensitivity is the ratio of the scale response change to weight change and is usually expressed as scale-division deflection per mg. If a 1-mg weight produces a displacement of three scale divisions from the rest point, then the sensitivity is expressed as three scale divisions per mg. The precision of the instrument is expressed as the standard deviation of repetitive measurements of the same mass. The accuracy can be checked using National Bureau of Standards Certified Class S weights. The readability of the instrument is the smallest fraction of a division to which the index scale can be read with ease. When selecting an analytical balance for a particular weighing requirement, the capacity of the instrument should also be considered.

To ensure proper operation of an analytical balance, study the instruction manual provided by the manufacturer of the instrument. The balance should be placed on a solid support, either marble or concrete, and located away from sources of heat, draft, or vibration. Do not place objects on the pan that will overload the balance and exceed its capacity. The balance should be cleaned after each weighing. Do not place or use corrosive materials near an analytical balance. The beam support and pan arrest should always be engaged whenever loading or unloading the pan. When not in use, all weights should be returned to the zero position and the beams and pan placed in the support position.

For optimum balance performance, preventive maintenance and calibration should be done according to the manufacturer's instructions once a year. The accuracy of the balance should be checked monthly using National Bureau of Standards Certified Class S weights.

Suggested Reading

Bietry L: Balances and Weighing. Zurich, Mettler Instruments, 1975
Ewing GW: Electronic laboratory balances. J Chem Educ 53:A252–A257, 1976
Fritz JS, Schenk GH: Quantitative Analytical Chemistry. Boston, Allyn & Bacon, 1974
Skoog DA, West DM: Fundamentals of Analytical Chemistry. New York, Holt, Rinehart, Winston, 1969

3

CENTRIFUGES
Gene d'Allemand

Definitions

Adapters: Inserts used in large shields or cups to allow the use of smaller glassware, thereby giving the original shield or cup more versatility.

Angle Head: Another term for fixed angle rotor.

Brushes: In a centrifuge motor, the graphite plates that serve as the conductor between the electrical circuit and the commutator.

Centrifuge: A device used to apply a centrifugal force for separating substances of different densities, for removing moisture, or for simulating gravitational effects.

Centrifugal Force: The force that tends to impel matter outward from a center of rotation. It is dependent upon three variables: mass, speed, and radius. In the clinical laboratory, most work is done with aqueous solutions having a specific gravity of near 1.000; therefore, mass is generally not considered in calculations.

Commutator: In a centrifuge motor, a revolving part that collects current from the brushes.

Cushions: Rubber pads positioned at the bottom of the inside cavity of the shields, cups, or adapters to minimize glassware breakage by distributing the effects of centrifugal force over a greater area.

Fixed Angle Rotor: A rotor with drilled holes that support the tubes at a fixed angle, generally 25° to 50°.

Gravity: The unit of measure for the rate of acceleration of gravity, equal to 9807 mm/s^2; abbreviated "g." For reference, the earth's force is expressed as $1 \times g$.

Horizontal Rotor: A rotor that allows tubes, shields, and cups to swing from a vertical to a horizontal position when subjected to centrifugation.

Relative Centrifugal Force (RCF): A method of comparing the forces generated by various centrifuges, considering the speed of rotation and the radius from the center of rotation. Relative centrifugal force is calculated according to the formula,

$$RCF = 1.12 \, r \left(\frac{rpm}{1000}\right)^2$$

where

r = the radius in millimeters
rpm = the number of revolutions per minute

The radius is measured from the center of rotation to the inside bottom of the tube when measuring maximum RCF (nomograms for computing RCF are usually included in the manufacturer's manual). Relative centrifugal force is expressed as some number times gravity, or some number × g.

Revolutions per Minute (rpm):   A unit for expressing the number of complete rotations occurring per minute in time; a measure of speed.

Rotor: The device used to hold the tubes, shields, and cups.

Shields, Cups, and Carriers: Metal containers used to hold the various sizes of glassware.

Stroboscope: A tachometer instrument for measuring the speed of rotation by matching rotation with the frequency of flashing light.

Swinging Bucket: Another term for horizontal rotor.

Trunnion Carrier: A metal carrier that holds the tubes upright for filling and balancing prior to centrifugation. It can act as a stand for the tubes after processing.

Ultracentrifuge: A very high-speed centrifuge capable of obtaining extremely high RCF values.

Introduction

Centrifuges are designed to accelerate the sedimentation process by utilizing centrifugal force. Various types of centrifuges are used in the clinical laboratory for separating suspended particles from a liquid in which the particles are not soluble. Liquids of differing specific gravities (density) may also be separated.

There are three general types of centrifuges: the horizontal rotor, the fixed-angle rotor, and the ultracentrifuge. Many variations of the horizontal and fixed-angle rotor units are found in the clinical laboratory. These include bench-top and floor-standing units, high-speed units, refrigerated units, and such special-purpose instruments as the microhematocrit, cell washer, cytospin, and continuous-flow systems.

Principles

In the clinical laboratory, the centrifuge functions as a filtration or packing device. The development of large-batch centrifuges and continuous-flow systems that can sediment a precipitate from a large volume of solution in a short time have tended to replace the tedious process of filtration in most clinical and research laboratories. This development has not only speeded up the process of separation but, when coupled with refrigeration, has also reduced sample lability to a minimum.

General applications include the separation of serum or plasma from red blood cells, the separation of precipitated solids from the liquid phase of a mixture, or the separation of liquids of varying density. Special-purpose units include such applications as quantitative red blood cell packing for measuring hematocrit, automatic cell washing, and component preparation for blood banking. Ultracentrifuges employ very high speed and force to achieve difficult and precise quantitative separations of ultrasmall particles or macromolecules.

The horizontal rotor centrifuge shields or cups are in a vertical position when the centrifuge is at rest and assume a horizontal position when the centrifuge is operating. The horizontal rotor unit will operate at speeds up to about 3000 revolutions per minute (rpm). Speeds higher than this can be attained but are not generally practical because of the excess heat developed by air friction. Depending upon the radius of the rotor, these units attain forces of approximately 1650 $\times$ g.

The fixed-angle rotor centrifuge shields or cups are positioned rigidly at a fixed angle, generally 25° to 50°, to the shaft around which they rotate. Angle-rotor units may attain much higher speeds. This is due to the special construction of the rotor, which exhibits very low friction with air. The cups of the fixed-angle rotor are enclosed by a metal case that reduces wind resistance, minimizing the increase of sample temperature commonly exhibited by the horizontal-rotor centrifuge. Thus the fixed-angle units can reach speeds of about 7000 rpm and can exhibit forces of over 9000 $\times$ g.

In the horizontal-rotor centrifuge, the particles being sedimented must travel the entire length of the column of liquid to reach the bottom of the tube. As the containers fall from the horizontal to the vertical position when the centrifuge stops, a remixing of the sediment and solution can occur. In the fixed-angle rotor centrifuge, this is not the case. With the shields and cups at a fixed angle, the particles have a shorter distance to travel; that is, across the column of liquid to the side of the container. These particles form clusters and move to the bottom of the container very rapidly. The fixed-angle rotor centrifuge is a more efficient means of sedimentation.

High-speed microcentrifuges are common in many laboratories. These units incorporate either fixed-angle or horizontal rotors of small radius. With sample volumes up to 2 ml, they are capable of speeds to 15,000 rpm and forces up to 15,000 $\times$ g. Refrigerated centrifuges are available in both bench-type and floor models. They have internal refrigeration systems capable of maintaining temperatures ranging from $-15°$ to 25°C during centrifugation; they may incorporate either fixed-angle or horizontal rotors. Refrigeration permits separation at higher speeds by protecting samples from heat generated during centrifugation.

Centrifuges capable of producing speeds up to 100,000 rpm with relative centrifugal force (RCF) values to 600,000 $\times$ g are referred to as ultracentrifuges. Both fixed-angle and horizontal rotors are used in these units. In addition, some instruments have vertical rotors in which the axis of the tubes is fixed parallel to the rotor's axis of rotation. Even with the high forces produced, several hours or even days are often required to obtain complex separations under controlled temperatures. The general centrifugation techniques utilizing the ultracentrifuge include differential, rate zonal, and isopyknic separations. Differential centrifugation separates particles from a mixture by sedimenting those of larger mass to the bottom, leaving a portion of the small particles in the supernatant. The rate zonal technique separates particles based on differences in sedimentation rate in a density gradient, such as sucrose. The isopyknic technique separates particles based on differences in density (composition) in a density gradient, such as cesium chloride. The large ultracentrifuge is significantly more complex than general laboratory centrifuges and has not as yet found widespread use in the clinical laboratory. The information included under components, operation, and maintenance does not strictly apply.

One variation of the ultracentrifuge that is being used in the clinical laboratory is the Airfuge (Beckman Instruments). This unit is a miniature ultracentrifuge that uses a small turbine rotor driven by air pressure. It is capable of speeds up to 95,000 rpm and forces up to 178,000 $\times$ g. The rotor spins nearly friction-free on a cushion of air and temperature can be controlled by the temperature of the drive air. A variety of rotors are available. General applications include receptor assays, protein fractionation, and drug-binding assays. Perhaps the most common clinical laboratory application is the clarification of lipemic sera.

Selection of a centrifuge for the laboratory should involve careful review of several factors. The number and volume of samples to be separated during a run, and at what RCF, are central to the choice. Other considerations include physical size, rotor versatility, timing and refrigeration needs, frequency of use, and maintenance requirements. By consulting the manufacturer's literature, a wide variety of rotors, adapters, and other accessories can generally be found to improve the versatility of a particular centrifuge model.

Components

The parts of a common centrifuge include the chamber, which encloses the internal parts, a cover with latch, the centrifuge rotor with shields or cups, and the motor-drive assembly. Most centrifuges will include a power switch, a braking device, speed control, a timer, and possibly a tachometer.

Centrifuge motors are either series-wound dc motors that turn faster as voltage is increased or ac motors in which speed adjustment is achieved through stepwise reduction of the number of poles in the magnetic field. Both types are high-speed motors that generally employ direct-drive systems to the rotor through the motor shaft.

Electrical contact to the commutator in nearly all centrifuge motors is provided by graphite brushes, which gradually wear down as they press against the commutator turning at high speed. If the graphite is allowed to completely wear away, the retainer spring of the brush will make contact with the smooth surface of the commutator and will cut grooves or scratches in its surface. A rough commutator surface will cause excessively fast wear of new brushes. The graphite that is worn away may deposit around the contacts, causing arcing and burning, both of which decrease the efficiency of the motor and may damage it or, in extreme cases, may even start a fire in the motor. The shaft of the motor turns through sleeve bearings located at the top and bottom of the motor. Most units contain sealed bearings that are permanently lubricated, whereas others require periodic oil or grease. Many centrifuges contain an internal imbalance switch that turns the unit off before vibrations from load imbalance can damage bearings on the drive shaft. Knowledge of basic operating principles is important for establishing and performing proper maintenance on the centrifuge.

The speed of the centrifuge is controlled by a potentiometer, which raises and lowers the voltage supplied to the motor. The calibrations furnished on the speed control of a centrifuge are often only relative voltage increments and can never be taken as accurate indicators of speed. Because speed is dependent upon voltage in most centrifuges, as resistance is increased, speed is lost. Air resistance and turbulence, brush friction, and electrical inefficiency of the centrifuge itself are sources of resistance. Those resistances can cause a centrifuge to operate at differing speeds on the same speed-control setting. Different accessories, loads, and varying states of repair will also result in the same speed-control problems. Calibration and periodic recalibration of centrifuge speed is extremely important.

Operating a centrifuge with the lid raised is dangerous and must be discouraged. In addition to being hazardous and reducing the centrifuge's speed through increased air resistance, it also causes the revolving parts of the centrifuge to vibrate excessively. Vibrations cause extensive wear on the centrifuge and a remixing of the sedimented particles.

Tachometers are provided on many centrifuges to indicate the speed in rpm. On mechanical tachometers, a flexible shaft or cable attached to the motor spindle turns inside a flexible housing to which the meter movement is attached at the other end. As the cable turns, it causes the needle to move up scale. Modern centrifuges use electric tachometers in which a magnet rotates around a coil, producing a current that may be measured. If a tachometer is not attached to the centrifuge, a stroboscope or an electronic meter can be used to determine the actual rpm of each centrifuge setting. For any given setting, the speed of the centrifuge will vary with the specimen load. The rpm determined for each centrifuge setting should be recorded and attached to the centrifuge for easy reference.

The value of rpm is only one factor involved in determining centrifugal force. The true efficiency of a particular centrifuge is expressed in relative centrifugal force, some number times gravity. The relative centrifugal force is calculated from the experimentally determined rpm and the radius of the rotor plus carrier (see formula under Definitions). The RCF value for various speed settings is also generally listed in tabular or graphic form in the manufacturer's instruction manual for the instrument.

The term *rpm*, when applied to a centrifuge, does not give any indication of the force applied to samples in that centrifuge. All comparisons made between centrifuges should be in relative centrifugal force. When an RCF value specified in a procedure cannot be obtained on a particular centrifuge, it is possible to adjust the length of time in which samples are centrifuged to achieve equivalent centrifugal force. Time required would be calculated as follows:

$$T = \frac{T_s \times RCF_s}{RCF}$$

where

$$T = \text{run time needed}$$
$$T_s = \text{run time specified in a procedure}$$
$$RCF = \text{RCF obtainable}$$
$$RCF_s = \text{RCF specified in a procedure}$$

A timer device is commonly employed in many centrifuges. Some are spring-driven clock mechanisms that turn the unit off after a preset time cycle. Others are electronic timers that perform the same function. Many units have switches that allow the units to be operated continuously without using the timer device.

Braking devices are incorporated to provide rapid deceleration of the unit. Two general types of brake mechanisms are found on centrifuges. One type is mechanical and functions by physically applying pressure to the rotor at some point when a lever is pressed. The other type, found on most units, is electrical in nature and functions by reversing the polarity of the current to the motor.

General Operation and Maintenance

Daily inspection along with periodic function verification and proper preventive maintenance are vital to the efficiency and longevity of the centrifuge. A regular schedule for checks must be established and followed to ensure proper operation of the instrument. Always consult the manufacturer's instruction manual for specific operating and maintenance procedures.

DAILY OPERATION

Daily operation should include observation and inspection of the following:

1. The centrifuge should not be on the same circuit as sensitive electronic measuring devices, such as spectrophotometers, because it generates electrical noise and has a high current drain when started up. The unit should not be run near combustible fluids because ignition may occur from sparking motor brushes.
2. Check the cleanliness of the chamber, and immediately clean up all spills. Be aware of biohazardous materials (microbiologic, radioactive, chemical) that require specific decontamination procedures. Observe for gray or black dust buildup within the chamber; this can be a sign of sandblasting of the rotor chamber caused by glass particles and must be cleaned up. Refrigerated units will require periodic defrosting.
3. Always balance the load of the centrifuge before operating; use the correct tube sizes and types for the particular centrifuge. The load must be balanced both by equal mass and by centers of gravity across the center of rotation. Do not run the centrifuge with buckets, carriers, or shields missing from the unit.
4. Always make sure that the cover is closed while the unit is operating. This will help prevent the dangerous aerosolization of biohazardous and scattering of physically dangerous material into the environment where the operator and others may be exposed. Centrifuge only sealed or stoppered tubes if at all possible.
5. Observe for unusual noises or vibrations during operation. Do not operate the unit in excess of the maximum speed recommended by the manufacturer for the rotor in use. Vibration occurs naturally during acceleration and deceleration at low speeds. This is the critical speed range of the rotor and is

generally in the 500 to 1000 rpm range. Avoid prolonged operation of the unit within this range.

6. Never open the chamber until the rotor has come to a complete stop.

FUNCTION VERIFICATION

The frequency of function verification procedures should be appropriate for the application of the centrifuge. It is generally recommended that such procedures be performed at 1- to 3-month intervals, with the more frequent checks being on those units with critical application. All checks performed and data gathered should be recorded in such a fashion that the information is readily available to the operator. Correction factors for speed, timing, or temperature should be posted on the unit.

Tolerance limits for function checks should be established. The limits set will again depend on the application of the centrifuge. Include information for corrective action should tolerance limits be exceeded.

Function verification procedures should include the following:

1. *rpm calibration.* One of the best ways to check the function of a centrifuge is to check its speed. Depending upon how the unit is equipped, both the speed control and built-in tachometer should be checked with an external device. This may be accomplished with either a stroboscope or a mechanical or electronic tachometer of good accuracy. Several speeds used regularly on the unit should be checked. Values obtained with the external measuring device should agree within 5% of those from a built-in tachometer. Centrifuges that cannot be checked for speed without opening the chamber lid should be tested by factory-trained personnel only.

2. *Timer.* The timer should be set for common timing intervals and these intervals should be checked against an accurate stopwatch or electronic timer. The timing interval includes the period of acceleration and spin, but not the brake or stopping time. General laboratory centrifuges should be accurate to 10% of the total timed interval.

3. *Temperature.* The thermometer on refrigerated units should be checked against a certified thermometer, and a correction factor should be derived if necessary.

PREVENTIVE MAINTENANCE

Preventive maintenance should be performed on the same time schedule as function verification procedures. The preventive maintenance schedule should include the following:

1. *Lubrication.* Depending upon the type of centrifuge, bearings on the upper and lower end of the motor shaft may be permanently lubricated or sealed. If they are not sealed, the manufacturer's instructions must be followed for lubrication. Bearing wear may be checked at this time by determining the amount of side play in the shaft.

2. *Motor components.* Brushes should be removed and checked for wear. Replacement is recommended if they are worn to more than one-half their original

length. When reinserting used brushes, replace them in the same orientation and be certain that spring tension is adequate to maintain good contact with the commutator. New brushes should be broken in by accelerating the unloaded unit slowly to mid-speed and by allowing it to operate this way for a period of time. The condition of the commutator should be examined. To avoid electrical arcing, the commutator and brush holders must be free of dirt, oil, and dust. Severe arcing of new brushes can be a sign of a bad commutator. If the commutator is scratched or scored, it will have to be removed and machined smooth with a lathe or replaced. On refrigerated units, the manufacturer's instruction manual should be consulted for maintenance procedures on the refrigeration system.

3. *Electrical integrity.* Both grounding resistance and current leakage should be checked periodically on each centrifuge. The fuse should be checked for proper rating; if the unit has a circuit breaker, it should be checked for proper operation. In addition, the line cord, plug, lamps, and wiring should be examined for defects.

4. *Mechanical integrity.* If the unit is equipped with a safety interlock, this device should be checked for proper working order. Gaskets, latches, hinges, and control knobs should be examined to determine that all are functioning and in good condition. The rotor and shields or carriers should be examined for signs of mechanical stress (cracks, corrosion) and for cleanliness and balance.

Suggested Reading

A Centrifuge Primer, Beckman Instruments, Spinco Division, Palo Alto, CA, 1980

Kaplan LA, Pesce AP: Clinical Chemistry Theory, Analysis, and Correlation. St Louis, CV Mosby, 1984

Laboratory Instrument Maintenance and Function Verification. Chicago, College of American Pathologists, 1982

Lee LW, Schmidt DA: Elementary Principles of Laboratory Instruments, 5th ed. St Louis, CV Mosby, 1983

Strickland RD: Centrifuges and Centrifugation. In Werner M (ed): CRC Handbook of Clinical Chemistry, Vol 1. Boca Raton, FL, CRC Press, 1982

Tenczar FJ, Kowalski TA: The centrifuge: Maintenance and calibration. ASCP Technical Improvement Service 14:72, 1973

4

DILUTERS

M. Robert Hicks

Definitions

Calibration: A series of checks on the system to ensure correct and accurate diluent volume and dilution ratio.

Cycle: A series of events in the diluting process, such as the sampling cycle and the dispensing cycle. A sampling cycle would consist of the following series of events: closing of sample valve, opening of diluent valve, aspiration of sample, and aspiration of solution into diluent chamber.

Stepping Motor: The stepping motor is a permanent magnet motor that converts electronic signals into mechanical motion. Each time the direction of current in the motor windings is changed, the motor output shaft rotates a specific angular distance. The motor shaft can be driven in either direction and can be operated at high stepping rates.

System: The total group of units making up the diluter (diluting) system.

Unit: Any component part of the diluting system. The units are: motor, pneumatic cylinder, sample pump, diluent pump, fluid valves, and control valves.

Tare: The determination of a stable base weight of an object. An analytical method of determining the weight of a chemically clean vessel so that errors caused by temperature and humidity are cancelled.

Introduction

A *diluter* is a system for sampling, dispensing, and diluting a specimen with a predetermined solution or reagent. This system is also capable of dispensing preset volumes of reagent or solution. These systems consist of two power-driven precision syringes or pipetting devices. One of these pipetting devices is for the aliquoting of the sample. The other device is for measuring and dispensing the diluting solution. These two devices are connected through valving mechanisms so that a preset volume of sample is aspirated by the action of the sampling syringe, as the diluting syringe is loaded by its downward stroke. In the next step, the valving units allow the solution in the diluent syringe to be dispensed through the sampling tip, thereby dispensing and diluting the sample to a predetermined ratio.

The diluter system not only provides the accurate pipetting of a mechanical device but also saves considerable personnel time and eliminates problems associated with manual pipetting and diluting. Repetitive precision is important when performing procedures that require accurate measuring and dispensing of liquids, as in preparing reagent blank, standards, blood components for photometric readings, cell counts, and, especially, chemical determinations on automatic systems dealing with microliter volumes.

Principles

Diluters utilize two types of pipetting devices, although either of them can be driven by the same kind of power source. The pipetting devices are constructed from barrel and plunger components. In one device, the barrel is a simple fluid-holding chamber with a seal at the base around a precision plunger, which will displace fluid from within the barrel. The other device is of a syringe- or piston-type unit, which operates by sliding in and out of the barrel, forcing fluid into and out of the chamber.

Valves control the starting mechanism and the shunting of fluids, air, and vacuum. The valving of these systems may be automatic or manual. Manual valves are operated by hand and are usually composed of sliding surfaces of inert plastic. The automatic devices may be flat or round flipper valves or solenoid-releasing pinch valves controlled by microswitches. These microswitches regulate the opening and closing of the solenoid-operated fluid valves.

The power used to actuate these systems may be from an electric motor that drives eccentric cams, by air or vacuum cylinders, or by combined air and vacuum cylinders. These power sources are used to move the piston of the pipetting device in and out of its barrel, thereby causing movement of the fluids.

Components

The plungers of these diluting systems are moved by two main sources of energy. This is supplied by a 115-volt (V) motor that may be operated continuously or intermittently. A cam-type mechanism, activated by an intermittently operated motor, can drive the unit as it is operated.

Pneumatic cylinders (Fig. 4-1) activated by air, vacuum, or both can also be used to operate the diluter plungers. In this case, a continuously operating motor drives an air or vacuum pump. When air is shunted into port *B* of the system (Fig. 4-1), the pneumatic piston is forced up, and solution from the diluent chamber is displaced. When air is shunted into port *A*, the pneumatic piston is lowered, and solution is forced into the diluent chamber. If vacuum activation is used, the opposite shunting is necessary to accomplish this same action. By using both air and vacuum activation, the same function may be obtained by the alternative shunting of these two forces into port *B* and leaving port *A* open for venting. In

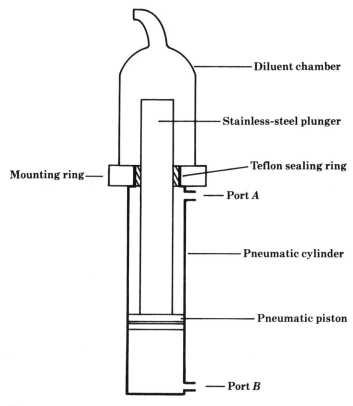

Figure 4-1. Pneumatic-powered pump unit.

this case, shunting air pressure into port *B* will raise the pneumatic piston, and by using vacuum, the opposite action will occur.

By adjusting the eccentric cams, the syringe volumes can be changed to provide various dilution ratios. These adjustments are made by varying the radius of the cam action and are generally accomplished by the fine settings of a locking screw. The locking action of this mechanism is mandatory, so that the micrometer settings will not change after adjustments are made. The stroke adjustment of the pneumatic cylinder units are also of the screw type and have special locking devices to hold the settings. These adjustments function by limiting the stroke of the pneumatic cylinders. Some diluting systems are permanently set and cannot be adjusted.

VALVE CONTROL UNITS

The pneumatic-powered diluters utilize air and vacuum valves to actuate the systems. These valves function by shunting the pneumatics of the system to the correct port to get the desired cylinder action; that is, these valves are used to supply air pressure to the bottom of the piston on the dispense cycle and to the top of the piston on the intake cycle. This valve action may be manual or automatic, depending upon the sophistication of the system.

The direct motor-driven systems are actuated by an electric switch. The ensuing functions of these systems are automatic and are controlled by micro-switches that are actuated by the cam wheels. The action of the fluid valves of these systems is also controlled by microswitches that are actuated by these same cams. With this system, it is possible to operate on single cycle or to run on automatic continuous cycling.

PUMP UNITS

The sampling units of diluters are syringe-type fluid pumps that are driven by the power supply. These dispensing units may be composed of either piston-type (Fig. 4-2) or plunger-type mechanisms (Fig. 4-1). There is a diluent and a sample pump unit in each diluter. These pumps are interconnected with fluid valves (Fig. 4-2).

The fluid control valves of these systems are used to control the direction of flow and to give positive sampling on the aspiration cycle. These valves must be synchronized to the particular cycle of the diluter system (Fig. 4-2). On the intake or sampling cycle, solenoid valve A is closed and solenoid valve B is open. Therefore, on this cycle, diluent is drawn into the diluent pump chamber, and sample is aspirated up into the sampling tip as the pump plungers are lowered. On the dispensing cycle, solenoid A opens, and solenoid B closes. As the pump cylinders raise to the top position, the sample is delivered and diluted with the solution from the diluent pump.

Operation

The operation of a diluting system requires two actions by the operator. The first is to place the sampling tip into the liquid sample and activate the starting valve. This automatically closes the sampling valve, opens the diluent valve, and shunts air to the top of the pneumatic cylinder. The air pressure applied to the top of the cylinder lowers the pistons in the sampling and diluent chambers, causing the sample to be aspirated into the sample tip and the diluent solution to be drawn into the diluent chamber. This is known as the *sample cycle*. The second step is to place the sampling tip into a recipient vessel and to activate the start switch. This opens the sample valve, closes the diluent valve, and shunts air to the bottom of the air cylinder, which dispenses the sample and diluent through the sample tip into the recipient vessel. This is the *dispensing cycle*.

The power used to actuate these systems may be created by a synchronous electric motor that drives eccentric cams, by off-center shaft systems, by dc-powered stepping motors, by air or vacuum cylinders, or by combined air and vacuum cylinders. These power sources are used to move the piston of the pipetting device in and out of its barrel, thereby causing movement of fluids.

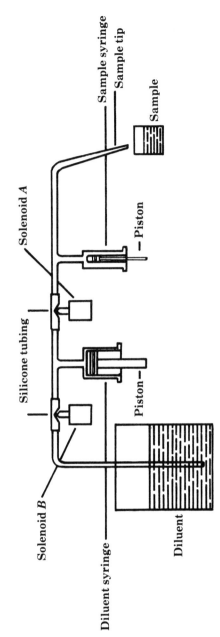

Figure 4-2. Pump and fluid valve units of diluter system.

PRECISION SAMPLERS

Precision samplers are primarily small-bore precision syringes powered by dc stepping motors that are coupled together through a threaded drive shaft and nut system such that the syringe plunger is moved as the motor turns forward and backward, thereby providing very precise sampling and dispensing action.

The *stepping motor* is a very special type of electric motor powered by pulses of dc current to produce mechanical motion. Each time the direction of the current in the motor windings is changed, the motor output shaft rotates a specific angular distance. The motor shaft can be driven in either direction and can be operated at high stepping rates. These motors are also available in different stepping angles with a step accuracy of 3%. Common full-step angles are 0.72°, 1.8°, 5°, 7.5°, and 15°. These step angles divide one revolution into 500, 200, 72, 48, and 24 angular distances.

The *digital stepping motor* rotates precisely as determined by an energizing current pulse from a step driver that is microprocessor controlled. If this power controller is monitored by a power control computer, this sampling and dispensing system can be engineered to handle 1 μl of solution per step, and any other volume by repeated steps. This control computer can be programmed to change the number of steps and, consequently, the volumes from one cycle to another.

This extremely accurate and precise sampling system is the heart of most of the discrete automatic chemistry analyzers used in the clinical laboratories today. The precision of this sampler is governed by the design of this motor to approach instant starting and stopping; therefore, when coupled by a screw drive shaft and nut, the precision syringe sampler is capable of very precise measurements of sample, reagent, and diluent.

Only valving, connections, and sampling tips need to be added to this system to finish the sampler. The movement of the sample probes to sample cups and reaction vessels will be discussed with the various analyzers.

Calibration

The calibration of diluters includes certain checks made to determine the diluent volume and the dilution ratio. The most commonly used and the best method of determining the diluent volume is by gravimetric measurement. To check the dilution ratio, dilute a dye solution (Evans blue, BSP, or bathophenanthroline) with the diluter, and make the same dilution using volumetric pipettes and flasks. (This glassware must be of National Bureau of Standard certified class A quality.) Mix both and read the absorbances at the desired wavelength for the particular solution, using a precision spectrophotometer and calibrated cuvettes. If the diluter volumes are preset, the absorbance values for the manual method should compare closely with the values for the diluter. This reading should be noted and all following checks should be compared to the original reading.

Multiple dilutions, both manual and with the diluter, may be made and the average absorbance reading calculated for each group. Alternatively, repetitive dilutions may be made into a larger recipient vessel that will average out dilution variations for both the manual and the diluter methods. Both methods are recommended because precision is best evaluated using multiple, separate dilutions, and accuracy is best measured using a single, larger recipient vessel. If the volumes are adjustable, this process must be repeated each time adjustments are made.

Before the dilution ratio check is made, gravimetric calibration of the diluent dispenser must be made. This is done by using distilled water as the diluent and cycling the system many times to completely flush the system so that only distilled water is present within the diluter. An aliquot of water should then be dispensed into a tared narrow-mouthed flask and weighed immediately. This should be repeated several times so that the average weight of a single dispensing of the diluent can be determined. If the weight of the water dispensed and the weight of a given volume of distilled water at a certain temperature is known (Table 4-1), the volume of water dispensed can be determined if the temperature of that water is also known.

For example, if the temperature of water is 25°C,

Weight of 10 ml volumetric flask	21.00 g
Weight of flask + diluent	31.00 g
Net weight of dispensed diluent	10.00 g
Volume dispensed	10.00/0.9970
	= 10.03 ml

A simple practical method for calibration is to calculate the weight that a given volume of water should weigh at its temperature. The adjustable diluter can then be set to deliver that weight of water. This set volume can then be checked daily with a class A volumetric flask (if the volume dispensed is one for which a volumetric flask is available). The dilution ratio should also be checked as confirmation of the calibration of the sampler unit.

Table 4-1
Weight in Grams of 1 ml Water at Specified Temperature

Temperature (°C)	Weight (g)
20	0.9982
21	0.9980
22	0.9977
23	0.9975
24	0.9974
25	0.9970
26	0.9968
27	0.9965
28	0.9962
29	0.9959
30	0.9956

Suggested Reading

Bermes EW, Forman DT: Basic laboratory principles and procedures. In Tietz N (ed): Fundamentals of Clinical Chemistry, 2nd ed. Philadelphia, WB Saunders, 1976
Tietz NW: Textbook of Clinical Chemistry. Philadelphia, WB Saunders, 1986
Varley H: Practical Clinical Biochemistry, 4th ed. New York, Interscience, 1967
Winstead M: Instrument Check Systems. Philadelphia, Lea & Febiger, 1971

5

SPECTROPHOTOMETRY

M. Robert Hicks

Definitions

Absorbance A: Same as optical density (OD) or A = 2 − log%T (percent transmittance).

Filter Photometer: Similar to spectrophotometer, but uses a filter instead of a dispersing device.

Half-bandpass (Bandpass):   The half-bandpass width is the range of wavelengths between the two points at which the transmittance is one-half the peak transmittance of the various wavelengths included in a monochromator's transmitted light.

Micron, μ: One millionth of a meter (10^{-6} m).

Monochromator: Any system or component that will emit monochromatic light, whether it be a filter or a dispersing system.

Nanometer, nm: The preferred term for the designation of 10^{-9} m; also referred to as millimicron, or mμ.

Nephelometry: The detection of light scattered and leaving the solution at some angle other than that of the incident beam.

Nominal Wavelength: The wavelength at which peak transmittance occurs.

Peak Transmittance: The maximal percent emission at the nominal wavelength.

Photometer: An instrument for measuring relative radiant power or some function of this quantity (as measured by receptors such as photocells, and so on).

Photometric Accuracy: Photometric accuracy states the ability of a spectrophotometer to correctly indicate the energy level presented to the detector.

Photometric Linearity: This is the general check of the instrument's performance to confirm that a solution known to conform to the Beer-Lambert Law will give a linear absorbance response to that solution.

Spectrometer, Optical: An instrument with an entrance slit, a dispersing device, and one or more exit slits, with which measurements are made at selected wavelengths within the spectral range or by scanning over the range.

Spectrophotometer: A spectrometer with associated equipment, so that it furnishes the ratio or a function of the ratio of the radiant power of two beams as a function of the spectral wavelength. These two beams may be separated in time, space, or both.

Spectrophotometry (Spectrophotometric Measurement):   Making light intensity measurement in a narrow wavelength range of the spectrum to determine the degree of radiant energy absorption by a solution.

Stray Radiant Energy (Stray Light):   All radiant energy that reaches the detector at wavelengths that do not correspond to the spectral position under consideration.

Turbidimetry: The measurement of the transmitted light at the same wavelength and direction as incident light.

Wavelength Accuracy: This measurement is the deviation of the average wavelength reading at an absorption-band peak or emission line from a recognized standard.

Wavelength Repeatability: This is a measure of the ability of a spectrophotometer to return to the same spectral position as determined by an absorption band or emission line of known wavelength when the instrument is reset or is read at a given wavelength.

Introduction

Because of the similarity of function and use, both spectrophotometers and photoelectric colorimeters will be presented here. These instruments that are similar in design with respect to having many identical components can be markedly different in application and versatility. The colorimeter, which utilizes a filter as a monochromator, has proven to be a most rugged and stable instrument requiring very little maintenance. Nevertheless, these systems are of limited or specialized usage because of the fixed wavelength of the monochromatic system. This wavelength can be changed only by changing the filter. The spectrophotometers, on the other hand, are more versatile but require much more maintenance. This is because the conditions of the light source and the dispersing element are directly related to the quality of the monochromatic light; therefore, this system requires closer monitoring and more maintenance. However, the dispersion element enables the selection of a continuously variable source of monochromatic light with either a simple manual or automatic adjustment.

It seems that as the efficiency of the monochromatic system to produce a narrow half-bandpass with a relative high percentage of light transmitted increases, the complexity of the associated optics and light source also increases. As the sensitivity of the detectors increases, the requirements for a more stable power supply and meter system also increase. Because of the interrelation of the aforementioned, it must be understood that a good knowledge of the component parts, and their functions as a part of that system, is a prerequisite to understanding the system. With a knowledge of these systems, principles of operations, and of the laws that govern the absorption of light, the student is better able to cope with the problems of photometry.

Principles

In relation to analytical chemistry, *photometry* refers to the measurement of the light-transmitting power of a solution in order to determine the concentration of light-absorbing substances present within. Photometry can, of course, be applied to measure the transmission of energy in the ultraviolet, infrared, and visible regions of the radiant energy spectrum. Instruments that are used to measure transmittance at various wavelengths are called spectrophotometers or photo-electric colorimeters, depending upon certain essential differences in construction, particularly the method of producing monochromatic light.

In all such instruments, monochromatic light is passed through an absorbing column of an often colored solution of a fixed depth and directed upon a photo-sensitive device that converts the radiant energy into electrical energy. The current produced under these conditions is measured by means of a galvanometer or a sensitive voltmeter.

Absorbance as measured in photometers (Fig. 5-1) involves not only the absorbance of the solute in the solution being evaluated, but also all of the molecules of the liquid through which the light passes. It is necessary, therefore, to adjust the instrument by means of a "blank." This blank is prepared by placing in the absorption cell (cuvette) all of the constituents of the unknown solution (solvents, reagents, and so forth), but under conditions that will not permit the color reaction to take place. The blank solution is used to set the meter of the instrument at a fixed point (100% transmittance [T] or zero absorbance). After adjusting the meter, the cuvette containing the unknown is placed in the instrument and read. By this means, the absorbance of the reagents used can be cancelled. It follows that the reading of the meter with the unknown cuvette in place is a measure of the amount of absorbance of monochromatic light by the unknown. The greater the number of molecules or ions of absorbing substance present, the greater is the absorption of light. In other words, the deeper the color, the greater is the deflection of the galvanometer from its original setting. Therefore, the concentration of the absorbing component present in a solution may be accurately measured by a photometer, provided that the necessary monochromatic light is used.

Beer's Law

Although the laws of photometry have been referred to as *Beer's Law* (for convenience sake), they are actually laws derived by five different individuals. Bouguer showed (in 1729) that when light passes through an absorbing body, there

Figure 5-1.   Schematic diagram of single-beam system.

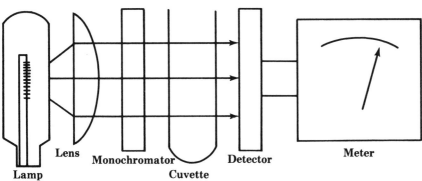

Lamp   Lens   Monochromator   Cuvette   Detector   Meter

is always the same difference between the logarithms of the amount of light entering and the amount of light leaving any section of the same thickness; or, as Lambert expressed it (in 1760), if one-half the amount of light entering leaves the first section, then $\frac{1}{2} \times \frac{1}{2}$ of the original light will leave the second section. Beer (in 1852) found that one solution of copper sulfate will absorb the same amount as another if the concentration of the first is twice that of the second and the length of the light path of the first is one-half that of the second.

These laws then state that light, in passing through a colored medium, is absorbed in direct proportion to the amount of the colored substance in the light path. Therefore, the strength of the observed "color" is directly proportional to the concentration of the absorbing chromagen in solution.

If we let P equal the transmitted energy and P_0 the incident energy, then the ratio P/P_0 represents the transmittance (T) of the absorbing material. If the material does not absorb at all, then P and P_0 are the same, $P/P_0 = T$, and $\%T = 100$. By using the negative logarithm of T, measurements are transformed to the energy absorbed $1/T$. The equation now becomes $A = -\log T$; because 2 is the log of 100, the $\%T$ formula becomes $A = 2 - \log \%T$. In practice, we adjust the photometer to read $100\%\ T$ with a cuvette containing a blank solution. We then substitute a standard or unknown solution and read the meter. Thus, we may use $\%T$ and semilog paper (Fig. 5-2), or A with regular (Cartesian) graph paper (Fig.

Figure 5-2. Calibration curve: $\%\ T$ versus concentration plotted on semilog paper.

$$C_u = A_u/A_s \times C_s$$

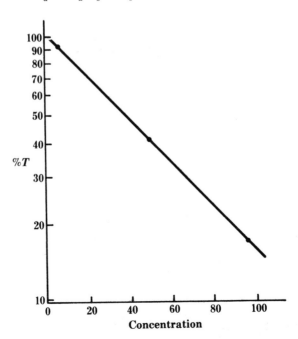

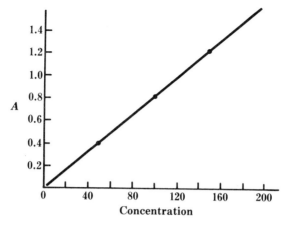

Figure 5-3. Calibration curve: *A* versus concentration.

5-3) to get a straight line when plotting against concentration as the abscissa. When a straight line is obtained on one of the above graphs, we may also calculate the unknown from the formula: Concentration of the unknown equals *A* of unknown divided by *A* of standard times the concentration of the standard.

Nephelometry and Turbidimetry

When a beam of radiant energy is directed through particles in solution (suspension), the intensity of the transmitted radiation is decreased. As this happens, reradiation will occur in all directions at the same time, at the same frequency, and in the same phase with the incident radiation.[11] This phase–coherence relationship between incident and reradiated energy may be destroyed by the physical effects of the surrounding medium.

The intensity of the scattered light at any particular angle from a particle is a function of the wavelength of the incident light, the size and shape of the particle, and the difference in the refractive indices of the particle and of the medium. As the size of the scattering particle increases, more of the incident radiation is scattered in the forward direction, resulting in an asymmetrical scatter of light. Therefore, the amount of light scatter is nearly linear to the concentration of particles in solution and the angular distribution of the scattered light indicates the size and shape of the scattering particle.[28] This system of photometric measurement has provided a means of studying and quantitating crystals, human cells, and precipitated protein in solution. The antigen–antibody reactions to drugs and specific proteins are of primary interest in the clinical laboratory.[6,7,22,24,25,26]

In order to prepare a standard for turbidity measurements, either an arbitrary standard or a pure compound is used. Arbitrary standards, such as latex particles, give a stable turbid solution but no actual standard value can be applied. If pure solutions of the compounds in question can be precipitated by physical or chemical means, then these compounds can be treated in the same way as an unknown solution and the turbidities can be compared, thereby providing standards for quantitation.

NEPHELOMETRIC MEASUREMENT

Nephelometry refers to the detection of light scattered and leaving a solution at some angle other than that of the incident beam.[14] This type of measurement is best performed in dilute suspensions of particles where self-absorption and reflection are minimal. For greater sensitivity, incident light of short wavelength (ultraviolet and visional) should be used.[29] Reradiated light at this same wavelength is measured at a shorter angle than 90° or greater than 0° for greater sensitivity.[11]

TURBIDIMETRIC MEASUREMENT

Turbidimetry refers to the measurement of the transmitted light through a turbid solution, at the same wavelength, and direction as the incident beam. For a very simple definition, let us consider that nephelometry measures scattered light and turbidity measures the light remaining after scatter.[14] Turbidimetric methods are similar to colorimetric methods in that both involve measurement of the intensity of light transmitted through a medium and both employ similar apparatus. As with absorption, the scattering of light by a turbid sample may be used analytically. When a light beam passes through a turbid sample, the energy that is lost from the incident beam is a reflection of the number of particles in solution. In order to make this measurement meaningful, as to a protein concentration, a specific protein of known concentrations must be precipitated and measured. When this standard protein is treated and measured in the same way as in unknown samples, the results are comparable. Again, for greatest sensitivity, light of short wavelength should be used.

Component Parts

POWER SUPPLIES

The commercial power supply is adequate for most general uses, and the usual fluctuations of voltage and current do not significantly upset the equilibrium of lamps, heaters, or motors. Nevertheless, no stable operation of light-measuring instruments is possible without better control of the power source. Therefore, a power supply capable of furnishing adequately regulated electrical energy for the particular need of the instrument must be utilized. These power supplies fall into three general categories: batteries, voltage-regulating transformers (Sola), and electronic power supplies.

Batteries, either wet-cell or dry-cell, produce quite stable voltages and are relatively inexpensive. Dry-cell batteries are mainly used for the operation of some small photometers, Wheatstone bridges, and radiation detectors, or wherever portability is necessary and a low direct current supply can be used. The wet-cell (lead-acid) battery, as used in automobiles, also produces a fairly stable current supply; however, it is also limited to being a source of low voltage and direct current. In addition, it requires regular maintenance consisting of frequent recharging and addition of water. After charging, the battery must go through a short period of discharging before stable current is obtained.

The constant-voltage transformers (such as Sola) will regulate power output very closely as long as the input remains between 95 and 125 V and at 60 Hz (cps). These devices are essentially trouble-free and have no moving parts.

The electronic power supplies will give more precise regulation than can be easily obtained from the "Sola-type" transformer. Situations may be encountered in which frequency variations must be taken into account. This necessitates the use of an electronic device to regulate and supply the desired voltage. These devices are complex and expensive; however, they are becoming more common and it is known that they are dependable. Nevertheless, it should be remembered that no inexperienced person should even try to tinker with solid state components. These solid state power supplies are also subject to erratic behavior from unstable line voltage. Low voltage can cause complete component failure, and voltage spikes can burn out components as well as produce erratic results.

RADIANT ENERGY SOURCES

The function of the light source is to provide incident light of sufficient intensity for measurement. For work in the visible, near-infrared, and near-ultraviolet regions, the most common source is the glass-enclosed, tungsten filament, incandescent lamp. These lamps with prefocused bases are most useful with respect to easy replacement in an optical system; however, when used with a grating or prism monochromator, wavelength calibration must be checked when lamps are changed. Although these lamps produce a continuous spectrum over a wide range, they do have some shortcomings. Most of their energy is emitted in the near-infrared region of the spectrum, about 15% in the visible, when operated normally. Operating temperatures can be increased to produce a greater percentage of short-wavelength energy, but this drastically shortens lamp life.

For work in the ultraviolet region, the high-pressure hydrogen (or deuterium) discharge lamp is adequate from 200 nm to an upper limit extending to about 375 nm. At longer wavelengths the emission is no longer continuous. When deuterium is used instead of hydrogen, the light intensity is tripled.

For very high levels of ultraviolet illumination, the xenon arc or high-pressure mercury vapor lamps provide a large amount of continuous radiation plus high energies at the spectral lines of these elements. These lamps become very hot in operation and may even require thermal insulation, with or without auxiliary cooling, to protect the surrounding components.

Although these special lamps are available and can be used, they usually require special power supplies and mountings. When planning to use these types of energy sources, it is better to purchase the equipment as a unit so that the light source will be properly set up and the necessary insulation will be in place.

MONOCHROMATOR

When measuring the absorption or emission of radiant energy by an absorbing solution, it is necessary to be able to isolate the desired wavelength of that energy and exclude the rest. In other words, by restricting the band of wavelengths passing through the sample to those absorbed by the substance of interest, the sensitivity of the instrumental measurements to concentration changes is greatly enhanced. Thus, the important characteristics of a monochromator (dispersing device) are its bandpass width, the nominal wavelength, and peak transmittance.

There are numerous ways of isolating the desired spectrum. The simplest device is a *filter* (glass, Wratten, or interference) placed just in front of the sample holder. The usual glass and Wratten filters are of relative wide bandwidths and low peak emission. Because the function of the filter is to absorb unwanted energy, the dissipation of the heat produced in the filter must be considered. The filter must resist change in the spectral characteristics over long periods of usage. For these reasons, the gelatin (Wratten) filter is now seldom used because it tends to deteriorate quickly with time.

Narrower bandwidths are obtained with *interference filters* (Fig. 5-4). This type of filter consists of an evaporated coating of a transparent dielectric spacer of low refractive index sandwiched between semitransparent silver films. Sharp cutoff filters are placed on each side of these films to eliminate other than first-order effects. These filters have a bandwidth of 10 to 17 nm and a peak transmittance of 40% to 60%.

Multilayer interference filters consist of successive layers of high and low refractive index dielectrics on alternating layers. These filters are characterized by a bandpass width of 8 nm or less and a peak transmittance of 60% to 90%. These multilayer interference filters will only transmit light with a wavelength two times the distance between the silver films (in phase); that is, with complete constructive interference. All other wavelengths will show partial or complete destructive interference as the reflected light rays are retransmitted out of phase with those of the same wavelength which are transmitted directly. These interference filters can be used with high-intensity light sources because they remove unwanted radiation by transmission and reflection and not by absorption.

Figure 5-4.   Interference filter.

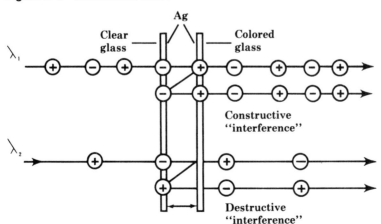

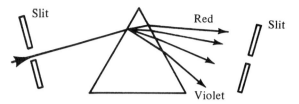

Figure 5-5. Light dispersion by prism.

Many instruments use *prisms* (Fig. 5-5) or *diffraction gratings* (Fig. 5-6) as monochromators. These devices separate the various wavelengths of radiant energy as produced by a tungsten lamp by refraction or diffraction, and present them as a spectrum from which the desired wavelengths may be selected. The action of a prism in dispersing a polychromatic beam of radiation into a spectrum depends upon the variation of the index of refraction with wavelength. As used in spectrometers, the light from the source is directed through a convergent lens into an entrance slit at the focal point of the lens, then through the prism and a second convergent lens. At an air–prism interface, an entering light ray at an angle of incidence will be bent toward the vertical to the surface and, at the prism–air interface, it is bent away from the vertical. The image of the entrance slit is projected onto the exit slit as a series of colored images arranged next to each other. Violet light is refracted (bent) farther than red.

The actual separation between two wavelengths depends upon the dispersive power of the prism and the apical angle of the prism; a nonlinear wavelength scale

Figure 5-6. Light dispersion by diffraction grating, showing possible second- and third-order interference.

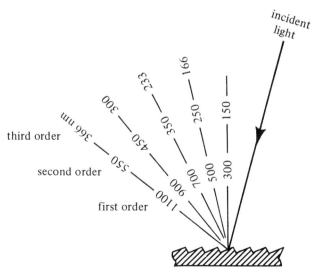

results. The longer wavelengths are not refracted as much and are therefore crowded. Dispersion by glass is about three times that of quartz. Quartz or fused silica is mandatory for inclusion of the spectra below 350 nm.

Diffraction gratings, on the other hand, produce a linear noncurved spectrum. A diffraction grating is based upon the principle that light rays of radiant energy will bend around a sharp corner, the degree of bending depending upon the wavelength. Therefore, with a beam of energy containing many wavelengths striking a grating, many tiny spectra are produced, one for each line of the grating. As the wavelengths move past the corners, wavefronts are formed. Where these cross, those that are in phase reinforce one another, and those that are not cancel out and disappear, thereby leaving a complete spectrum to display upon the exit slit, much the same as with the prisms. Some grating monochromators have a half-bandwidth as high as 35 nm, whereas other more expensive units have half-bandwidths of less than 0.5 nm.

Despite the good dispersive qualities and the linear spectrum presentation, diffraction gratings have problems with stray light. This stray light may be defined as radiant energy at unwanted wavelengths reaching the detector. One problem with stray light is that slight imperfections exist in the ruling. Another problem is caused by second-order effects of the grating. Part of this trouble can be eliminated by using a double monochromator or by using a special mounting such as the Ebert system.

The holographic grating, on the other hand, has no ghosts and a much lower stray light level. This grating is blazed by the action of monochromatic laser light on a photosensitive material coating the surface of optical glass. This portion of the photoresistant material is then washed away, leaving a groove structure in relief. The grating is then coated with an appropriate reflective layer and can be used in the same manner as a ruled grating. When this type of grating is produced on a concave optical glass surface, it becomes the only form of optics necessary in a simple monochromator.[29] With this type of monochromator, a spectrophotometer may not need a powerful exciter lamp to work well in the near-ultraviolet range, because excess light is not lost on many optical surfaces.

SAMPLE CELL (CUVETTE)

Absorption spectrophotometry usually evaluates the absorption of a solute in a liquid solvent. The square or rectangular absorption cells have plane parallel faces and a light path of constant length. They are free of optical aberrations. Sets of cuvettes may be matched to very close tolerances. This type of cuvette is rather expensive and is usually utilized in the more expensive instruments. For ultraviolet work (below 340 nm) it is mandatory that this type of cell, constructed from silica or quartz, be used.

For most work in the visual range, the cylindrical test tube type is sufficiently accurate. These cuvettes are prone to variable reflection and refraction errors as well as lens effect. Glass tubing (from which cuvettes are made) is rarely round and is not polished, so there are considerably more surface irregularities. For this reason, round tube-typed absorption cells require close calibration and segregation into matched groups. Because these cells are generally somewhat oval, it is necessary that they be marked in front for proper light-path orientation.

Another solution to this problem would be to use a flow-through cuvette. Because the same cuvette is in the light path at all times, cuvette errors would be compensated for by the blank. Highly reproducible results can be obtained, provided the cuvette does not become dirty and no bubbles are introduced and/or trapped in the cell. A source of vacuum is needed to empty the cell. Filling is often a very real problem because of the small tops. This may lead to spillage into the instrument and resultant corrosion.

ASSOCIATED OPTICS

The range of transmittance of materials for construction of windows and lenses is a critical factor. The absorbance of any material should be less than 0.2 at the wavelength of use. Ordinary silica glass transmits satisfactorily from 350 to 3000 nm. Special Corex glass will extend the ultraviolet range to about 300 nm. Quartz or fused silica must be used below this. Beam reduction is accomplished by condensers that can reduce the beam size by a factor of 25 without loss of appreciable energy.

In colorimeters and economically priced spectrophotometers, simple lenses are used to focus or collimate the light beams. In the more expensive instruments, front-surfaced mirrors are used to reduce energy loss. These mirrors are aluminized on their front surfaces because other metallic surfaces show selective absorption at certain wavelengths. The surfaces of these mirrors are coated with a thin film of magnesium fluoride to reduce light scattering.

DETECTORS

Any photosensitive device may be of use as a detector of radiant energy, provided that it has a linear response in the part of the spectrum to be used and is sensitive enough for the task at hand. These devices must first convert electromagnetic energy to a different type of energy, namely electrical energy. The electrical energy produced can then be measured.

The most common of these devices are the photocells (barrier layer cells, Fig. 5-7). These require no external voltage source, but rely on internal electron transfers to produce a current in an external circuit. These cells are composed of an iron back plate and a layer of crystalline selenium or cadmium on one surface. Electrical contacts are made with the iron plate and an electrical conductive transparent film on the front active layer. The cells are then sealed to prevent physical or chemical damage.

A photon striking one of the selenium or cadmium atoms transfers its energy to an electron and raises it into a conduction band. This electron now travels from the front to the back of the photocell and through the external circuit for measurement. These cells are simple, quite inexpensive, and, in general, very dependable. However, they have certain faults that should be understood. These cells can become "light blinded," a condition similar to that of the human eye. They need time to rest. Their response is temperature-sensitive, requiring some

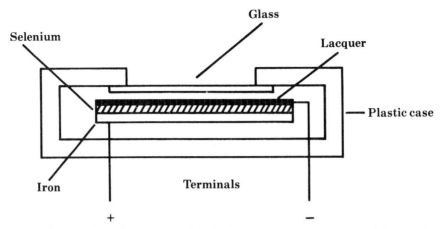

Figure 5-7. Photocell. (Tammes AR: Electronics for Medical and Biology Laboratory Personnel. Baltimore, Williams & Wilkins, 1971)

warm-up time for temperature stability. Because of their low internal resistance and low output of electrical energy, the signals are not easily amplified.

Phototubes are constructed of a negatively charged cathode and a wirelike, positively charged anode. The cathode is coated with a photoemissive substance such as cesium oxide. When a photon strikes this layer, electrons are emitted and jump through the vacuum over to the anode, where they are collected and return via the external circuit. The output from these tubes can be amplified and then fed into external circuits for greater sensitivity. For this reason, this type of detector is used on all precise instruments that have a close restriction on the slit and, thereby, the wavelength presentation.

The photomultiplier tube combines photocathode emission with multiple cascade stages of electron amplification of primary photocurrent within the tube itself. The tube is constructed so that the primary photoelectrons from the cathode are attracted and accelerated to several succeeding dynodes. These dynodes are constructed of a material that will give off several secondary electrons when hit by other high-energy electrons. Therefore, the photomultiplier tube can measure light intensities about 200 times weaker than the ordinary phototube.

READOUT DEVICES

A *galvanometer* (Fig. 5-8) is an instrument used to detect or measure currents. A flat suspended coil lies in the plane between the poles of a permanent magnet. When the current to be detected or compared passes through the coil, it sets up a magnetic field whose poles are at the front and back, or 90° away from the permanent magnet poles. In trying to set its lines of force in line with those of the magnet, the coil turns as far as the magnetic forces can twist the wire. The stronger the current, the stronger the magnetic field and the farther the coil turns. The iron core makes a uniform field for the coil to turn in; a beam of light reflected from the mirror on the coil serves as a pointer.

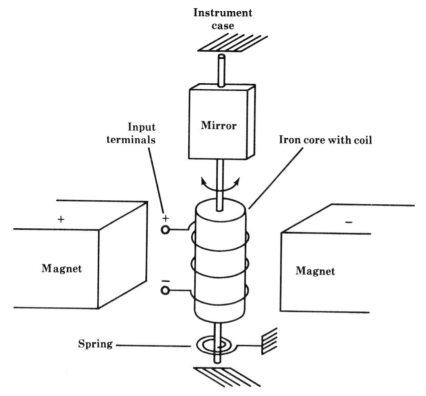

Figure 5-8. Galvanometer schematic with terminals.

When an arbitrary readout device, such as a percent scale or optical density scale, is incorporated into this system, we have what is called a *direct readout meter*. Actually, this readout could be in millivolts, milliamps, mg%, mEq/liter, or any other arbitrary unitage, provided the scales take into consideration the linear relation of milliamps and %T and the log relationship between millivolts and absorbance. Therefore, this type of readout is generally considered to be the fastest, simplest, and the easiest to use.

If, on the other hand, an electrical force governed by the action of a variable resister (potentiometer) is used to bring the meter to null point, the system is said to be a *null-point system*. In this case, an arbitrary scale is fitted to the potentiometer scale. This scale may carry the same arbitrary type of unitage as the first. This slide wire potentiometer may also be connected to a servomotor of a digital readout system or of a recorder.

Types of Instruments

Although the filter photometer is not to be considered as a spectrophotometer because it does not give a continuous source of monochromatic radiant energy, the two must be considered together when it comes to function and system design.

Colorimeters that use the regular glass filter will also use a simple low-energy light source. In fact, this type of filter dictates the use of this type of source, as well as eliminating the need for even a single lens. Therefore, the simplest system would require a power supply, light source, filter, sample holder, detector, and a meter, in that order; however, when an interference filter, prism, or diffraction grating is used, a more elaborate system is necessary. These types of monochromators require that radiant energy be focused into the system in parallel lines. Diffraction gratings and prisms also require the use of entrance and exit slits to limit the spectrum and exclude stray light. In fact, most grating monochromators require that sharp cutoff filters be placed at the entrance to eliminate second-order spectrum. When you add to this a sample holder, a detector, and a meter, you then have a single-beam spectrophotometer.

In a double-beam system (Fig. 5-9), monochromatic light from either a single or double monochromator is focused through both a reference and a sample compartment. The intensity of these two beams of light is then measured by either one or two detectors, and the sample beam is compared to the reference side as a ratio. This ratio may then be fed into a meter or directly into a ratio recording

Figure 5-9. Double-beam system with optics.

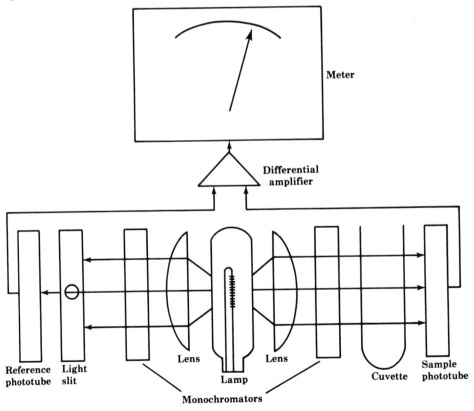

and a beam splitting and reuniting system of choppers to overcome the problem of balancing two phototubes to an exactly equal spectral response.

Instrument Quality Control

Spectrophotometric analysis is generally used in two types of measurement. The first is a quantitative determination of chemical constituents, achieved by comparing the optical transmittance of one solution to that of a pure solution of known concentration. In this way, the system is calibrated in known units of specific chemical concentration; therefore, the accuracy of the analysis is directly related to the quality of the standard solution, the spectrophotometric method, and the instrument used.

The second type of measurement used is the determination of the optical transmission values of a liquid solution followed by the calculation of molar absorptivities. In both cases, proven accuracy of the transmittance scale of the instrument is essential. For this reason, it is imperative that all spectrophotometer functions and settings be checked periodically.[9,12,13,20]

The most insidious problems of instrument malfunction have to do with the certainty of wavelength, bandwidth, linearity, stray light, and photometric accuracy.[1,2,3,21] These terms probably mean very little to the laboratory workers who rely completely on the colorimeters to perform, without a question as to how well they did or could function; but quality in instrument performance cannot be assumed, it must be proven. The monitoring of instrument performance is even more important in the spectrophotometer. This is especially true in the narrow bandpass units. These systems with their greater potential accuracy and sensitivity demand closer attention to their functional performance.[4,5,9,10,16]

Electrical malfunction will not be considered here, even though it is a part of instrument quality control. This type of problem is usually covered in detail by the instrument handbook and requires a specially trained individual to make repairs.

WAVELENGTH CALIBRATION

Wavelength calibration is a means of ensuring that the radiant energy being emitted from the exit slit of the monochromator is the same as that specified by the wavelength selector and within the tolerances of the instrument. This simple check should be made whenever a new lamp is installed and routinely thereafter. This is to ensure that the slight changes in lamp filament position during usage are corrected and do not lead to gross analytical errors. Minor errors in wavelength settings are of relatively little importance in wide bandpass spectrophotometers, and these units may be checked less often. Wavelength calibration of the more sophisticated narrow bandpass instruments are of the utmost importance, and no scan of any substance is worth doing if the monochromator is not in calibration.

Didymium and holmium oxide glass filters have been used for many years on the general laboratory instruments.[17] More recently, the combination of the didymium glass filter and an acid solution of nickel sulfate[8] has been used. This solution gives a peak transmission at 510 nm. A solution of cobalt chloride has a peak absorbance at this wavelength. This solution may be helpful as a secondary check on the nickel sulfate when it is not in agreement with the didymium filter.

Precision instruments require a more precise means of wavelength calibration. The emission bands of mercury arc or deuterium lamps are good sources of radiant energy with specific emission spectra.[2,21] The quartz mercury arc lamp, with its multiple emission bands, provides the best source for accurate wavelength calibration from 205 to 1014 nm.[30] The deuterium lamp in ultraviolet instruments has two major emission lines, 486 and 656.2 nm, that provide a good source of wavelength calibration in the visual range. This lamp provides the most practical means of wavelength calibration of a grating instrument, because only two lines are needed when light dispersion is linear.

STRAY LIGHT

Stray light is any radiant energy measured by the detector that is outside the spectral region isolated by the monochromator of the instrument. It can be caused by dirty optics, poor baffling, or faulty grating in the monochromator, as well as fluorescence of the sample itself. Because stray light may be independent of sample concentration, its relative effect is usually greatest at low transmittance, where instrument errors are also greater.

The American Society of Testing Material E-13 Committee Standards[3] have been adopted for the measurement of stray radiant energy in spectrophotometers and provides a good means of instrument evaluation; however, for ease of understanding and routine checking, a common sense approach may be more practical. Scattered light can be of any wavelength, and in grating instruments it may also be of second-order reflection.[23] This may also be true of old and poorly constructed interference filters. Therefore, this light may well be of a wavelength far removed from that selected and will not be absorbed by the test solution. From this information, it is easy to reason that scattered light can cause nonlinearity and insensitivity.

Sharp cutoff filters may be used to directly assess the amount of stray light at the extremes of the instrument range.[21] These filters have the unique ability to stop all light above or below a certain range. Thus, by the proper selection of filters, it is possible to check the apparent stray light of any instrument. This may be done by setting the wavelength selector at the desired wavelength (400 or 700 nm) and then adjusting the instrument meter to read 100% transmission. Place a filter in the sample compartment and note the meter reading. This reading is an indication of stray light and must be considered as an instrumental error.

If one is performing time rate analyses, one of the simplest checks to make is to measure the absorbance of NADH at 340 nm with the tungsten and deuterium light source. If the absorbance of the solution is greater with the deuterium lamp, stray light was present when the tungsten lamp was used and this has been corrected by employing the deuterium radiation source. This is because the deuterium lamp is a discontinuous radiant energy source in the visual range, and therefore does not emit radiation at 680 nm, the wavelength of light that is of primary importance in second-order effect. Also, very little energy is emitted by this lamp above 400 nm, so that scattered-light problems are greatly diminished when working in the ultraviolet range.

Nickel sulfate solution has also been used for this purpose over the visual range. This solution shows maximum absorption at 400 and 700 nm, and under certain circumstances no light should be transmitted at these wavelengths. Any deviation from this on repeated checks is an indication of stray light.

PHOTOMETRIC ACCURACY

Provided that the stray-light check is negligible, the linearity check tests the ability of the photocell to produce a signal proportional to the light intensity and of the instrument's meter system to measure this signal accurately. A linearity check can be made by reading the absorbance of standard solutions of various salt solutions that have major absorption peaks at certain wavelengths or by using neutral density filters that absorb energy over a broad range.

Solutions of potassium chromate[19] and potassium dichromate[15,19] have been used for evaluating photometric accuracy in the ultraviolet range. A solution of 0.04 g/liter of potassium chromate dissolved in 0.05N potassium hydroxide will show maximum absorbance at 273 and 373 nm. The absorbance range reported for this solution[30] is 0.189 to 0.199A and 0.247 to 0.249A, respectively, for these two wavelengths. When measuring absorbance below 260 nm, this solution should not be more than 6 months old. This may be the reason for the wide range in absorbance values at 273 nm. A solution of potassium dichromate, 0.05 g/liter dissolved in 0.01N sulfuric acid, also exhibits two absorbance peaks that may be used. These are at 257 and 350 nm and should read 27.6% transmission at the latter wavelength. Absorbance patterns of this solution are varied by changes in acidity; therefore, the pH should be carefully controlled. Cobalt ammonium sulfate[8] and Thompson's solution[27] have been used for this evaluation in the visual range. These solutions require great care in preparation and handling. The absorbance cells used must be cleaned and matched before use. Although these materials are relatively stable, they may react with contaminants and deteriorate. The solvent solution must also be checked for absorbance in the ultraviolet range when these solutions are to be analyzed. Frings and colleagues[12,13] have proposed using French's green food coloring for monitoring detector response at three wavelengths. This dye solution has absorbance maxima at 257 nm, 410 nm, and 630 nm. The advantage of this solution is that it provides a means of response verification in both visual and ultraviolet ranges with one solution at a very modest cost.

The National Bureau of Standards developed a set of neutral density glass filters[18] for the specific purpose of checking the photometric scale of spectrophotometers. These filters are premounted in holders ready for use in the standard 10-mm cell compartment. They are not readily affected by temperature change nor do they require a critical wavelength adjustment. These standard reference materials (SRM) come as a set of three individual filters calibrated and certified to ±0.5% transmittance over four different wavelengths of the visual range. These filters were the forerunners of other sets manufactured by Bausch and Lomb as well as Chemetrics Corporation. All of the later filter sets have a filter that will fit a standard 10-mm cell compartment. These sets provide a means of checking for stray light, bandpass, and wavelength as well as photometric accuracy.

References

1. AACC Committee on Standards: Guideline for photometric instruments for measuring enzyme reaction rates. Clin Chem 23:2160, 1977
2. American Society of Testing Materials Committee E-13: Annual Book of ASTM Standards, pp 193–302. Philadelphia, American Society of Testing Materials, 1974
3. American Society of Testing Materials Committee E-13: Recommended Practices in Spectrophotometry, pp 63–83. Philadelphia, American Society of Testing Materials, 1967
4. Beeler MF: Laboratory Performance of Spectrophotometers. Am J Clin Pathol 61:789, 1974
5. Beeler MF, Lancaster RG: CAP survey to assess the extent of stray light problems in precision spectrophotometry. Am J Clin Pathol 63:953, 1975
6. Buffone GJ, Savory J, Cross RE: Use of a laser-equipped centrifugal analyzer for kinetic measurement of serum IgG. Clin Chem 20:1320, 1974
7. Buffone GJ, Savory J, Cross RE, Hammond JE: Evaluation of kinetic light scattering as an approach to the measurement of specific proteins with the centrifugal analyzer: Methodology. Clin Chem 21:1731, 1975
8. Burke RW, Mavodineau R, Smith MV: Standard reference materials for verifying the accuracy of spectrophotometers. American Clinical Products Review 3:12 (August), 1984
9. Chamron M, Keiser R: Maintaining optimum spectrophotometer performance, Part 1. American Laboratory 9:33, 1978
10. Chamron M, Keiser R: Maintaining optimum spectrophotometric performance, Part 2. American Laboratory 9:35, 1978
11. Finley PR: Nephelometry: Principles and clinical laboratory applications. Laboratory Management 20:34 (Sept), 1982
12. Frings CS, Broussard LA: Calibration and monitoring of spectrometers and spectrophotometers. Clin Chem 25:1013, 1979
13. Frings CS, Vincent I, Waldrop NT: Convenient method for checking detector response of spectrophotometers at three wavelengths. Clin Chem 22:101, 1976
14. Hills LP, Tiffany TO: Comparison of turbidimetric and light-scattering measurements of immunoglobulins by use of a centrifugal analyzer with absorbance and fluorescence light-scattering optics. Clin Chem 26:1459, 1980
15. Johnson EA: Potassium dichromate as an absorbence standard. Photo Spect Group Bull 17:505, 1967
16. Lucas DH, Blank RE: Spectrophotometric Standards in the Clinical Laboratory. American Laboratory 8:77, 1977
17. MacDonald RP: Uses of holmium oxide filter in spectrometry. Clin Chem 10:1117, 1964
18. Meinke WW: Standard reference materials for clinical measurement. Anal Chem 43:28a, 1971
19. Natl Bur Std Circ 4C929, 1948
20. NCCLS: Standard for Relating Spectrophotometer Performance Characteristics to Analytical Goals: NCCLS Approved Standard, AS1-3, 1980
21. Rand RN: Spectrophotometric standards. Clin Chem 15:839, 1969
22. Savory J, Buffone GJ, Rerch R: Kinetics of IgG-anti-IgG reaction as evaluated by conventional and stopped-flow nephelometry. Clin Chem 20:1078, 1974
23. Slavin W: Stray light in ultraviolet, visible, and near-infrared spectrophotometry. Anal Chem 35:561, 1963
24. Sternberg JC: A rate nephelometer for measuring specific proteins by immunoprecipitin reactions. Clin Chem 23:1456, 1977
25. Sternburg JC: Monitoring the precipitin reaction using rate nephelometry. Am Clin Prod Rev 3:24 (April), 1984
26. Thomson LC: An inorganic gray solution. Tran Faraday Soc 42:663, 1946

27. Tiffany TO, Parella JM, Johnson WF, Burtis CA: Specific protein analysis by light-scatter measurement with a miniature centrifugal fast analyzer. Clin Chem 20:1055, 1974
28. Whicher JT, Price CP, Spencer K, Ward AM: Immunonephelometric and immunoturbidimetric assays for proteins: CRC Crit Rev Clin Lab Sci 18:213, 1982–1983
29. Willard HH, Merritt LL Jr, Dean JA, Settle FA Jr: Instrumental Methods of Analysis, 6th ed. Princeton, NJ, Van Nostrand, 1981
30. Winstead M: Instrument Check Systems. Philadelphia, Lea & Febiger, 1971

6

FLAME PHOTOMETRY

Martin R. Lohff

Definitions

Emission Spectra: The characteristic spectra or color given off by atoms, ions, or molecules when excited by heat or other means.

Excitation Potential: The relative ease with which atoms entering a flame of constant temperature can be excited.

Excited State: The elevation of orbiting electrons from their ground or resting energy level to higher levels by the addition of thermal energy.

Flame Background (Background Interference):   The formation of continuous emission spectra by unknown substances in the solution to be analyzed, adding to the overall intensity of emission of light spectra.

Ground State: The unexcited state of the atom or molecule, according to Rutherford's and Bohr's concepts, in which orbital electrons have their normal unexcited energy potential and orbital planes.

Ionization Potential: The relative ease with which atoms in a gaseous state undergo ionization.

Interference: Changes in emission intensity from the expected of a standard or unknown due to the presence of certain anions, cations, overlapping emission spectra, or suppression of ionization through mass action.

Resonance Line: The return of an excited orbital electron to the unexcited or ground state, resulting in the release of radiation of a specific wavelength characteristic for a specific element.

Self-Absorption: The absorption by an atom of emitted radiation from a similar atom in quantum fashion.

Introduction

This chapter will explore the principles of flame photometry with expansion of the definitions by specific examples. Components of a typical flame photometer will be explained and examples will be given. The principle of internal standards will be explored. Typical routine maintenance will be covered, followed by a bibliography and suggested reading list to provide the reader with further information.

Principles

Flame photometry is the quantitation of specific atoms, ions, or molecules that have been brought to excitation in a flame. Emission spectra generated by this excitation are characteristic for each substance to be measured. Emission spectra may be continuous, band, or line spectra. A continuous spectrum contains light energy of approximately the same intensity over a wide range of wavelengths. Incandescent solids exhibit this phenomenon. A continuous spectrum is emitted without sharply defined lines. This type of spectral emission is used primarily as a radiant energy source for absorption spectroscopy and spectrophotometry. A band spectrum is generally caused by excited molecules such as metal oxides, and involves groups of emission lines (isolated energy maxima) that come closer and closer together until they approach the limits of resolution and merge, forming a band of spectral energy. Line spectra are definite, widely and irregularly spaced lines (sharply delineated energy maxima) of spectral emission caused generally by excited atoms or ions. Being spectral emission lines, they are essentially of the same wavelength (monochromatic).

General emission photometry is performed using a carbon arc, electrical discharge, or flame as the source of thermal excitation. Because of the higher temperatures generated (up to 6000K) by the first two methods, a greater number of elements can be excited, the radiation spectra that are emitted will be richer in energy, and a greater number of emission lines will be given off. These forms of emission spectrography are used primarily for research purposes.

Flame photometry, a subdivision of emission photometry, involves excitation by use of a flame. Because lower energies are involved, only those elements with lower excitation potential can be excited. Some elements (such as the alkaline metals of sodium, potassium, cesium, and lithium) have a relatively low excitation potential. Other metals (such as the alkaline earth elements of calcium and magnesium) have a higher excitation potential and therefore require greater temperatures for adequate thermal excitation. The excitation potential is a function of the energy levels of orbital electrons, and this in turn is related to the difference in number of orbital electrons and increasing nuclear charge.

Certain orbiting electrons may be raised from their ground or resting energy level to higher levels by the addition of thermal energy. The orbital electrons in this excited state are unstable and rapidly drop back to the unexcited or ground state. If this occurs in one jump, a quantum of energy is given off and a line spectrum is formed (Fig. 6-1). The energy may be given off in the ultraviolet, visible, or infrared regions. With the addition of greater amounts of energy (*i.e.*, increased flame temperature) the excitation potential of a greater number of atoms is overcome, and a larger number of elements are thereby excited. The emission intensity is greater, and the emission spectra are more complex. If the electron loses its acquired energy in several steps while returning to its original orbit, multiple line spectra may be generated.

The external form of the flame from a mixture of a combustible substance

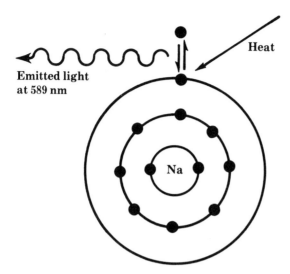

Figure 6-1.   Excited state of an atom.

and an oxidant depends upon the quantitative ratio of the components. With decreased air or oxygen ratio, a luminous yellow flame is obtained. This is produced by the presence of incandescent carbon particles. An example is the bunsen flame.

  With an increase in the air or oxygen ratio, the brightness of the flame decreases and finally disappears to become a clear, blue, nonluminous flame. This results in a flame with two cones: an inner, bright blue-green cone and an outer blue-violet cone. An intermediate zone is also discernible. The typical structure of a flame resulting from acetylene-oxygen is shown in Figure 6-2. The inner cone

Figure 6-2.   Temperature distribution in flame zones: (*A*) illuminating gas–air flame; (*B*) acetylene–oxygen flame.

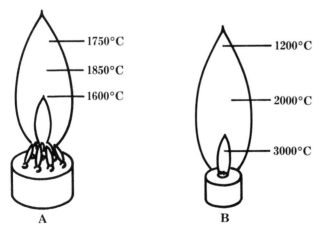

is hollow and the thickness of the layer forming the inner cone varies according to the reactants used. It consists of an inner reaction zone and an outer luminous zone. The merging gases enter the inner cone and are heated to the ignition temperature. Primary combustion proceeds with a deficiency of oxidant and occurs over a period of approximately 10^{-4} seconds. Molecules and radicals are formed in the combustion area. No reaction occurs in the intermediate zone although the flame has its maximum temperature here.

The outer zone (secondary combustion zone) results in complete combustion of hydrogen and those carbon monoxide molecules formed by the reaction in the inner cone. Oxygen for the oxidation of these molecules is obtained by diffusion from the surrounding atmosphere. The flame temperature in this reaction zone is close to, but slightly below, that of the intermediate zone.

It must be emphasized that the greater the thermal energy of any particular flame used, the greater the number of elements that will be excited. Increased emission intensity will result in increased sensitivity. However, increased background noise is often an unwanted by-product.

Flame photometry is rapid, uses relatively inexpensive apparatus, and requires a small volume of sample. Major disadvantages may include spectral interference between two or more substances in the solution to be analyzed, background interference, anionic and cationic interference, ionization, and self-absorption.

Spectral interference is that interference resulting when two or more elements having emission spectra in adjacent or overlapping wavelengths are present in a solution under analysis. The difficulty can be considerably lessened by use of a monochromator with more precise spectral isolation characteristics (narrow bandpass). Another way to avoid the effects of spectral interference is to use another wavelength, preferably toward the ultraviolet region, and one not associated with spectral line emissions from other atoms in solution.

Another disadvantage is flame background (background interference) (Fig. 6-3). *Flame background* is the formation of continuous emission spectra by unknown substances in the solution to be analyzed, adding to the overall emission intensity of light spectra. The maximum intensity of the line spectra generated by the elements under analysis, however, remains unchanged. Electronic correction for this background noise can be accomplished, provided it does not exceed the level of the line spectrum under analysis.

Other sources of interference include anionic and cationic interference. Anionic interference is the change in emission intensity from that expected of a standard or unknown due to the presence of certain anions in solution in the form of salts or acids. It generally has a negative effect. An example is the presence of hydrochloric acid in the flame photometric analysis of sodium and potassium. A $0.01M$ concentration results in a 15% decrease of sodium and 40% decrease in potassium emission intensity. Phosphoric acid shows even greater effect at a concentration as low as $0.01M$. The degree of reduction in emission depends not only upon the nature of the acid and its concentration, but also upon the nature of the alkali metal. It increases with increasing atomic number.

A more practical problem involves the marked decrease in emission intensity

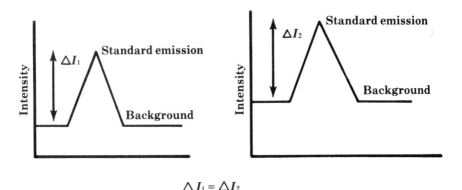

$$\triangle I_1 = \triangle I_2$$

Figure 6-3.   Correction of standard emission with variable flame background.

of calcium in the presence of sulfates and phosphates. The degree of effect is also related to flame temperature. For example, a 92% reduction in emission intensity of calcium is noted in a hydrogen-air flame. However, with hydrogen-oxygen flame, the reduction in intensity is only 30%. The practical effects of this are quite apparent when attempts at calcium or magnesium determinations are made by flame photometry.

The nature of the anion effect is complex and involves the formation of poorly dissociable compounds, formation of nonvolatile compounds, or hindrance of the evaporation of metal from the aerosol particles with reduction of the number of free metal atoms. In the case of phosphates and calcium determination, the effect is primarily that of formation of calcium phosphate ($Ca_3[PO_4]_2$).

The presence of certain cations in a solution under analysis may result in radiation interference, again generally having a negative effect. For example, the presence of aluminum in the same solution causes a decreased emission intensity of the alkaline earth metals such as calcium. Again, the formation of compounds that volatilize poorly is probably the reason. The magnitude of interference is inversely related to the ionization potential of the interfering cation. The postulated mechanism involves a shift in ionization equilibria in the flame between emissive, un-ionized atoms and nonemissive ions and electrons. The literature is somewhat more confusing on the interaction of cations such as sodium and potassium in routine analysis. Both positive and negative interferences have been described. These differences were felt to be a function of the bandpass of the instrument used in analysis (spectral interference). However, it now appears more likely that the directions and magnitude of interferences depend primarily on flame temperature, being negative for low temperatures and positive for high temperatures.

Ionization is another cause of interference. Those elements with low ionization potentials are more readily ionized in the flame, especially at low concentration. With few atoms in solution, all the energy available can go to them, and ionization results. With increasing concentrations, the energy is spread over more atoms, less ionization occurs, and greater spectral emission occurs. This is most noticeable in such metals as potassium, rubidium, and cesium. Lithium, having a some-what higher ionization potential, actually does not show such a phenomenon at the concentrations usually used in flame photometry.

Through the law of mass action, the introduction of two ionizable metals in a flame results in an increase in the concentration of free electrons and, conse-quently, the suppression of the degree of ionization of each individual atom. This leads to an increase in the concentration of neutral atoms and their particular emission spectra. The increase in emission is most clearly seen with cesium and decreases through increasing atomic number of the alkali metals to sodium and lithium, where it is almost unnoticeable. The size of increase is also directly related to flame temperature. Increasing concentration of the other alkali metals also increases the effect by suppression of ionization.

Self-absorption is another form of interference. Emitted radiation from one atom may be at the right energy levels to be absorbed by a second atom. This radiation may then be lost by further collisions with similar atoms or may be reradiated. However, in the latter circumstance, the detector would count it as having originated from one atom and low results would be obtained. Therefore, self-absorption is a problem of high sample concentrations that can be decreased or eliminated by the use of more dilute solutions.

Use of Modules

The basic components of flame photometry apparatus include an atomizer, a burner with gas supply and regulators, a monochromator, and a detector with indicating instrument. These components are discussed in the following paragraphs.

PRESSURE REGULATORS

Minimum instrumental error requires a steady flame with constant thermal output. This depends upon a steady air or oxygen supply and gas pressure. Gen-erally, piped-in gas supplies vary in pressure and must be carefully monitored and/or regulated. If bottled gas and oxygen sources are used as a supply for the flame, it is essential that proper pressure reduction be accomplished. Most air or oxygen tanks work best with two-stage automatic reduction valves for pressure regulation.

FUEL

The composition of the various gas–oxidant combinations used in flame pho-tometry varies considerably. In Figure 6-2, the more commonly used fuels and the temperatures generated are given. As can be noted, these temperatures range generally from 1200°C to 3000°C. It is possible with the use of cyanogen and oxygen that flames up to 5000°C can be generated. However, toxic products of combustion are formed, which are potentially hazardous.

ATOMIZERS

Atomizers are generally of two types. The *gravity blast* type (Fig. 6-4) is made mostly of glass. A sample is introduced and flows via gravity into an air stream, where it is broken into small droplets.

The second type, known as the *direct sample aspiration* type (Fig. 6-5), uses the Venturi effect. In this type, a stream of gas passing over a capillary causes a reduced pressure; therefore, the sample is pushed up into the capillary tube, where the solution is broken into droplets and vapor by the stream of gas.

In the combined atomizer-burner (Fig. 6-6), the mist is introduced directly into the flame. With this type, all of the liquid aspirated passes directly into the flame, resulting in greater sensitivity. However, increased background interference due to the introduction of larger droplets is also observed. This results in a more turbulent and noisy flame.

Some atomizers use a spray chamber, which allows the larger particles to settle out and the finer aerosol mist to be drawn into the burner (Fig. 6-7). In this type, the amount of solution entering the flame is often not more than 2% of the total amount aspirated.

In either type of atomizer, it is imperative that the atomizer introduce a sample at a maximum, stable, and reproducible rate. If compressed air is used, the volume requires a compressor. Approximately 10 lb/in² is needed for optimum atomization. The optimum pressure is the highest one that can be used without causing any appreciable increase in background noise. It is also important to note that the viscosity, density, and surface tension of the solution to be analyzed also affect the rate of atomization and droplet size. These effects are generally minimized by the use of sufficiently high dilution. Another important requirement for reproducibility of analysis is uniformity of size and shape in the internal diameter of the aspirator. Prevention of protein buildup in the aspirator tube by use of

Figure 6-4.   Gravity blast.

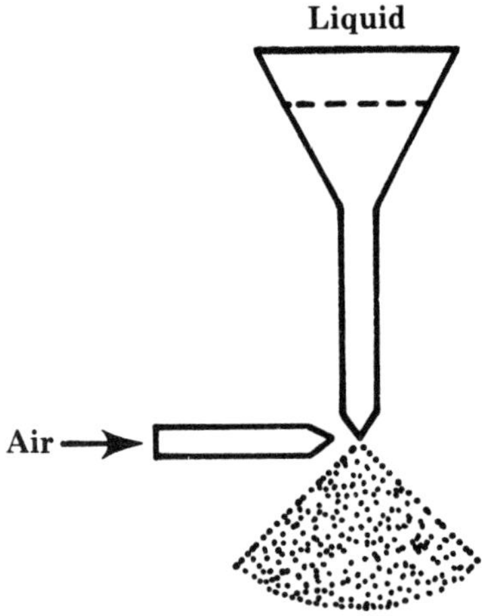

Liquid

Air →

Figure 6-5.   Sample aspiration.

Air

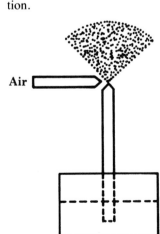

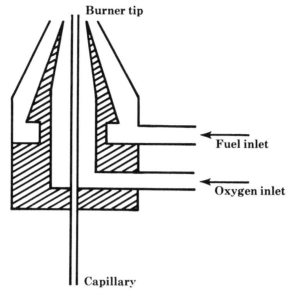

Figure 6-6. Combined atomizer-burner.

Figure 6-7. Indirect atomizer with mixing chamber and burner. (Van der Weij AD: Flame Photometry. In Krugers J, Keulemans AI [eds]: Practical Instrumental Analysis. New York, Elsevier, 1965)

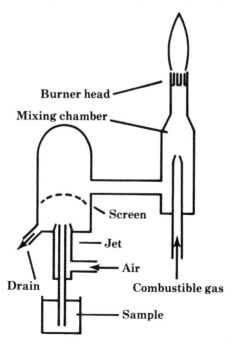

mechanical cleaning wires supplied with the instrument is, therefore, important. The use of incorrect wires could scratch and distort the internal bore of the aspirator tube, leading to nonuniformity of aspiration.

BURNERS

Burners may be made of glass, quartz, or metal. Glass is used only in work with relatively low-temperature flames, such as mixtures of illuminating gas or acetylene with air. Quartz is somewhat more widely used, but is difficult to manufacture. The most common types are made of metal; however, these corrode and plug up more often, particularly with heavy salt concentrations. Burners may be divided into two groups. In the first, there is preliminary mixing of the fuel with air or oxygen. An example is the normal laboratory bunsen burner.

In the second type, the gases are mixed only at the moment of combustion. Outside air is not used, but is supplied by the compressor and sprayer. As noted in the previous section, the sample may be introduced by a separate atomizer or may be aspirated directly into the flame (Fig. 6-7).

MONOCHROMATION

Once the sample has been aspirated, and introduced into the flame, and spectral emission lines have been generated, accurate optical analysis is required. This involves the use of collimation and a means of spectral isolation or monochromation.

Collimation is the use of lenses and mirrors for focusing the beams of emitted light. Through its use, increased sensitivity is obtained. An example is shown in Figure 6-8.

Monochromation is used in all flame photometers for spectral isolation. The principles, advantages, and disadvantages of each particular type are similar to those involved in absorption spectrophotometry. In one type, prisms are used with mechanical separation of the spectral lines (Fig. 6-9). The spectral dispersion is not linear with wavelength. Exit slits are, therefore, required to isolate that portion of the spectrum desired. The use of a diffraction grating (Fig. 6-10) has an advantage over a prism in that its spectrum is linear. Again, the separation of the spectral lines is mechanical.

The second and more commonly used method utilizes filters for spectral isolation. As in absorption spectrophotometry, these can be either interference or cutoff filters. An example is shown in Figure 6-11. The advantages of filters include ease of operation, reproducibility, durability, and relative inexpensiveness. The major disadvantage is possible decreased resolution. This is a function of the half-bandpass.

The advantages of a flame photometer with a spectrophotometric method of spectral isolation (*i.e.*, prism, grating, or both) are increased versatility, ease of operation, and the ability to analyze many spectral lines from any elements. Major disadvantages include increased cost, loss of light, the use of front surface reflectors that cannot be cleaned, and the danger of destruction of the optical alignment by either heat or mechanical damage. For these reasons, such systems of spectral isolation are generally reserved for emission spectrophotometry.

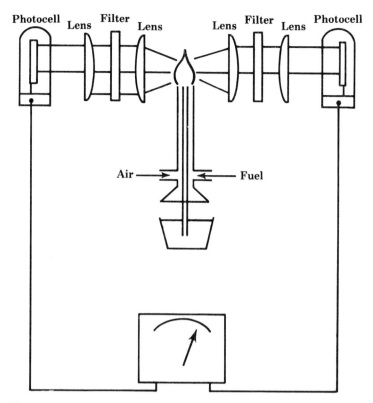

Figure 6-8. Basic flame photometer. (Corbett MB: ASCP Workshop on Instrumentation. Chicago, American Society of Clinical Pathologists, 1967)

DETECTION

Detection of the emission intensity is done in a fashion similar to absorption spectrophotometry. It is generally accomplished in one of two ways. In the first method, a photomultiplier tube is used. This tube converts incident light energy into electrical energy via multiple cathodes as a cascade effect. It has increased sensitivity, is somewhat less resistant to damage than a barrier layer cell, requires a power supply, and may need amplification.

Figure 6-9. Use of prism for monochromation.

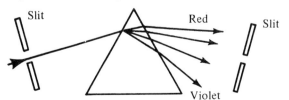

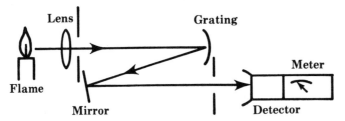

Figure 6-10. Use of diffraction grating for monochromation.

The second method of detection is the barrier layer (photovoltaic) photocell. This consists of a layer of metal insulated from, but coated by, a compound such as cadmium sulfate. Incident light energy strikes the compound and electron flow between the two layers is generated. This particular type of detection is relatively resistant to damage and requires no power supply but is less sensitive, exhibits fatigue, and is amplified with difficulty.

In either event, the current generated is reflected in a meter for direct readout or is amplified and sent to a digital converter for readout and/or printout.

INTERNAL STANDARD

The principle of internal standards was first used by Gerlich in 1925. It involves the addition to a sample of an element in known concentration and simultaneous analysis for both the added known and unknown elements. The intensity of the internal standard should be the same for all standard, unknown, and blank solutions. The ratio of the intensity of the spectral emission line of the unknown is compared to that of the known internal standard and is proportional to the concentration. The use of the internal standard principle helps to eliminate many of the sources of instrumental error because, theoretically, both internal standard and unknown would be affected in like fashion. Such things as variation in flame temperature, degree of atomization, oxygen and fuel flow and pressure, and voltage fluctuations would affect each in like fashion.

In establishing a constant relationship between the internal standard and the element under measurement, it is important that several principles and procedures be followed.

Figure 6-11. Use of filter for monochromation.

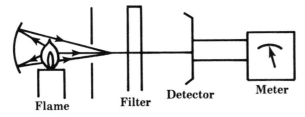

1. The concentration of the internal standard must be known precisely. The compound used must be pure, because the precision will be only as accurate as the known concentration of the internal solution.
2. The internal standard should have physical and chemical properties similar to unknowns under measurement.
3. The excitation potentials of the unknown element and the internal standard should be matched as closely as possible for previously stated reasons.
4. The emission lines should not lie close to each other, because spectral interference would result.
5. The concentration of the internal standard should be of the same order of magnitude as the unknown element.
6. The internal standard should not occur normally in significant concentrations in the unknown solution under analysis.

The most common internal standard used for sodium and potassium analysis involves the use of a lithium salt, usually lithium nitrate or lithium sulfate. Its physical and chemical properties are similar to sodium and potassium. The excitation potentials of sodium, potassium, and lithium are similar. However the use of lithium would be less desirable for flame photometric determination of the alkaline earth metals such as calcium and magnesium.

The lithium internal standard may be coupled with simultaneous potassium and sodium determination as in the IL flame photometer, AutoAnalyzer flame photometer, and SMA-12/60 Analyzer. A typical schematic diagram is shown in Figure 6-12. Newer flame photometers also allow measurement of lithium directly. In this case, potassium is used as the internal standard and lithium concentration is determined by direct readout, after the instrument is calibrated with appropriate standards.

Cesium has recently been introduced as an alternative internal standard. It shares many of the theoretical advantages of lithium, but unlike lithium, it is never

Figure 6-12. Plan of multichannel photometer—(1) flame, (2) light filters, (3) photocells, (4) meter.

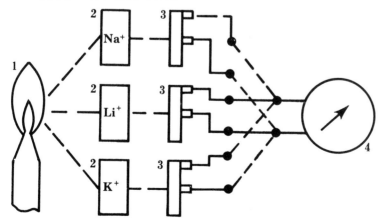

used as a therapeutic drug. Therefore, it does not occur in significant concentrations in patient samples. This permits direct determination of sodium, potassium, and lithium on the same sample.

Maintenance

Routine maintenance and function checks are required on flame photometers as for any other piece of laboratory equipment. The burner assembly, chimney, and appropriate optical services should be checked for dirt and film accumulation and cleaned at periodic intervals. The atomizer should be periodically cleaned and the flow rate should be optimized at regular intervals. The burner head and aspirator should be flushed thoroughly with water each day of use. The operator should refer to specific maintenance manuals pertinent to the instrument being used. Where lithium or cesium are used as the internal standard, the concentration should be maintained precisely. It is important that the same concentration of internal standard be used for establishing baseline or zero calibration, calibration of standards, and dilution of patient samples.

When manual dilutions of calibrators and patient samples are performed, precision is required. If automatic diluters are used, it is important to observe for possible viscosity effects. Calibrators are frequently aqueous and are readily aspirated whereas patient samples, containing varying concentrations of proteins, may be less readily aspirated. It is imperative that scrupulous quality control be performed to ensure that such viscosity effects are avoided.

Bibliography

Brown DE: Flame photometry. Am J Clin Pathol 26:807, 1956
Meloan CE: Instrumental Analysis Using Spectroscopy, Vol I. Philadelphia, Lea & Febiger, 1968
Morgoshes M, Vallee BL: In Glick D (ed): Methods of Biochemical Analysis, Vol III, p 353. New York, Interscience, 1956
Poleuktov NS: Techniques in Flame Photometric Analysis. Princeton, NJ, Van Nostrand, 1961

Suggested Reading

Henry RJ: Clinical Chemistry: Principles and Technics, 2nd ed. New York, Harper & Row, 1974
Van Der Weij AD, Krugers J, Keulemans AI (eds): Flame Photometry in Practical Instrumental Analysis. New York, Elsevier, 1965

7

ATOMIC ABSORPTION SPECTROSCOPY

Mary C. Haven

Definitions

Angstrom (Å):   A unit of length equal to 10^{-10} m.
Excited State: An atom with an orbiting electron in an unstable higher energy state.
Fluorescence: The emission of radiation by an excited atom or molecule.
Ground State: The lowest possible energy form of an atom.
I_i: Intensity of light transmitted after sample absorption.
I_0:   Intensity of the incident light.
Resonance Fluorescence: The return of an excited electron to its initial state by the emission of radiation of exactly the same frequency as that absorbed.
Resonance Line: The wavelength absorbed in exciting an atom from the ground state to the next highest energy state.

Principles

All elements have the capability of absorbing electromagnetic radiation at the same wavelength that the element emits radiation. This elemental property is the basis of atomic absorption spectrophotometry.

Recall that an atom is composed of a nucleus with electrons revolving around it in discrete orbits. If energy (thermal, electrical, or electromagnetic) is supplied to this atom, the electrons can move to an orbit of higher energy (Fig. 7-1). This is what occurs in atomic absorption. The atom in the ground state, the lowest possible energy form of the atom, absorbs a unit of energy. The absorption of this energy forces an electron to move to an orbit of higher energy. An excited atom is the result.

Atomic emission (flame photometry) is the reverse of this process. The excited atom, in returning to the ground state, releases a photon. The intensity of the emission line is proportional to the number of excited atoms.

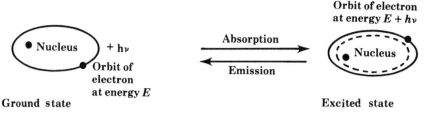

Figure 7-1. Atomic absorption or atomic emission.

Before going further in discussing atomic absorption, it would be wise to digress a few moments into line spectra in order to understand some definitions.

The hydrogen atom is usually used for the example: As it absorbs energy, the electrons can move to higher orbits; as the electron falls back to its original orbit, it emits radiation in specific lines (Fig. 7-2). The move of an electron from the ground state to the next higher orbit requires the least amount of energy.

Remember: $E = h v$, but $v = c/\lambda$, where
h = Planck's constant
  = 6.625×10^{-27} erg-sec
v = frequency
c = velocity of light
λ = wavelength

Therefore, the wavelength absorbed in exciting the atom from the ground state to the next higher orbit is the longest wavelength of the spectra and is called the *resonance line*.

Atomic absorption consists of three steps:

1. The sample is converted to an atomic vapor, usually by a flame.
2. The atomic vapor is irradiated at a wavelength characteristic of the element being sought.
3. Absorption of the light by the vaporized sample is related to the concentration of the desired element in it.

Although the principles of atomic absorption theoretically hold true for all the elements, present application of the technique has been limited to those metals whose resonance lines lie in the ultraviolet and visible regions of the spectrum.

Figure 7-2. Emissions from excited hydrogen electron.

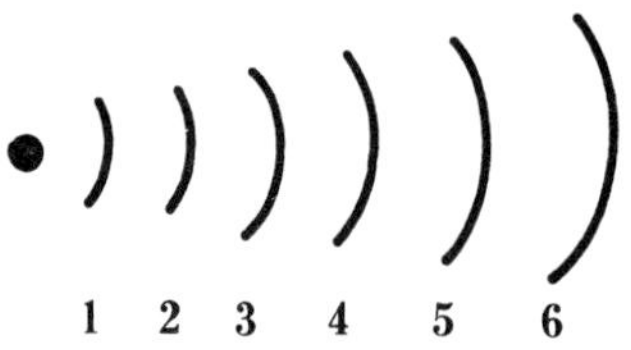

Orbits	Wavelength (Å)
2 to 1	1216
3 to 1	1025
4 to 1	973
5 to 1	950
6 to 1	938

The degree of absorption (dv) follows the following relationship:[5]

$$\Sigma \, Kv \, dv = (\pi e^2/mc) \, Nf$$

where

K = absorption coefficient at frequency v
e = charge on the electron
m = mass of an electron
c = speed of light
N = number of atoms in the ground state
f = oscillator strength of the absorbing line

K, e, m, c, and f are all constants for a given element. The only variable is N, the number of atoms in the ground state. The intensity of the emission line in flame photometry is proportional to the number of excited atoms, but the number of excited atoms is also a function of the wavelength of emission and the temperature of the system. An advantage of atomic absorption is that there are many more atoms in the ground state than the excited state. Even though sodium is easily excited, most of the sodium atoms in a flame remain in the ground state.

Na	1 excited	100 ground
Ca	1 excited	1000 ground
Zn	1 excited	1×10^9 ground

If we want to get very theoretical about it, the Beer–Lambert Law ($I_i = I_0 e^{-Kbc}$) does not really apply to atomic absorption spectroscopy. This is because the atoms are not in a steady state of homogeneous distribution. The sample is going from molecules, to ions, to atoms in the ground state, to oxides. Valid values for b and c cannot be obtained. However, in actual spectrophotometric work, these values are not calculated either. Standards and samples are run at the same time under the same conditions, canceling out all values except K (concentration).

From these principles of atomic absorption, we see the inherent advantages of this method over atomic emission:

1. A greater number of atoms are available for absorption because the majority of atoms are in the ground state.
2. Interferences from temperature and wavelength variation are slight whereas emission is quite dependent on these parameters.
3. A ratio of transmitted light to incident light can be used as the measurement of absorption; in emission, the absolute intensity of emitted light must be determined.

Instrumentation

The individual components of atomic absorption equipment are similar to other spectroscopic instrumentation. They are a radiation source, a sample cell, a monochromator, and a detector. A very simple diagram of a single-beam unit is shown in Figure 7-3.

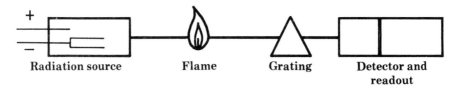

Figure 7-3. Single-beam absorption spectrophotometer.

HOLLOW CATHODE LAMP

The most common radiation source is a hollow cathode lamp with the element of interest as the cathode filament. This lamp is filled with either argon or neon gas. When voltage is applied, the gas becomes charged and bombards the metal atoms of the filament. This bombardment causes excited metal atoms to be dislodged into the atmosphere of the lamp. The excited metal atoms emit light of characteristic wavelengths as they return to the unexcited state. In other words, as the excited atoms, which can only exist for 10^{-6} to 10^{-8} seconds, return to the ground state, a photon is given off. So the principle of atomic emission is the principle of the hollow cathode lamp. This photon of energy $h\nu$ is the exact energy that the metallic atom in the sample absorbs.

The high-intensity hollow cathode lamps are an improvement over the conventional hollow cathode. The high-intensity lamps contain two extra electrodes that are coated with an easily excited material. A direct current flows between these auxiliary electrodes, causing more gas atoms to become ionized and bombard the sputtering metal atoms from the cathode. This causes an increase in the number of excited atoms, thereby increasing the intensity of the lamp. An additional power supply is required for the high-brightness lamps.

Another type of lamp, the vapor discharge lamp, is most often used for the determination of the alkali metals (sodium, potassium, cesium, and rubidium). This lamp is filled with a vapor at least partially composed of the element of interest. A current is passed through the vapor and emission results. These lamps require special mounts and a special power supply.

BURNERS AND FURNACES

The function of the atomizer, whether flame or furnace, is likened to the sample cuvette. The atomizer takes up the sample and reduces the metal being determined from an ion or molecule to the neutral atomic state (*i.e.*, the ground state). This is the most difficult and least efficient step in the atomic absorption process. In Robinson's work on atomic absorption,[5] he states that the conversion of elements from chemical compounds to their atomic state involves physics, chemistry, and voodoo, but mostly voodoo. Calculations show that the flame atomization step may only reduce one atom per million in the sample. Furnace atomization has vastly increased the efficiency in reducing elements to their ground state.

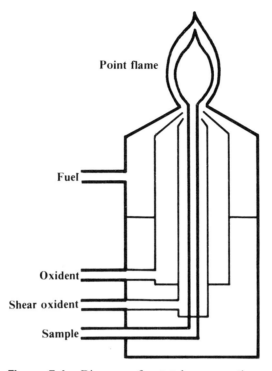

Figure 7-4. Diagram of a total consumption burner.

Flame atomizers can accommodate only liquid samples. The two most common burners are the total consumption burner and the Lundegardh burner. In the total consumption burner, all the sample that is aspirated is injected into the flame (Fig. 7-4).

The advantages of this burner are the following:

1. It is relatively easy to clean.
2. An aliquot of the entire sample passes into the flame.
3. It has a rapid response.

Its chief disadvantages include the following:

1. The viscosity of the sample affects the aspiration rate.
2. The droplet size varies over a wide range, with many unburned droplets scattering incident light.
3. The burner tip can become partially blocked, resulting in a decrease in absorption caused by lower aspiration rate.
4. Turbulence makes these burners noisy, both physically and electronically.

The Lundegardh burner, or premix burner, is shown in Figure 7-5. The oxidants and fuel are premixed in the barrel of the burner. The sample is aspirated

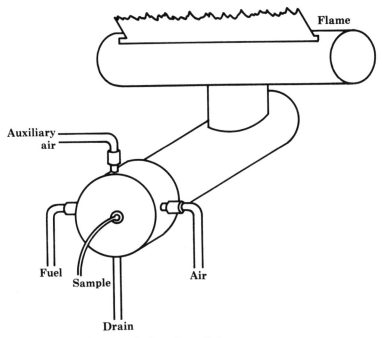

Figure 7-5.   Diagram of a Lundegardh burner.

into the same bowl, and an appreciable part of the sample evaporates on the fuel oxidant mixture. The excess sample is drained off.

Advantages are as follows:

1. Improved sensitivity results from the elongated burner putting more atoms in the light path.
2. Clogging of the burner is reduced because the larger droplets are drained off.
3. Less turbulence makes this burner quiet.

Figure 7-6.   Composition of the flame.

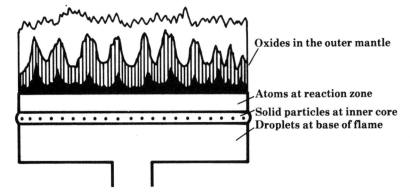

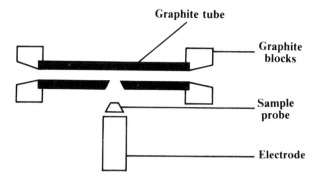

Figure 7-7. Diagram of a L'Vov graphite cuvette.

Disadvantages are as follows:

1. The burner is more difficult to clean.
2. Explosions can occur from the unburned mixtures of fuel and oxidant.

The light absorbed, by passage through different parts of the flame, is not constant. This is because the number of neutral atoms varies in different parts of the flame. Basically, the flame is composed of four parts (Fig. 7-6).

The use of high-temperature furnaces has significantly increased the number of ground-state atoms in the light path, which has increased sensitivity and lowered the detection limit. However, with increased sensitivity comes increased interference from the sample matrix (*e.g.*, nonselective molecular absorption and light scattering), and some method of background correction is therefore necessary when using a furnace. These background corrections will be discussed later in the chapter. Commercially available furnaces are generally of two types: the L'Vov graphite cuvette and the Massman furnace.

The L'Vov graphite cuvette (as shown in Fig. 7-7) is a 30- to 50-mm cylinder lined with pyrographite, which ensures a uniform heating of the tube and is resistant to oxidation. The sample is placed on an auxiliary carbon rod electrode, 6 mm in diameter; the sample unit is then purged with nitrogen or argon gas, and the rod is heated to dry and ash the sample. The auxiliary electrode is then introduced into the center of the graphite cuvette. The sample is rapidly vaporized by heating the electrode by an independent current, and a pulsed signal of maximum absorption is obtained and recorded. Analytical results can be calculated by peak height or peak integration.[6]

Figure 7-8 shows a Massman furnace, a hollow graphite cylinder about 8 mm in diameter and about 28 mm long. The hollow cathode beam passes through this cylinder, and the sample (1 to 100 μl) is introduced through a hole in the center of the cylinder. Solid samples can also be introduced through the end of the cylinder. The system is purged with argon or nitrogen and the cylinder is heated in three stages: The first stage dries the sample, the second chars and ashes the sample, and the third vaporizes the sample. Again the absorption signal is monitored by a recorder.

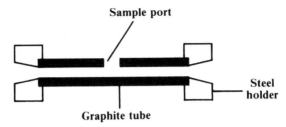

Figure 7-8. Diagram of a Massman furnace.

Advantages of furnace over flame atomizers are as follows:

1. They have high concentrations of ground-state atoms within a well-defined volume.
2. Small samples can be used.
3. They have high sensitivity (10^{-8} to 10^{-11} g absolute).[10]
4. No pretreatment of biological samples is necessary.

Disadvantages are as follows:

1. Precision is not as good as with flame atomizers.
2. Because matrix interferences are so severe, background correction is necessary.
3. The number of samples analyzed per unit time is less than with flame atomizers as furnaces must cool down between samples.

MONOCHROMATOR

The monochromator is used to separate the resonance line from other spectral lines in the immediate vicinity. These spectral lines originate from other metals in the hollow cathode and the filler gas. The wavelength range of this monochromator is the same as that of flame emission or ultraviolet-visible spectrophotometry, approximately 1900 to 8600 Å. The bandpass must be able to transmit the resonance lines. For some elements whose resonance lines are closely surrounded by other lines, a bandpass of 2 Å is required. Yet it is also desirable when working with other elements to increase the available light. This can be done by increasing the slit width, thereby widening the bandpass to as high as 40 Å. A good monochromator for atomic absorption should then be capable of being operated at wide slit widths. The wavelength accuracy for atomic absorption need not be greater than 10 Å, because the exact wavelength desired is "tuned in" with the hollow cathode as the source.

Figure 7-9. Single-beam modulated atomic absorption spectrophotometer.

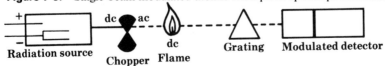

The detector is usually a photomultiplier tube, generally either a Bi-O-Ag or a Cs-Sb type of cathode. The most widely used is the Cs-Sb, but the more expensive Bi-O-Ag material has advantages in the far ultraviolet and red ends of the spectrum.

SYSTEMS

The first atomic absorption spectrophotometers were made with direct current components, lamp source, flame, monochromator, and detector. However, certain problems arose and modifications were made. The first modification was modulated equipment.[9] If the source of radiation is considered I_0, then I_0 is reduced to I_i after passing through the flame. However, the element of interest emits radiation at exactly the wavelength it absorbs. As the atom that has absorbed radiation returns to the ground state, it emits the same energy it had just absorbed. Therefore, the detector would see $(I_0 - I_i) + S$, where S is the emission signal. The absorption signal, which should be $I_0 - I_i$, would now be reduced and equal to $(I_0 - I_i) + S$. This would cause a reduction in sensitivity. Also, S is the same signal used in flame photometry and the process would then be subject to errors of both atomic absorption and flame spectroscopy. Modulation of the instrument is brought about by electrical or mechanical means. In the mechanical method, the output of the lamp, which is a dc signal, is modified to an ac signal with a chopper (Fig. 7-9). The detector is then synchronized to the same frequency. In this manner, the detector sees only the ac signal from the radiation source and the absorption thereof. The emission signal from the flame is dc; the detector is unable to register it, and only $(I_0 - I_i)$ is detected.

After a stable and instrumentally quiet burner was manufactured, it was noted that the weakest link in the system was the hollow cathode lamp. Lamps may need a considerable warmup time to give a constant emission. For this reason, the second modification, the double-beam (Fig. 7-10), was made. With the double-beam system, the light, from the source of radiation through the flame to the photodetector, is split into two paths: a sample path and a reference path. The reference path goes directly to the detector. The sample path goes through the sample to the detector. In this system, the ratio between the reference and the

Figure 7-10. Double-beam atomic absorption spectrophotometer.

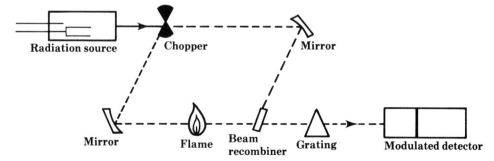

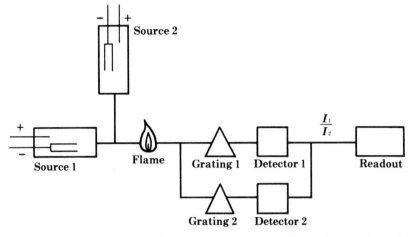

Figure 7-11. Atomic absorption spectrophotometer with monitoring channel.

sample beams is determined; thus, the absorbed light is monitored. The double-beam instrument usually yields a steadier base line; less time is necessary for lamp warmup, but this does not compensate for variations in the flame because the reference beam does not go through the flame.

A further modification found in some atomic absorption instruments attempts to eliminate signal changes caused by flame variations. For this purpose, a second hollow cathode, monochromator, and detector are used as a monitoring channel. The light paths of both lamps go through the flame and the ratio of the monitoring channel signal to the measuring channel signal is computed (Fig. 7-11). Instead of using the second channel for monitoring, it can also be used for determining a second element.

BACKGROUND CORRECTION

When using the graphite furnaces, it becomes very important to correct for background absorption in the sample cuvette. This background absorbance can be caused by molecules, salt particles, or smoke. If no correction is made, erroneously high results will be computed. Background correction can be accomplished by means of a monitoring channel as explained in the previous paragraph, a deuterium arc, or the Zeeman effect. With the deuterium background corrector, light from the hollow cathode lamp and light from the deuterium arc pass alternately through the graphite tube or the flame. Absorption of radiation from the deuterium source by ground-state atoms being determined will be negligible, but background absorption should be the same for both beams, hollow cathode and deuterium. The ratio of the two beams is determined in the double-beam instrument electronics and background absorption is automatically compensated. With the deuterium arc, compensation for background levels of 0.5 to 0.7 absorbance units can be achieved.

Correction by taking advantage of the splitting of spectral lines under the influence of a magnetic field (Zeeman effect) can compensate for background

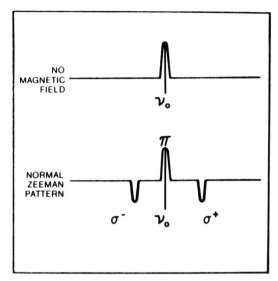

Figure 7-12. Zeeman effect: normal pattern. (Courtesy of Perkin-Elmer Corp, Norwalk, CT)

levels up to 2 absorbance units.[1] When a magnetic field is applied to an atomic spectral line, the line is split into a π component at the original wavelength and two σ components equidistant from the original line; one of slightly longer wavelength, the other of slightly shorter wavelength (Fig. 7-12). The magnetic field also causes polarization of these lines; the π component is polarized in the plane parallel to the magnetic field, the σ components are polarized perpendicular to the magnetic field. More complicated splitting of the spectral line occurs with some elements, but the simple form is the easiest to use when explaining the background correction.

Because background absorption is largely broadbase molecular scattering or absorption and, usually, only atoms are affected by the Zeeman effect, instrument manufacturers have used this type of background correction in two ways, by placing the magnetic field around the source (source-shifted Zeeman correction) or around the furnace (analyte-shifted Zeeman correction).

When the hollow cathode is placed in the magnetic field, polarized light is passed through the atomized sample. Background correction is made with a rotating polarizer added to the system before the detector (Fig. 7-13). When polarized parallel to the magnetic field, only the π component is absorbed; thus, absorption

Figure 7-13. Source-shifted Zeeman background correction.

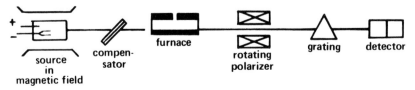

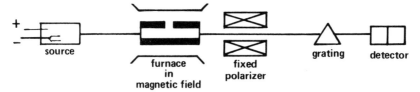

Figure 7-14. Analyte-shifted Zeeman background correction; fixed polarizer after magnetic field.

of analyte and background occurs. When polarized perpendicular to the magnetic field, only the ± σ component is absorbed, (*i.e.*, background only). Subtraction of the perpendicular component from the parallel component yields absorption due to the analyte.

By placing the magnetic field around the furnace, the signal from the analyte is shifted. If the polarizer is fixed for the vertical component after the furnace (Fig. 7-14), application of the magnetic field measures the ± σ component or background only. When the magnetic field is off, both background and sample are measured. Subtraction yields a background correction a slight distance (≈ 0.01 nm) from the absorbing line. If the polarizer is fixed before the furnace (Fig. 7-15), allowing only the vertical component to pass, the application of the magnetic field does not allow the horizontal π component of the analyte to absorb any of the vertical incident light. Therefore, any absorption when the magnetic field is on is due to background. Without the magnetic field, both analyte and background can absorb the horizontally polarized incident light. Background is corrected at the exact wavelength of the absorbing line.

READOUT DEVICES

The commercial instruments may differ in their readout devices. All readout devices are based on the fact that, in atomic absorption, the concentration is proportional to the negative logarithm of transmittance. The formula for converting percent absorption to absorbance is the same as for percent transmittance to absorbance.

$$A = 2 - \log \% T$$
$$= 2 - \log (100 - \% \text{ absorption), where } A = \text{absorbance}$$

Figure 7-15. Analyte-shifted Zeeman background correction; fixed polarizer before magnetic field.

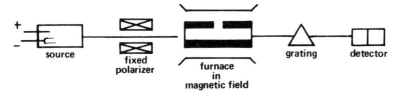

Most instruments are now microprocessor controlled, with multistandard calibration programs that allow direct readout in concentration. The microprocessors may also control an automated sampling system and the programming for the furnace.

INTERFERENCES

There are three major types of interference in atomic absorption spectroscopy: chemical, ionization, and matrix.

Chemical interference is quite common in atomic absorption but can generally be overcome. The number of atoms in the ground state depends on the stability of the metal compounds in the flame atomizer. If the compound is readily dissociated, many neutral atoms are formed; however, if the compound remains partially undissociated, fewer neutral atoms are the result. Then, the predominant anion can have an effect on the number of neutral atoms if this anion binds strongly to the element of interest. This interference can be overcome by the addition of another metal that binds preferentially with the interfering anion. For example, in calcium and magnesium procedures, lanthanum is added in excess to complex the phosphate anion.[7,8,11]

Ionization interference results when a substantial number of atoms in the sample become ionized and no longer absorb at the atom resonance line. These ionized atoms are lost to the determination. A decrease in flame temperature may solve the problem as may the addition of a large excess of a more easily ionized element. For example, in determination of lithium, excess sodium ions are added to decrease the ionization of lithium.[3]

A matrix interference is noted in solutions of high salt concentration, resulting in a decrease in signal. This interference is caused by a decrease in atomizing efficiency of the flame, because much of the available flame energy will be utilized decomposing the other salts present. This effect can be overcome by simple dilution or by extraction. A viscosity effect can also be called a matrix effect. If the viscosity of samples and standards varies greatly, the amount of sample reaching the burner will not be the same as that of the standard. An apparent decrease in absorption will occur in the more viscous samples. This can be overcome by matching the viscosity of the standards to that of the samples[4] or by forcing the samples and standards into the burner at the same rate by using a peristaltic pump.[2]

References

1. Brown SD: Zeeman effect-based background correction in atomic absorption spectrometry. Anal Chem 49:1269A, 1977
2. Hicks R, Haven M: Use of positive pressure sampling to minimize errors in atomic absorption spectrophotometry. Am J Clin Pathol 54:235, 1970
3. Kahn HL: Instrumentation for atomic absorption. J Chem Ed 43:No 1, 2, 1966
4. Parker MM, Humoller FW, Mahler DJ: Determination of copper and zinc in biological material. Clin Chem 13:40, 1967
5. Robinson JW: Atomic Absorption Spectroscopy. New York, Dekker, 1966

6. Sturgeon RE: Factors affecting atomization and measurement in graphite furnace atomic absorption spectrometry. Anal Chem 49:1255A, 1977

7. Sunderman FW, Carroll JE: Measurements of serum calcium and magnesium by atomic absorption spectrometry. Am J Clin Pathol 43:302, 1965

8. Trudeau DL, Freier EF: Determination of calcium in urine and serum by atomic absorption spectrophotometry. Clin Chem 13:101, 1967

9. Walsh A: Application of atomic absorption spectra to chemical analysis. Spectrochim Acta 7:108, 1955

10. Willard HH, Merritt LL, Jr, Dean JA, Settle FA, Jr: Instrumental Methods of Analysis, 6th ed. Princeton, Van Nostrand, 1981

11. Zettner A, Seligson D: Application of atomic absorption spectrophotometry in the determination of calcium in serum. Clin Chem 10:869, 1964

8

FLUOROMETRY AND FLUORESCENCE POLARIZATION

Jeffrey A. Huth

Definitions

Emission Spectrum: The wavelengths at which a fluorescent compound will emit energy in the form of light.

Excitation Spectrum: The wavelengths at which a fluorescent compound will absorb energy in the form of light.

Filter: A device that will pass only light from a particular portion of the spectrum while absorbing other wavelengths.

Fluorescence: The emission of light energy from an excited molecule as it returns to the ground state.

Fluorescence Polarization: The emission of polarized light from a fluorophor that has been excited with polarized light.

Fluorometer: An instrument that is used to measure the intensity of fluorescence produced from a fluorophor. The fluorometer uses filters for wavelength selection.

Fluorophor: A molecule or portion of a molecule that is capable of being excited with high-energy radiation and that will subsequently emit low-energy radiation.

Monochromator: A device used to selectively pass light at only specific wavelengths.

Photomultiplier Tube: A vacuum tube containing a light-sensitive screen that generates an electrical signal proportional to the intensity of light striking the screen. Through the use of several electron emitter/collector cells, the tube amplifies the signal.

Polarizer: A crystal that filters the electronic component of electromagnetic radiation so that the radiation that passes through the crystal lies in a single plane.

Quantum Yield: The efficiency at which a fluorophor emits light.

Spectrofluorometer: An instrument that is used to measure intensity of fluorescence produced from a fluorophor. The spectrofluorometer can select wavelengths continuously because it uses dispersion monochromators for wavelength selection.

Introduction

In the natural environment of a chemical substance, that substance will exist in what is called the *ground state*. As electromagnetic radiation or light energy impinges upon that substance, enough energy may be absorbed to cause the substance to alter its electron configuration and place it in an excited state. The excited state is only short lived, however, and the substance quickly returns to the ground state. If the substance is of unique chemical nature, energy may be given off in the form of emitted light as the transition from excited state to ground state occurs. This emitted light that is produced as the substance passes from an excited state to the ground state is called *fluorescence.*

Historically, *fluorometry* may be defined as the quantitative measurement of the intensity of light produced by an excited fluorescent substance, and the relationship between the measured intensity and the concentration of that substance. Although this definition still holds true, it must be emphasized that fluorometry is now recognized as a single facet in a group of techniques recently coined *multiparameter techniques* or *multidimensional luminescence measurements.*[8] Due to the widespread use of fluorometry and fluorescence polarization in the clinical area, this chapter will focus only on these two multiparameter techniques. For further reading on other multiparameter techniques, the article by Warner, Patonay, and Thomas is recommended.[8]

Principles

As previously mentioned, for fluorescence to occur, a molecule must first be placed in an excited state through the absorption of light energy. Although the absorption process is not as complex or competitive as the emission process (see below), the proper energy requirements must be met for the electronic transition to occur. Most often for organic molecules, the excitation process involves π electrons in a π-to-π^* transition. Although other electron transitions may occur, it is this difference in energy levels that favors fluorescence. These transitions are common for aromatic or highly conjugated double bonds in an organic molecule.

During the excitation process, both electronic energy and vibrational energy are absorbed from the photons of light hitting the molecule. However, during the emission process, only electronic energy is given off in the form of light. Because the emission energy is less than the total excitation energy, the emission spectrum is shifted to longer wavelengths (less energy) as compared to the excitation spectrum of shorter wavelengths (higher energy).

The excitation of an organic molecule to a higher energy level is a rather simple process involving the absorption of electromagnetic radiation. The return to the ground state, or deactivation, however, is not quite so simple and involves a competition between several different pathways. The emission process found in fluorescence is only one mechanism through which the excited molecule may return. Skoog and West give complete descriptions of the many other pathways that may be involved in the deactivation process of an excited molecule. See

Deactivation Processes for Excited Molecules, below, for a list of these other processes, and the reader should consult reference 7 for a complete description. Of important concern in the evaluation of all these deactivation processes is the concept of quantum efficiency or quantum yield, ϕ. The *quantum yield* may be defined as the number of molecules that fluoresce divided by the total number of excited molecules.

$$\phi = \frac{\text{number of fluorescent molecules}}{\text{total number of excited molecules}}$$

Accordingly, the total number of molecules that are excited includes molecules that fluoresce plus all those excited molecules that deactivate by other processes. Therefore, a molecule whose quantum yield approaches 1 would have a high degree of fluorescence due to less competing deactivating processes, whereas a quantum yield that approaches 0 indicates that a competing process would be more favored and would produce less fluorescence.

From the discussion above, it is evident that a number of molecular events may occur, reducing the probability that fluorescence will be produced. Many of these events may be the result of the chemical nature of the molecule itself, or may be produced because of an incompatible environment. The importance of π-to-π^* transitions has already been discussed. Those molecules that fluoresce are most likely highly conjugated organic molecules, aromatic hydrocarbons, and heterocyclics with fused benzene rings. Other important parameters that affect fluorescence are chemical substitution, structural rigidity, and polarity. Environmental parameters that may affect fluorescence are solvent viscosity, temperature, pH, heavy atoms, and dissolved oxygen. Table 8-1 lists the parameters and whether they tend to enhance ($\uparrow$) or decrease ($\downarrow$) fluorescence.

In fluorometry, it is common practice to develop a standard curve for measured fluorescence intensity versus solute concentration. A linear curve is obtained with an equation of

$$F = kc$$

where F is fluorescence, k is a constant, and c is the concentration of the species being measured. Mathematically, this equation is derived from the Beer–Lambert law. Similar to absorption methods, the fluorescence-concentration curve deviates from linearity at high concentration. In fluorometry, the deviation may occur for

Deactivation Processes for Excited Molecules[7]
Emission (fluorescence)
Vibrational relaxation
Internal conversion
Predissociation
Dissociation
External conversion
Intersystem crossing (phosphorescence)

Table 8-1
Factors That May Affect Fluorescence

Factor	Fluorescence
Chemical substitution	↑ or ↓
Rigidity/chelation	↑
Polarity	↑
Viscosity	↑
Temperature (low)	↑
pH	↑ or ↓
Heavy atoms (Cl)	↓
Oxygen	↓

several reasons. First, at high concentrations in which the absorption approaches 0.02, the mathematical equation derived from Beer's law for fluorometry cannot be simplified to $F = kc$. Therefore, a linear equation for the curve is not obtained. High absorption of the solution also promotes a phenomenon called the *inner filter effect*. As light impinges on the front of the cuvette containing the fluorescent sample, those molecules in the front will absorb the incident radiation. Because of this, the molecules at the back of the cuvette will be exposed to less radiation resulting in less fluorescence. Another problem encountered at high concentrations is self-quenching. If an abundant amount of excited molecules are in solution, collisions between the molecules occur more frequently. Radiationless energy is then given off as heat energy to the solvent molecules, which results in decreased fluorescence. In each of these cases, appropriate dilution of the concentrated solution would eliminate these problems and would result in a linear fluorescence-concentration curve. One instrumental technique to eliminate absorption problems has been designed by Adamsons and associates.[1] Through the use of cell rotation methods, absorption-corrected fluorescence measurements have produced linear curves from solutions with absorbances as high as 2.5.

The excitation/emission phenomenon that occurs in molecular fluorescence also occurs in fluorescence polarization. The added feature in fluorescence polarization is that the excitation source is modulated (polarized) so that the light energy that impinges upon the molecules does so in a well-defined plane. The resultant emission is then measured in the dimension of a well-defined plane relative to the excitation source.

Two different instrumental techniques are utilized in fluorescence polarization. In the first system, the excitation source is polarized only in one direction. The resultant emission is measured in planes both parallel to and perpendicular to the excitation source. The other system is the reverse of the first. The excitation source is polarized alternatingly in horizontal and vertical planes. The emission is measured only in the vertical plane.

In both of the above systems, horizontal (perpendicular) fluorescent intensity and vertical (parallel) fluorescent intensity are measured. The resultant degree of polarization (P) is calculated as follows:

$$P = \frac{I_{\parallel} - I_{\perp}}{I_{\parallel} + I_{\perp}}$$

where P is the degree of polarization and $I_{\parallel}$ and $I_{\perp}$ are the fluorescent intensities measured in the vertical and horizontal planes, respectively.

On a molecular level, if polarized light is used to excite a fluorescent substance, only those molecules that are electronically aligned properly will be excited and have potential for fluorescence. Should these aligned molecules be in a fixed state (no molecular rotation), the fluorescence produced would be emitted in the same polarized plane as the excitation source. However, in solution, molecules are free to rotate, and do so. Because fluorescence is not an instantaneous process, some time will elapse between the moment that the molecule becomes excited and the emission of light. This time lapse is sufficiently long for molecular rotation to occur, causing the emitted fluorescence to deviate from the excitation-polarized plane. As a result, depolarized fluorescence is emitted in all directions.

From the above discussion, it is evident that depolarization is dependent upon molecular rotation. Because of this dependency, small molecules with a greater freedom of rotation will produce less polarized fluorescence as compared to a larger, slower rotating molecule. The use of this principle is the key to fluorescence polarization assays. In these assays, a competitive immunoassay is performed in which a substrate and a fluorescent-labelled substrate compete for binding on an antibody. The binding of the fluorescent-labelled substrate to the antibody causes the fluorescent tag to be part of a large molecule that rotates slowly. Thus, the fluorescence produced by this bound fluorescent tag would be highly polarized. Conversely, the fluorescent-labelled substrate that is unbound is free to rotate and would produce depolarized fluorescence. In using the competitive binding assay in fluorescence polarization, the presence of large amounts of natural substrate causes less binding of labelled substrate and results in less fluorescence polarization. If the natural substrate concentration is low, more labelled substrate binds to the antibody and results in a high degree of polarization.

Basic Components of a Fluorometer

The basic components of a fluorometer are essentially identical to those of a spectrophotometer. These components include a light source, a primary (excitation) monochromator, a cell, a secondary (emission) monochromator, a detector, and a readout device. In addition to these components, a fluorescence polarization instrument has both excitation and emission polarizers.

Generally, fluorometers and fluorescence polarization instruments are designed such that the emitted fluorescence is measured from a light path that is at a 90° angle from the excitation light path (Fig. 8-1). Because fluorescence is emitted in all directions, the fluorescent signal could theoretically be measured at any angle. However, at 90°, stray light from different scattering mechanisms is at a minimum; thus, the fluorescent signal at this point has less background interference. One system has been described in which the optical path has a "straight-

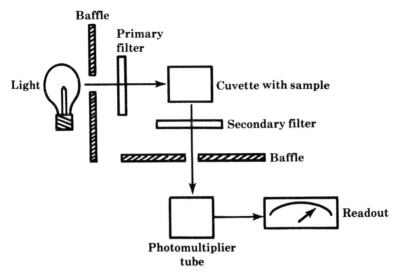

Figure 8-1.   Simple right-angle fluorometric system.

through'' geometry.[4] Through the use of special filters and an attenuated light source, stray light and high background problems are eliminated.

SOURCE

The light source used for fluorescence measurements serves the purpose of supplying the radiant energy that is necessary to excite the fluorescent molecule or fluorophor. In consideration of the desired features for a source, the intensity, stability, and wavelength variability are of utmost concern.[10] The source must be a supply of intense radiant energy. Because fluorescence is a function of source intensity, a more intense source is desired in that it will produce greater fluorescence. Stability is the second characteristic of concern. If source flicker is a problem, fluorescence measurements will not be reproducible. The third area to be considered is the spectral range of the source. Fluorescent molecules are generally excited at specific wavelengths. The source must supply energy for excitation at these wavelengths if any fluorescence is to occur.

Lasers are a source of very intense radiation and high stability. Although these light sources have great potential for molecular excitation, the wavelength variability is a major drawback in that these sources are monochromatic. The fluorophor must be able to be excited at the specific wavelength to which the laser has been "tuned," or no fluorescence is observed. The high cost of these sources is another major drawback.

The more commonly used sources in fluorometry are the deuterium lamp, the xenon arc, and the mercury vapor lamp. The deuterium lamp provides for an intense source; however, its wavelength range is limited to the 200- to 350-nm range.

The mercury vapor lamp provides a very intense and stable source. The major drawback is that this source does not provide a continuous spectrum. The mercury lamp emits radiation only at well-defined wavelengths; therefore, it is called a line source. This source will give off light at the following wavelengths: 257.7 nm, 313.0 nm, 365 nm, 404.7 nm, 407.8 nm, 435.8 nm, 546.1 nm, 577.0 nm, and 579.1 nm.[10] The advantage of this source is its intensity and stability. In addition, the mercury lines provide a monochromatic beam at each wavelength. If other lines are efficiently filtered, stray light is minimized. As a result, mercury lamps are quite often used in filter fluorometers. Although this source is discontinuous, most fluorescing molecules will absorb some radiation at one of the mercury lines. By setting the excitation source at the line nearest to the absorption maximum, fluorescence can be achieved.

The xenon arc is the other commonly used source in fluorescence. This source produces a continuous spectrum from 250 to 600 nm; however, the intensity varies with wavelength. Peak intensity is at 470 nm. The major advantage of the xenon source is its continuous spectrum. Through this, optimal fluorescence can be obtained by setting the source at the wavelength at which absorption is a maximum. The disadvantages are that some lamp designs need cooling apparatus for proper operation. The removal of ozone that may be produced by the xenon arc also poses instrumental limitations. Use of this source over the deuterium lamp extends the working excitation wavelength range and considerably adds more selectivity.[9]

As with fluorescence, the source in fluorescence polarization must supply the intensity and proper wavelength for excitation of the fluorophor. However, the use of intensity ratios for polarization calculations permits less sophistication in lamp design. Through the use of ratios, lamp instability as a source of error is significantly reduced. Generally, a tungsten lamp is used as the source for fluorescence polarization. This source provides a continuous spectrum in the visible range. The use of highly efficient fluorophors (high quantum yield) facilitates use of this less intense source while retaining accurate fluorescent measurements. One wavelength in the range is optimally chosen to match the excitation maximum of the fluorescent tag chosen. The major advantages of the tungsten lamp in fluorescence polarization are the instrumental simplicity required for operation and its low cost.

MONOCHROMATORS

At this point, a distinction between fluorometers (fluorimeters) and spectrofluorometers must be made. Fluorometers use filters for the selection of monochromatic light, whereas spectrofluorometers use prisms or gratings (monochromators) for monochromatic light selection. As a result, spectrofluorometers permit continuous wavelength selection whereas fluorometers do not.

Filters may be defined as either short-pass, long-pass, or bandpass filters. A short-pass filter will permit light at wavelengths below that given for the filter to pass. Similarly, long-pass filters permit light at wavelengths above that given for the filter to pass. A bandpass filter permits light between two given wavelengths to pass and performs similarly to a monochromator. Each of these types of filters is good for eliminating different sources of interfering light. Weinberger and Sapp describe these in detail.[9]

As stated previously, the mercury vapor lamp is most often used in fluorometers. Because the lamp supplies narrow lines of radiation, a bandpass filter is often used to select the desired wavelength for excitation. Other undesired wavelengths are excluded. On the emission side of the fluorometer, a long-pass filter is commonly used. Of importance is that the excitation bandpass filter and the long-pass emission filter have no wavelengths in common. Through this, stray light is essentially eliminated.

Filters are often made of glass or are dye-containing Wratten filters. Through proper selection of the glass or dye, optical transmission can be regulated. The glass or dye acts by absorbing those wavelengths that are not desired. In other words, the undesired wavelengths are filtered out. Accordingly, those wavelengths that are desired are not absorbed and pass through the filters.

The monochromators used in spectrofluorometers are the same as those used in spectrophotometers (see Chap. 5). Although prisms were used in early instruments, gratings are more prominent today. Gratings may be classified as either ruled or holographic, with the ruled type being more common. Generally, the holographic gratings are better at reducing stray light, but the efficiency of these is less than that of the ruled gratings.[9] The ruled gratings permit greater intensity to pass for a given wavelength as compared to holographic gratings.

The monochromators operate by adjusting the angle at which the incident radiation strikes the surface of the grating. By rotating the gratings, the monochromator separates the incident light into its component wavelengths and focuses it onto the sample through the use of slits. In the case of emission, the fluorescent sample serves as the light source and the gratings are used in the same manner for selection of the emission wavelength.

CUVETTES

Generally, glass cuvettes can be used when the excitation wavelength is greater than 320 nm. At wavelengths below this, the glass cuvette itself will absorb significant amounts of radiation; therefore, glass cuvettes are used mainly in the visible range. For ultraviolet excitation or for very sensitive fluorescent measurements, quartz cuvettes should be used. In addition, matched quartz cuvettes are available so that both the reference and the sample are contained in identical cuvettes. Elimination of cuvette variability is obtained and enables sensitive measurements to be made.

In the clinical laboratory, matched quartz cuvettes are seldom required. In fact, for routine fluorescent measurements using a filter fluorometer, round glass test tubes are satisfactory. Stray light may cause significant problems with round tubes; however, the optical and electronic null of the instrument usually permits compensation for this. In addition, appropriate use of baffles blocks stray radiation and permits only the radiation emitted from the sample to be focused onto the detector.

DETECTORS

The photomultiplier tube is the detector commonly used in fluorometry. Generally, for emission that is measured in the visible range, a glass-encased tube is sufficient. In the ultraviolet range, glass absorbs the radiation; therefore, special ultraviolet-responsive tubes are required for ultraviolet fluorescence measurements.

The photomultiplier tube operates on an amplification process. As light strikes the surface of a light-sensitive screen in the detector, a potential proportional to the intensity of the light is generated. This potential is magnified through the use of several electron emitter/collector cells. As an electronic signal passes from one cell to the next, it is amplified until the end-stage collector is reached. At this point, the potential is measured and recorded on a meter, digital display, or other recording device.

Many instruments are now equipped with microprocessors that permit concentration calculations and direct printouts. The instrument is calibrated with a series of standards and stores the concentration-fluorescence curve. Subsequent samples are analyzed and compared to the curve for the concentration calculation.

POLARIZERS

Electromagnetic radiation consists of both electronic and magnetic components. Only the electronic component of electromagnetic radiation interacts with electrons during the absorption process. This electronic component is made of radiation vibrating in two planes perpendicular to each other. Thus, for any given radiation beam, the electronic component may be defined in terms of two planes perpendicular to each other.

Certain, noncubic (anisotropic) crystals are used as polarizers because they have the capability of filtering one of the two perpendicular planes. Depending on the orientation of the crystal to the incident beam, one plane of light will pass directly through the crystal while the other plane of light is absorbed. The resultant light that passes through the crystal is plane-polarized. Polarizers essentially permit passage of 50% of incident radiation as a plane-polarized beam, while the other 50% is absorbed.[7]

SYSTEMS

As discussed previously, fluorometers employ a mercury vapor lamp with wavelength selection achieved by the use of filters. In the simplest form, the instrumentation design of a fluorometer would follow the schematic in Figure 8-1. This simple fluorometer utilizes single-beam design. The advantage of such a system is its simplicity and low cost. In addition, the stability of the mercury lamp provides for accurate measurements. Extreme sensitivity can be achieved if the maximum excitation wavelength of the fluorophor coincides with one of the mercury lines. The major disadvantage of this system arises from its lack of versatility.

Spectrofluorometers, like spectrophotometers, can be used in either the single-beam or double-beam mode. Generally, these instruments use the xenon arc lamp for the source. The use of monochromators in these instruments adds versatility. One area of concern in the single-beam spectrofluorometer is the error caused by xenon arc lamp flicker. To compensate for this instability, the single-beam instrument is operated in the ratio mode. In the ratio mode of operation, the source light is focused onto a rotating chopper. This device alternates the direction of the beam between the sample and a reference photomultiplier tube. The signal from the sample photomultiplier tube is compared with the signal from the reference photomultiplier tube. Through the use of this ratio mode, any alteration of the fluorescence as a result of a change in source intensity is corrected. In other words, any change in the source would be detected by both photomultiplier tubes. Because a ratio is employed, error due to an unstable source would be minimized. Filter fluorometers may also be operated in a ratio mode.

Spectrofluorometers are also available as double-beam instruments. Essentially, the design is very similar to the double-beam spectrophotometers. The beam of light from the source is focused onto a rotating chopper. The source light is then split between a sample cell and a reference cell, and the fluorescence produced by each cell is monitored by a single photomultiplier tube synchronized with the chopper. The synchronization permits distinction between sample and reference signals. Use of the double-beam design permits correction of background fluorescence that may be produced by the sample matrix. The double-beam design also compensates for source flicker in the same manner as the single-beam design in the ratio mode. For very sensitive measurements, matched quartz cuvettes are used to eliminate any difference that may result from cuvette variances.

Fluorescence polarization instruments are basically filter fluorometers to which a set of excitation and emission polarizers have been added. Generally, the fluorescent tag used in fluorescent polarization immunoassays is fluoroscein. As a result, narrow-width bandpass filters are used for both excitation and emission wavelength selection. The excitation filter permits light at 485 nm to pass for excitation whereas the emission filter permits a light at 525 nm to pass for subsequent measurements. Because fluoroscein absorbs light in the visible range, a tungsten lamp can be utilized as the source.

Figure 8-2 illustrates the schematic diagram for the optics of a fluorescence polarization instrument.[6] The beam of light from the tungsten lamp is split and passes to both a sample and a reference detector. The reference detector is used to monitor the intensity of the source. The other portion of the beam strikes a polarizer/liquid crystal device. Here, the beam is polarized in the horizontal plane. The liquid crystal serves to rotate the polarized beam 90°. When a voltage is applied to the crystal, no rotation occurs. When no voltage is applied, the plane is rotated 90°. Therefore, by turning the voltage to the crystal on and off repeatedly, the excitation beam alternates between horizontal- and vertical-plane-polarized light.

The polarized light next strikes the sample. Baffles surround the sample to prevent excitation light from hitting the detector. Upon excitation, the sample emits its fluorescence. The fluorescent beam passes through the emission filter and onto an analyzer polarizer. This polarizer only passes light in the vertical plane and enables measurement of polarized fluorescence relative to the excitation

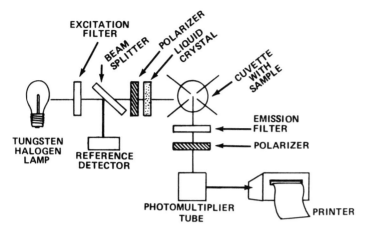

Figure 8-2. Optical components of a polarization instrument.

polarization. Depending upon the relative binding of the native analyte and the fluorescent-tagged analyte (see Principles earlier in this chapter), different degrees of polarized fluorescence are obtained.

The photomultiplier senses the vertical fluorescent intensity produced by both the horizontal and vertical excitation beams. Through the use of a microprocessor and a counter-timer device, the fluorescent intensities for each excitation component are determined and used to calculate the degree of polarization obtained for a particular sample. For quantitative purposes, a curve, as shown in Figure 8-3, is obtained. Through the use of the microprocessor, the curve is mathematically stored and can be used for subsequent sample analysis with direct concentration printout.

An automated system of the above design has been described and is commercially available.[2] This system is commonly used for the measurement of various drugs in serum. In addition, various hormones are becoming measurable entities by this automated technique. Curves as shown in Figure 8-3 are obtained and are quite reproducible. Of interest in the shape of the curve is the high degree of polarization at low analyte concentration. This phenomenon tends to give fluorescence polarization increased sensitivity and precision.[3]

The instrument design above utilizes a rotating excitation polarizer controlled by an electric signal, and a fixed emission polarizer. Another type of instrument is available that uses a different orientation of the polarizers.[5] The fluorometric components of the system operate similarly to the previously described system and produce similar data; however, operation of the polarizers is different.

The excitation polarizer is fixed so that the excitation beam is modulated to permit only polarized light in one plane to strike the sample. The emission or analyzer polarizer is variable and used to pass alternatively horizontal- and vertical-plane-polarized light for subsequent detection by the photomultiplier tube. The analyzer polarizer is varied in direction through the use of a motor that mechanically turns the crystal. The motor is synchronously driven so that fluo-

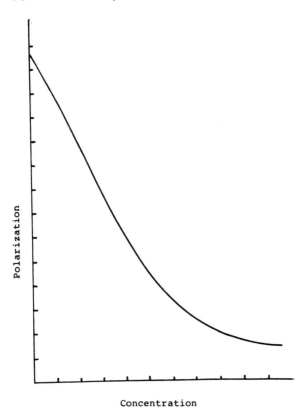

Figure 8-3. Calibration curve for a fluorescence polarization immunoassay.

rescence measurements coincide with the horizontal and vertical orientation of the crystal. A microprocessor collects the fluorescence data and calculates polarization values.

Routine Operation

In the development of a fluorometric assay, optimization of fluorescent intensity is desired to achieve maximum sensitivity. To optimize the fluorescence for a given analyte, some understanding of the absorption spectrum is helpful. With an analyte standard placed in the instrument, the emission wavelength is set at the absorption maximum for the analyte. The emission spectrum is scanned to find the wavelength at which fluorescence intensity is maximum. The emission monochromator is then set at this wavelength and the excitation spectrum is scanned to check for maximum fluorescence. For subsequent analyses, the excitation and emission monochromators are at the wavelengths found for maximum fluorescence.

If little is known about the absorption spectrum before checking for fluorescence maximum, a good starting place for the excitation wavelength adjustment may be nonspecific wavelengths of 254, 280, or 340 nm. Subsequent increases of 25 or 50 nm may be needed until a fluorescent signal is obtained, after which the above procedure may be followed.

Another point of consideration in finding optimum wavelengths is the specificity. Although maximum fluorescent intensity is found at one set of wavelengths for a standard, possible interferences in the sample matrix may prohibit use of these. By choosing a secondary set of wavelengths, fluorescence for the desired analyte may still be obtained, but the new wavelengths exclude the interference through lack of excitation or through filtering of the interferent emission.

Once the desired wavelengths are obtained, a fluorescent assay may be performed. Because fluorescent measurements are relative numbers and are not absolute, a reference must be established. Generally, a calibration curve is generated using standards in an appropriate matrix. The background of the matrix is subtracted using a blank consisting of the matrix. Once the curve is established, samples may be read relative to the standards. Concentration of the sample is determined from the calibration curve.

For polarization operation, the instrument generally performs all functions through microprocessor control.[2] Because only one fluorescent compound is analyzed (fluorescein), wavelengths need no adjustments. The instrument also performs the calibration curves through the use of a standard set. Background fluorescence for each sample is measured and stored for subsequent subtraction. Calculations are performed by the instrument and a direct printout of concentration is obtained.

Advantages

The use of fluorescence over absorption has several advantages. The first is the increase in sensitivity. In fluorescence, measurements are not based on difference as in absorption. Generally, a signal is obtained on a very low background. If increased sensitivity is desired, increasing the lamp intensity will increase fluorescence. Similarly, an increase in the voltage to the photomultiplier tube will increase sensitivity. Both of these adjustments increase fluorescence without significant alteration in the background intensity. Electronic noise and stray light may become a problem if the components are set near their respective limits. Adjustments to the source and detector tube in absorptivity measurements also increase the background, rendering the absorption measurement to be less sensitive. Fluorescence measurements are generally 10 to 1000 times more sensitive than absorption measurements.

Specificity is also an advantage of fluorometry. Through the use of two wavelengths, various interferences are eliminated. The emission of light in fluorescence adds inherent specificity. Many substances may absorb at a given wavelength, including the fluorophor; however, not as many substances will fluoresce. This limited degree of fluorescence coupled with the variance of the emission wavelengths greatly adds specificity to this technique.

For fluorescence polarization, sensitivity and specificity are also achieved.

Through the use of a highly efficient fluorophor, fluoroscein, and the utilization of polarization values (see Systems), sensitivity in the nanogram range is obtained. In addition, specificity is significantly increased from several factors. Sample background subtraction ensures that analytical measurements result only from the desired analyte. The use of narrow-bandwidth bandpass filters reduces stray light and potential fluorescent interferences. Utilization of specific antibodies directed only to the analyte of interest ensures that the polarization values obtained are from the competitive binding assay between the analyte of interest and its fluorescent-tagged analogue.

Disadvantages

Several disadvantages of fluorometry exist, owing to the unique nature of fluorescence. Interferences are a problem from both a positive- and negative-bias standpoint. Drugs that may be present in the sample matrix may fluoresce at the same wavelengths as the analyte of interest does, thereby giving an abnormally high measurement. From a negative approach, quenching of fluorescence for various reasons (*i.e.*, chloride ions) may occur and reduce the measured intensity (see Principles). In fluorescence polarization, interferences may result from the binding of substances that have a similar immunoreactivity as the analyte of interest. The interference would decrease binding of the fluorescent tag and would produce analyte concentrations that were abnormally high.

A second disadvantage is the environmental sensitivity of fluorescence and fluorescence polarization. The solvent and *p*H are important and should be kept as constant as possible to minimize errors. Temperature is important, particularly in polarization measurements. Usually, the instruments have a thermoregulated sample chamber to eliminate this variable.

Another potential problem in fluorescence is self-absorption. This phenomenon occurs when the excitation band and emission band overlap. As some molecules are excited and fluoresce, the emitted fluorescence is of a wavelength that may cause excitation of other fluorophors. As a result, emitted fluorescence is absorbed, causing an overall decrease in fluorescence intensity. Finally, as discussed in the Principles section, high fluorophor concentrations result in several problems and result in decreased fluorescence as well. Nonlinearity of the fluorescence-concentration curve occurs.

Applications

Fluorescence is used to measure various drugs, catecholamines, and porphyrins. Increased specificity is obtained through the use of fluorescence coupled to high-performance liquid chromatography. Many examples exist in the literature for various applications using such systems.

Fluorescence polarization is commonly used to measure various drugs. In addition, some hormones are currently measurable using this technique, with new applications constantly being developed.

References

1. Adamsons K, Sell JE, Holland JF, Timnick A: Absorption corrected measurements in molecular fluorescence. Am Lab 16:16, 1984
2. Jolley ME, Stroupe SD, Schwenzer KS et al: Fluorescence polarization immunoassay. III, An automated system for therapeutic drug determination. Clin Chem 27:1575, 1981
3. Jolley ME, Stroupe SD, Wang CJ et al: Fluorescence polarization immunoassay. I, Monitoring aminoglycoside antibiotics in serum and plasma. Clin Chem 27:1190, 1981
4. Khalil OS, Routh WS, Lingenfelter K, Can DB, Ladouceur P: Automated in-line ratio-correcting filter fluorometer. Clin Chem 27:1586, 1981
5. Muira H: Application of fluorescence polarization to the determination of urinary lysozyme activity. Clin Biochem 18:40, 1985
6. Popelka SR, Miller DM, Holen JT, Kelso DM: Fluorescence polarization immunoassay. II, Analyzer for rapid, precise measurement of fluorescence polarization with use of disposable cuvettes. Clin Chem 27:1198, 1981
7. Skoog DA, West DM: Principles of Instrumental Analysis. New York, Holt, Rinehart & Winston, 1971
8. Warner IM, Patonay G, Thomas MP: Multidimensional luminescence measurements. Anal Chem 57:463A, 1985
9. Weinberger R, Sapp E: Fluorescence detection in liquid chromatography. Am Lab 16:121, 1984
10. Willard HH, Merritt LL, Jr, Dean JA, Settle FA Jr: Instrumental methods of analysis, 6th ed. Princeton, Van Nostrand, 1981

9

ELECTROCHEMICAL METHODS OF ANALYSIS

Steven M. Faynor

Definitions

Acid: A hydrogen ion donor. An acid dissociates to a hydrogen ion plus a conjugate base. Example: hydrochloric acid.

$$\underset{\text{acid}}{\text{HCl}} \rightarrow \text{H}^+ + \underset{\text{conjugate base}}{\text{Cl}^-}$$

Activity: The thermodynamic expression for the effective concentration of a substance in solution. Activity (a) is equal to the concentration (C) times an activity coefficient (γ).

$$a = \gamma\text{C}$$

The activity coefficient varies with the ionic strength of the solution. In dilute solutions (most biologic systems), the activity coefficient approaches 1, so activity is roughly equivalent to concentration.

Ampere: The unit of current. One ampere (A) is one coulomb of charge per second.

Amperometry: An electrochemical technique that determines the concentration of a substance by measuring the amount of current produced by an oxidation or reduction of that substance at an electrode that is maintained at a single applied potential. In coulometry, amperometry is used to determine the endpoint of the titration by signaling the appearance of an excess of titrant.

Anode: The electrode where oxidation takes place.

Automatic Temperature Compensation: A device used to automatically change the gain of a pH meter to compensate for changes in sample temperature.[15]

Cathode: The electrode where reduction takes place.

CO_2 Content: The sum of the concentrations of all CO_2 species in solution. Although CO_2 is present in plasma in many ways, including that physically dissolved as well as attached to proteins and hemoglobin (carbamino groups), for practical purposes, the CO_2

content is approximately equal to the sum in millimoles per liter of the bicarbonate plus carbonic acid.

Combination Electrode: An electrode where the indicator and reference electrodes are combined into a single unit.

Coulomb: The unit of charge. One coulomb is equivalent to the charge on 6.24×10^{18} electrons.

Coulometry: A titration that utilizes an electrochemically generated titrant.

Direct-Reading Electrode: An electrode that is exposed to an undiluted specimen as the sample. It is usually applied to sodium and potassium electrodes.

Dissociation Constant: An acid present in dilute aqueous solution will dissociate predictably. The constant (K) is calculated by multiplying the hydrogen ion concentration by the conjugate base concentration and dividing this by the undissociated acid concentration.

$$K = \frac{[H^+] [HCO_3^-]}{[H_2CO_3]}$$

Electrode: The site of an oxidation or reduction reaction in solution.

Electrode Response: The change in potential of an ion-selective electrode in response to changes in the concentration of the ion the electrode is designed to measure. Predicted by the Nernst equation (q.v.).

Electrolyte: An aqueous solution containing ions and capable of conducting electricity.

Equivalence Point: That point in the titration at which stoichiometrically equivalent amounts of the main reactants have been brought together. It is the point at which there is no excess of either reactant.

Faraday: The charge carried by an equivalent weight of an ion. One faraday (1 F) = 96,487 C/equivalent.

Faraday's Law: The passage of one faraday of electricity (96,487 C) will oxidize or reduce one gram-equivalent of the substance under investigation.

Henderson-Hasselbalch Equation: In a weak aqueous solution such as blood, the *p*H can be predicted on the basis of the following equation utilizing the observed *p*K' (q.v.) of 6.1 for the most active plasma buffer, bicarbonate.

$$pH = pK' + \log \frac{[HCO_3^-]}{[H_2CO_3]}$$

where $[H_2CO_3] = 0.03 \, pCO_2$.

Indicator Electrode: The electrode designed to respond to a change in the concentration of some substance in solution; also called the *working electrode.*

Indirect-Reading Electrode: An electrode that is exposed to a diluted serum specimen as the sample. It is usually applied to sodium and potassium electrodes.

Ion-Selective Electrode: An electrode whose potential varies with the concentration of some ion in solution. The *p*H electrode is a hydrogen-ion-selective electrode.

Isopotential Point: The *p*H at which the combined potential of the *p*H and reference electrode is 0 mV and at which the response is relatively insensitive to changes in temperature. For most *p*H meter–electrode combinations, the isopotential point is approximately *p*H 7.

Liquid-Junction Potential: The electrical potential developing at a junction[19] between solutions composed of different ions, not necessarily related to *p*H. Factors affecting the liquid-junction potential include physical structure of the junction, types of salts in solution (ionic strength), temperature, and colloidal particles. For reproducibility, the two solutions should be brought together under the same conditions on each occasion. Apparent *p*H drift may be caused by diffusion of the two electrolyte solutions, one into the other.

   Nernst Equation: An expression relating the electrode response to the activity (or concentration) of an ion in solution.

$$E = E^0 + \frac{2.3\ RT}{nF} \log a$$

See text for explanation.

   Oxidation: The process of losing electrons.

   Partial Pressure: For a mixture of gases, the pressure contribution by any single gas will be equal to the mole-fraction of the gas times the total pressure. For example, for a gas at 760 mm Hg and containing 5% CO_2, the partial pressure of the CO_2 will be 38 mm Hg.

   pH: The negative common (base 10) logarithm of the hydrogen ion concentration or activity. In practice, hydrogen ion concentration and activity are used interchangeably.

   pK: The negative common (base 10) logarithm of the dissociation constant (q.v.).

   pK' (6.1):   The empirically determined *p*K for the bicarbonate buffer system of whole blood at 37°C. In practice, the actual *p*K' has been found to vary in patients from 5.8 to 6.4. It is unclear whether this variation is prevalent enough to introduce errors in parameters derived from the Henderson-Hasselbalch equation.[21,24]

   Polarography: An electrochemical technique for determining the concentration of a substance in solution by measuring the current produced from a polarized electrode when the substance undergoes oxidation or reduction at the electrode.

   Potentiometry: An electrochemical technique for determining the concentration of a substance in solution by measuring the potential of an electrode in response to changes in the concentration under conditions of no net current flow and at equilibrium.

   Reference Electrode: The electrode against which the potential change created in an ion-specific electrode is measured. These electrodes are generally silver–silver chloride (Ag/AgCl) or calomel (Hg/Hg_2Cl_2). The potential of the reference electrode remains constant in the face of changing ion concentrations of the test solutions.

   Salt Bridge: That solution used to connect the reference electrode with the test electrode and the intervening unknown solution. The salt bridge most commonly used is saturated potassium chloride, (KCl), although 0.1 N, 3.0 N, 3.5 N, and 4.5 N solutions of KCl, 0.15 N NaCl, and other concentrations of NaCl have also been utilized.

   Temperature Coefficient: The measurable millivolt change per *p*H unit at the various temperatures utilized for *p*H measurement (mV/*p*H unit). It is predicted by the Nernst equation to be equal to 2.3 RT/nF or 59.16 mV for the hydrogen electrode at 25°C. This is not to be confused with the temperature coefficient of buffer solutions, in which their measurable *p*H changes with temperature (*p*H/°C). (For example, whole blood *p*H changes 0.015 *p*H unit/°C, whereas plasma changes 0.01 *p*H unit/°C.)

Introduction

   The principles of electrochemistry have been used to develop several analytic techniques used in the modern clinical laboratory. The first major clinical electrochemical methods included the measurements of blood *p*H, pCO_2, and pO_2. In the last 20 years, refinements in electrode manufacturing have caused changes resulting in an increased use of analytic techniques based on measuring the flow of electricity. Now the electrolytes and some trace metals, as well as other analytes (*e.g.*, glucose), can be measured using electrochemical methods. This chapter will describe the clinical laboratory use of electrodes, specific-ion electrodes, coulometry, potentiometry, and anodic stripping voltammetry.

Principles

A metal rod, inserted into a solution of its own metallic ions, will develop an electrical potential (voltage) between the metal and the solution. This voltage results from the production of electrons as some of the metal atoms become dissolved in the solution. Free electrons are produced by this reaction.

$$M^0 \rightarrow M^+ + e^-$$

where

$$M^0 = \text{metal atom}$$
$$M^+ = \text{metallic ion}$$
$$e^- = \text{electron}$$

This system is a half-cell and the metal rod can be considered the electrode. Because oxidation is occurring at this electrode, it is also the anode.

The ions of another metal in solutions and in contact with their metal atom may favor formation of metal atoms with acceptance of an electron.

$$M^+ + e^- \rightarrow M^0$$

This second electrode would then be the cathode because reduction is taking place. This, too, is a half-cell. The two half-cells can be connected by means of a conducting solution (salt bridge). This establishes the circuit and enables a current to flow. Thus, a complete cell is formed.

A comparison of the voltage of one half-cell to another half-cell can be made. The International Union of Pure and Applied Chemistry in 1953 adopted the method of comparing all half-cell potentials to the standard hydrogen electrode, the potential of which they arbitrarily assigned as 0.0000 V. The standard electrode potential (E^0) for each half-cell is determined by a comparison to the standard hydrogen electrode. This standard electrode potential is defined as the emf of the half-cell when all activities are unity and is usually given at 25°C. A few examples follow:

Half-cell	*Reaction*	*emf*
$1/2H_2$	$H^+ + e^-$	0.0000 V
Ca	$Ca^{2+} + 2e^-$	+2.87 V
Fe	$Fe^{2+} + 2e^-$	+0.441 V
Cu	$Cu^{2+} + 2e^-$	−0.337 V

If the ions in the cells are not at unit activity, the potential E is given by the Nernst equation.

$$E = E^0 + \frac{RT}{nF} \ln a$$

where

E = observed potential (emf)
E^0 = standard electrode potential (emf)
R = molar gas constant (8.314 J/mole per °K)
T = absolute T in °K (25°C = 298°K)
n = number of electrons transferred
F = Faraday's constant (96,500 C/Eq weight)
ln = log to the base e (natural log)
a = activity of the ion

At 25°C, with conversion of the natural $\log_e$ to $\log_{10}$ and insertion of the values for R and F, this equation simplifies to

$$E = E^0 + \frac{0.0591}{n} \log_{10} a$$

For the pH electrode,

$$E = E^0 - 0.198\, T\, pH$$

From this equation, it can be seen that voltage is dependent upon the activity of the ion. Because a change in ion activity will change the measurable voltage, pH can be determined by a difference in voltage. A pH measurement is an indirect measurement of the hydrogen ion activity. The hydrogen ion activity coefficient approaches unity in very dilute solutions. Therefore, this activity measurement can become a workable approximation for concentration.

Electrodes

CALOMEL REFERENCE ELECTRODE

This electrode consists of a combination of mercury (Hg), mercurous chloride (Hg_2Cl_2), and KCl paste in a saturated KCl solution. The chloride ions become saturated with mercury at the surface of the mercury. Under these conditions, a typical calomel electrode will produce a constant reference potential of 224 mV to which other electrodes may be compared. For proper operation, the surface of the electrode tip must be completely immersed in the electrolyte.

It is best to have the electrode's electrolyte and the bridge salt solution identical; in this case, saturated KCl is used. Other bridge solutions are less satisfactory. With dilute bridging salt solutions, liquid junction potentials are much less predictable. The calomel electrode should be separated from the KCl salt bridge by a porous ceramic plug, which will reduce the chance of back diffusion and contamination.

Potential contaminating factors for the calomel electrode include the following:

Bromide contamination.   Concentration of bromide in KCl should be less than 0.005%.
Thermal instability.   The calomel reference electrode system contains at least

nine thermal-sensitive equilibrium sites with possible junction potentials. Thermal stability with $\pm 0.05°C$ is necessary.

Calomel potential. The calomel electrode provides a potential independent of *p*H when connected to a glass electrode by a KCl bridge whenever the *p*H is greater than 1.5 and less than 12. For best operation, the calomel electrode should be intact, appear silver gray, and have an open air vent during the time of use. The electrolyte level should be kept full using the fill hole on the side.

SILVER–SILVER CHLORIDE ELECTRODE

This electrode usually consists of a platinum wire on which silver and then silver chloride are deposited. The potential developed at the electrode surface can be described by the following equation:

$$AgCl + e^- \rightleftharpoons Ag^0 + Cl^-$$

This may be used as a reference electrode. However, KCl may not then be used as an electrolyte or salt bridge because silver chloride is soluble in KCl. Both HCl and NaCl may be used.

HYDROGEN ELECTRODE

This so-called ultimate standard electrode is created by bubbling pure hydrogen gas through a solution in which a platinum electrode is immersed and establishing an equilibrium between the hydrogen ion and the hydrogen gas in that solution.

$$H^+ + e^- \rightleftharpoons 1/2 H_2(g)$$

The platinum electrode is covered by a surface catalyst such as platinum or palladium black, which reduces the energy barrier, increases the equilibrium pressure of hydrogen, and makes the electrode reversible in response to the hydrogen ion. The electrode has disadvantages of working with hydrogen gas, having a slow equilibrium, and requiring large volumes of solution. This electrode has a potential of 199 mV when saturated KCl is used. It has better thermal stability than the calomel electrode, so it is used when measurement must be made at elevated temperatures.

GLASS ELECTRODE

Certain thin glass membranes will develop a potential difference when ionic solutions of differing *p*H are present on the membrane's two sides. The thin glass membrane separates an unknown solution from a reference electrode (AgCl electrode) immersed in a solution of a known *p*H. The electrode will reversibly respond to changes in *p*H within this solution. The electrolyte is usually HCl. These ion-selective electrodes measure hydrogen ion activity, not hydrogen ion concentration.

Each surface of the glass membrane (of the electrode) develops a hydrated glass lattice consisting of a network of oxygen atoms held together in an irregular chain by silicon atoms. This lattice contains anionic sites capable of attracting cations of appropriate size-to-charge ratio.

The mineral composition of the glass is critical. Minor changes in composition will produce major changes in the electrode sensitivity. Three types of glass electrodes (the *p*H type, the cation type, and the sodium type) are available. The general formula for all includes approximately 72% SiO_2, 6% CaO, and 21% Na_2O. One percent Al_2O_3 produces a good *p*H-sensitive glass membrane with little metal response. The concentration of oxides of sodium and aluminum is varied to make all three electrode types.

At the hydrated glass surface, exchange of alkaline metal ions in the lattice for hydrogen ions in solution plays a major part in the development of the *p*H response. Hydration generally occurs to the extent of 50 to 100 mg of water per cm^3 of glass, producing an average membrane with a dry glass thickness of 50 μ and an overlying hydrated layer on each surface of 50 to 100 Å. The hydration process causes swelling of the glass, but constant dissolution of the surface of the hydrated area maintains the glass membrane's total thickness at a steady state. The glass needs to be of relatively high chemical durability, or alkaline earths within the glass will dissolve too rapidly and, in solution, will erode glass and electrode alike over a period of months. The rate of dissolution of glass is one major factor determining the electrode's life.

For best performance, *p*H-sensitive glass electrodes should be

1. Stored in a buffer solution near the *p*H at which the electrode will be used
2. Never scratched
3. Never cleaned with chromic acid
4. Cleaned when the response is slow or erratic. For electrodes used with blood samples, protein is usually the offending agent. This can be removed with protein-denaturing agents such as 8 molar urea or pepsin. Most electrodes will show improved response after soaking in 0.1 N HCl for 15 minutes followed by reconditioning in *p*H 7 buffer for 30 minutes before use.

PRECIPITATE ELECTRODE

These anionic-sensitive electrodes exchange anions through a membrane containing cationic sites. One type uses polymerized silicon rubber diffusely permeated with small grains (5–10 μ) of a silver halide such as AgI. Each electrode exchanges best for the anion in common with its precipitate; that is, I^- for AgI-impregnated electrodes, Cl^- for AgCl, and Br^- for AgBr. The electrodes are relatively insensitive to redox interferences and surface poisonings. They are relatively insensitive to cation effect.

SOLID-STATE ELECTRODE

These electrodes, similar to precipitate electrodes, separate an external (unknown) from an internal (standard solution containing) electrode by an inorganic single crystal "doped" with a rare earth. In the fluoride-sensitive electrode, this thin membrane consists of crystalline lanthanum fluoride doped with europium (II), added to reduce electrical resistance and facilitate ionic charge transport. These solid-state electrodes show remarkable specificity for fluoride ion. The hydroxyl ion offers the only major interference.

LIQUID-LIQUID ELECTRODE

In these electrodes, custom-made liquid ionic exchange solutions of high specificity are separated from the test solution by synthetic membrane or porous glass permeable to the ion in question. Transport of such ions across the membrane, to or from the liquid ion exchanger, causes the development of measurable potential difference. The ionic exchange solution must be in contact with the sample solution (via membrane), yet mixing must be minimal. The exchanger must be relatively insoluble in the sample to reduce contamination and must exhibit photochemical and thermal stability.

In a variation of this model, termed the *liquid-membrane design*, the ion exchanger is not contained in the liquid but is incorporated into the membrane itself. The membrane usually consists of polyvinylchloride. Unlike the precipitate electrode above, the ion exchanger is dispersed in a homogeneous fashion and is not present in crystalline form.

In the calcium electrode (Fig. 9-1), calcium organophosphorus is used as the ionic exchange compound. It is active between pH 5.5 and 11. Higher pH levels cause interference by calcium hydroxide formation. Reagents that complex calcium and prevent ionization, such as phosphate buffers, and so forth, cannot be used. A calomel reference electrode is used to develop a circuit. A standard of ionic calcium is used (which has sodium, potassium, and magnesium ions added at levels approximately those of the unknown).

Figure 9-1. Schematic diagram of calcium ion-specific electrode.

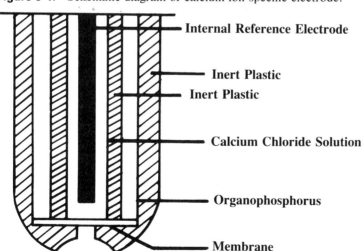

Internal Reference Electrode

Inert Plastic
Inert Plastic

Calcium Chloride Solution

Organophosphorus

Membrane

COMBINATION ELECTRODE

For measuring small volumes especially, a combination *p*H electrode can be used. This electrode combines the indicator and reference electrode in a single unit (Fig. 9-2).

SODIUM ELECTRODE

Sodium electrodes are similar in design to *p*H electrodes. By increasing the aluminum content of the glass at the tip, the electrode will show a preferential response to sodium over hydrogen ions. Actually, *p*H electrodes do respond to sodium ions to some extent, and at very high sodium concentrations, an appreciable *p*H error is induced.

Sodium ion-selective electrode (ISE) systems are of two kinds—direct-reading and indirect-reading. Direct-reading electrode systems use whole blood or serum as the sample, and the electrode is exposed to the undiluted sample. The electrode response is directly proportional to the sodium ion activity in the aqueous phase of the sample. In indirect-reading systems, a given volume of sample is first diluted

Figure 9-2.   Schematic diagram of a combination *p*H electrode.

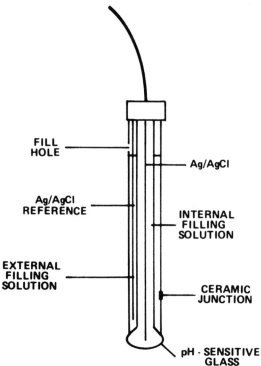

before being introduced into the measuring system. The electrode response is then proportional to the quantity of sodium ions delivered to the diluent.

The differences in these systems can have important implications for the interpretation of the results in clinical situations. In situations of high lipid content, such as severe lipemia, or high protein content, such as multiple myeloma, the lipid or protein will displace some water from the aqueous phase of the sample. In direct-reading systems, this makes no difference, because the electrode responds only to the ion activity of the aqueous phase, regardless of how much lipid or protein there is. The indirect-reading electrode will see fewer sodium ions, and will report a falsely lowered concentration. The biologic activity of sodium ions is related only to the concentration in the aqueous phase. The condition of a falsely lowered sodium concentration in the face of elevated lipid or protein is termed *pseudohyponatremia*.[10]

POTASSIUM ELECTRODE

The potassium electrode is a liquid-membrane design with a potassium ion exchanger incorporated into a solid plastic membrane. The ion exchanger is usually valinomycin, an ionophore with a particular affinity for monovalent cations with the ionic radius of potassium. These electrodes may be either of the direct-reading or indirect-reading types and are usually included on instruments along with a sodium electrode.

IONIZED CALCIUM ELECTRODE

The design of the ionized calcium electrode has been discussed above. Calcium exists in several forms in plasma. Approximately 46% is bound to serum proteins (most notably albumin), 6% is complexed to serum anions (citrate, oxalate, and so forth), and 47% exists as free, ionized calcium.[6]

Calcium is essential to neuromuscular activity and hemostasis, but it is only the ionized calcium that is active in this respect. In cases of decreased serum protein concentration, such as hypoalbuminemia due to liver failure, total calcium may be decreased but ionized calcium may be normal. Ionized calcium is elevated in persons with primary hyperparathyroidism. After a massive blood transfusion (*e.g.*, liver transplant), ionized calcium may fall owing to the infusion of the citrate anticoagulant. Ionized calcium levels are also affected by *p*H. In respiratory alkalosis, protein binding of calcium is increased and the ionized calcium falls.

Obviously, proper sample handling is essential for reliable results. Anaerobic handling is desired, because samples exposed to the atmosphere will lose CO_2 and the *p*H will rise. Some ionized calcium analyzers can add CO_2 to the sample before analysis. Others correct the ionized calcium concentration to *p*H 7.4. It should be remembered that this value will not be true in patients who have an acid–base disturbance. Clearly, specimens should not be collected in ethylenediaminetetraacetate (EDTA) or oxalate anticoagulants, because these will bind calcium.

Measurement of *p*H and Blood Gases

THE *p*H METER

The *p*H meter is an instrument for the potentiometric comparison of a change in emf (voltage) between a glass electrode and a reference electrode created by the relative hydrogen ion concentration in the unknown solution completing the circuit (Fig. 9-3).

The meter must be capable of measuring emf to 0.1 mV (equivalent to 0.002 *p*Hu). At this millivoltage an extremely small current will flow, in the neighborhood of 10^{-8} A, because of the high internal resistance of the glass electrode. In a direct-reading instrument, the actual emf produced by a change in *p*H is amplified and displayed digitally or on a meter. At any given temperature, the change in voltage resulting from a change in [H^+] will be directly proportional to the change in log [H^+]. Thus, the change in voltage is linear with respect to a change in *p*H. The instrument converts a change in millivoltage to a change in *p*H units at the various electrode temperatures. The instrument's temperature control knob alters the constant proportionally between voltage and scale reading. For example, an electrode that would reflect a change of 59.1 mV for a change of 1.00 *p*H units at 25°C would show a change of some 74 mV for the same change in *p*H, 1.00, at 100°C. In other words, the instrument's temperature control knob will accommodate the temperature coefficient. Temperature compensation therefore represents a slope adjustment relating the changes in *p*H to changes in millivolts.

Newer *p*H meters have automatic temperature compensators (ATC) built in. The ATC circuit consists of a temperature probe such as a platinum resistance thermometer, which is immersed into the test solution along with the reference and indicator electrodes. The resistance of the platinum element changes with

Figure 9-3. Schematic diagram of *p*H system.

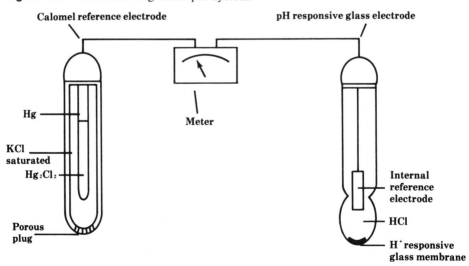

temperature, and the output of the probe is used to modify the gain of the *p*H meter's amplifier.

Some *p*H meters compensate directly for changes in temperature by measuring the change in resistance of the *p*H electrode's glass membrane. This resistance, like that of the platinum thermometer, varies with temperature. This eliminates the need for an extra ATC probe. This technique is termed *log R compensation.*[15]

All *p*H meters must be standardized before use so that the response and meter scale coincide. The first step is to immerse the electrodes into a *p*H 7.00 buffer and to adjust the meter to this value using the "zero," "standardize," or "calibrate" knob. For most *p*H meter–electrode combinations, *p*H 7 is the isopotential point so the output of the electrode pair should be 0 mV. The zero knob allows imposition of a small offset so the meter will read 7.00. This is roughly equivalent to a blank in a spectrophotometric assay.

The electrodes are then immmersed in a second buffer to adjust the slope. The second buffer is chosen so the *p*Hs of the buffers bracket the *p*H of the unknown solution. The meter is adjusted to the second *p*H using the "slope" knob. If all electrodes behaved as predicted by the Nernst equation, there would be no need for a slope adjustment. However, they don't always, so a slope correction is necessary for maximum accuracy. If no slope control is provided, the temperature control can be used for the same purpose, provided the electrodes, buffers, and samples are all at the same temperature.

Microprocessor-controlled *p*H meters modify the digital display so that it matches the values of the standardization buffers. To standardize these instruments successfully, the calibration algorithm must be followed exactly.

Glass electrodes operate best at *p*H between 2 and 12 and ionic strength between 0.01 and 0.1. Proper pH measurements require the following:

1. The sample and standard buffers must be treated identically.
2. The electrode must reflect the correct voltage to *p*H ratio at all times.
3. The *p*H meter must translate millivolts to *p*H units correctly regardless of the temperature at which the measurements are taken.
4. Meter standardization is best with buffers covering the entire useful range. Utilizing a buffer with temperature, *p*H, and ionic strength similar to that of the unknown will reduce the variables created by liquid junction potential difference and thermal effects.

LOCATION OF TROUBLE

Problems in *p*H meters are generally due to the following:

1. Scratched or cracked glass electrodes
2. Dirt on electrodes
3. Contaminated KCl
4. Clogged ceramic aperture
5. Inaccurate buffer
6. Unusable or improperly collected sample

Most of these problems should be avoided or detected prior to faulty use by an appropriate system of preventive maintenance and quality control.

Functional characteristics of a pH meter such as reproducibility, drift, noise, response time, and linearity should be periodically determined and can be utilized with advantage in any quality control program. A thorough review of check systems for pH meters should be consulted for guidance in setting up a quality control program.[25]

CARBON DIOXIDE PARTIAL PRESSURE MEASUREMENT

Carbon dioxide partial pressure (pCO_2) is measured as the change in pH of a weak bicarbonate buffer after it has reached equilibrium by dialysis across a semipermeable membrane with the CO_2 physically dissolved in an unknown solution, usually blood. The pCO_2 electrode takes advantage of the fact that pH has a linear relationship to the log pCO_2 over the range of 10 to 90 mm Hg (1.4%–11.4%). The following equilibrium exists in blood as well as in bicarbonate buffer.

$$H_2O + CO_2 \rightleftharpoons H_2CO_3 \rightleftharpoons HCO_3^- + H^+ \tag{1}$$

The dissociation equation can be written as follows:

$$K = \frac{[H^+] [HCO_3^-]}{[H_2CO_3]} \text{ or } K = \frac{[H^+][HCO_3^-]}{[k \times pCO_2]} \tag{2}$$

and, substituting into eq. (2),

$$\log [H^+] + \log [HCO_3^-] = \log K + \log k + \log pCO_2 \tag{3}$$

Because pH equals the negative log of the hydrogen ion concentration and pK equals the negative log of the dissociation constant K,

$$pH - \log [HCO_3^-] = pK - \log k - \log pCO_2 \tag{4}$$

pK and log k are constants. Therefore,

$$pH \cong \log [HCO_3^-] - \log pCO_2 \tag{5}$$

and pH has a linear dependence on log pCO_2 when equilibrium has been established.

The pCO_2 electrode (Fig. 9-4)[17,18] interposes a semipermeable (to CO_2 dissolved as a gas only) membrane between the unknown solution (usually blood) and a weak bicarbonate buffer into which is immersed both a pH-sensitive glass electrode and a reference electrode (usually silver–silver chloride).

After the CO_2, physically dissolved in the sample or as a calibrating gas or solution, reaches equilibrium with the bicarbonate buffer across the semipermeable membrane, some hydrogen ion concentration change within the buffer may occur. This will be detected by the pH-sensitive glass electrode. A potential difference will then exist between the glass electrode and the reference electrode and will be measured on the meter. The meter's scale is usually calibrated for pCO_2 in a semilogarithmic fashion, conforming to an observation that pH is inversely proportional to the log of the pCO_2 concentration.

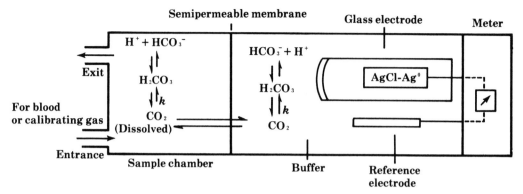

Figure 9-4.   Schematic diagram of pCO₂ electrode.

The semipermeable membranes utilized include tetrafluoroethylene resin (Teflon), silastic, or polyethylene. They are permeable to physically dissolved CO_2 but impermeable to anions and cations.

The electrode's response time is directly proportional to the type and thickness of the semipermeable membrane, the strength of the bicarbonate buffer, the depth of buffer layer separating the glass electrode from the semipermeable membrane, and the temperature. Teflon measuring 0.001 inch thick will respond to 99% of equilibrium within 120 seconds. For polyethylene of the same thickness, equilibrium time is 180 seconds.

Sodium chloride is added to the bicarbonate buffer to increase conductivity and thus facilitate the measurement. If KCl were added, the conductivity would be increased, but great drift would occur as a result of the silver chloride surface of the reference electrode dissolving into the buffer.

A chemically inert spacer is placed in the buffer between the membrane and the glass electrode's surface to prevent direct contact between the two, which could produce irregular readings. Nylon, fine glass paper, or porous ("Joseph") paper may be used. Air bubbles at this point produce irregular equilibrium development and irregular readings.

For example, one Radiometer system uses 12 μ thick Teflon, 40 μ thick Joseph paper, and a buffer of 0.005 to 0.01M bicarbonate with 0.02M sodium chloride. This produces a 99% response time in 120 seconds.

The calibration response of the pCO₂ electrodes appears identical for gas and liquid of the same pCO₂, provided the gas has been saturated with water vapor prior to the introduction into the pCO₂ cell. This facilitates calibration. The equilibration gases (low and high) should flow slowly so as to produce a slow, steady, regular stream of bubbles. This flow should be slow enough to allow thermal equilibrium to occur as well as vapor saturation.

Calibration

The method of calibration varies with the instrument and its sophistication. The following is an example of a general procedure:

1. Calculate the pCO_2 of the calibrating gases as in the following example: With barometric pressure at 760 mm Hg and the temperature at 37°C, the water vapor pressure will be 47 mm Hg, and the corrected barometric pressure equals $760 - 47 = 713$ mm Hg; for a 5% CO_2 gas, $0.05 \times 713 = 35.6$ mm Hg (the theoretical pCO_2 of this gas).
2. With the electrode in equilibrium with the low gas (pCO_2 equals 35.6 in this example), adjust the meter pCO_2 indicator by use of the calibration or balance control.
3. Now, equilibrate the electrode with the higher pCO_2 gas (10%). Adjust the meter indicator to the value of the high gas (71.3 mm Hg in this example) with the pCO_2 slope control.
4. Alternate methods of calibration are available from the manufacturers (see Semiautomated/Automated Instruments, below). The procedure recommended by the manufacturer should be used unless an undesirable or unreliable feature is identified by the user.

Total CO_2 Content Electrode

By mixing a serum sample with a suitable acidic buffer before analysis, the total CO_2 content can be measured. As can be seen from equation (1) above, the addition of acid will force all of the ionic species toward the direction of CO_2, which will diffuse across the semipermeable membrane. The Beckman Cl/CO_2 analyzer[1] measures the rate of the pH change in the pCO_2 electrode, which is directly proportional to the CO_2 concentration in the sample.

OXYGEN PARTIAL PRESSURE MEASUREMENT

Oxygen partial pressure (pO_2) is measured as the current flowing between a platinum and a silver–silver chloride electrode immersed in a buffer (phosphate and potassium chloride) which has been equilibrated with dissolved oxygen in an unknown solution by dialysis across a semipermeable membrane. The current results from oxygen reduction at the platinum electrode's surface after the electrode is polarized using a standard dc voltage, usually a mercury battery. This electrode differs from the other two in that it is polarographic and not potentiometric.

The Clark-type electrode,[4,5] a polarographic cell (Fig. 9-5), is the one most

Figure 9-5. Schematic diagram of pO_2 electrode.

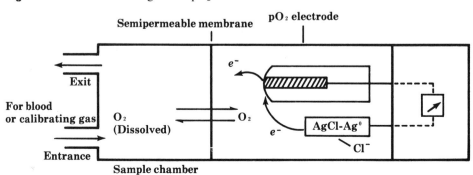

commonly used. It utilizes a silver chloride reference electrode (anode) and a glass-coated platinum electrode (cathode) connected to a small external voltage source, such as a 1.35-V mercury cell, to charge the circuit with a potential difference of 500 to 800 mV. This is called the *polarizing voltage*. The electrodes are connected by a buffer, generally saturated KCl with phosphate or sodium hydroxide added.

When the dissolved oxygen (pO_2) in the blood, gas, and so on is equilibrated with the buffer but separated from it by a semipermeable membrane, the following reaction occurs. At the platinum electrode (cathode) electroreduction occurs.

$$O_2 + 2H_2O + 4e^- \rightarrow 4OH^-$$

The electrons necessary for this electroreduction are produced at the reference electrode (anode) as follows:

$$4Ag + 4Cl^- \rightarrow 4\ AgCl + 4e^-$$

Therefore, the reaction is both polarographic and consumptive.

The current through the system is directly proportional to the pO_2 outside the membrane which has reached equilibrium with the buffer (provided oxygen consumption at the platinum electrode is low).

Solutions of high viscosity and low oxygen solubility may have difficulty reaching equilibrium with the buffer or may have a residual oxygen gradient between the sides of the membrane leading to faulty readings.

Equilibrium depends upon membrane permeability. Examples of membranes in use include the following:

1. Teflon. Highly permeable, but will respond differently to a gas and a liquid.
2. Mylar (also polypropylene and polyethylene). Less permeable but shows little difference in response to liquid and gas.

A background current can develop within the system when no oxygen is presented to the electrode. The background current is usually independent of this membrane but becomes important especially if Mylar is used. One must adjust the pO_2 meter to zero value with the calibration control when a solution of gas of known zero pO_2, such as CO_2 or N_2, is in equilibrium within the chamber. This cancels out the residual background current.

Oxygen utilization is proportional to the area of the platinum electrode available for electroreduction (usually held to a diameter of 20 μ) and the applied voltage.

1. Teflon membranes allow up to 1% per minute oxygen consumption with the chamber volume of 0.4 ml. This may lead to instrument drift.
2. Polyethylene membranes allow oxygen consumption up to 0.2% per minute with similar chamber volume and, therefore, show little tendency to drift.
3. Mylar membranes show drift and slow response. Time becomes a serious problem when this membrane is used.

The current flow is low (10^{-11} A/mm Hg at 37°C), when using a thin polyethylene or polypropylene membrane and a small platinum electrode. Reliable pO_2 reading requires the following:

1. A constant-temperature system must be capable of holding to $\pm 0.1°C$ tolerance.
2. Neither liquid nor gas should be introduced into the chamber under increased pressure.
3. Calibration must be made with a liquid standard or a gas standard that has been equilibrated with water vapor. Either standard must be equilibrated to the measuring temperature.
4. Reaction must occur anaerobically.
5. The electrode must have relatively rapid response time, in the neighborhood of 120 seconds.
6. Oxygen consumption by the platinum electrode must be low.
7. Adequate equilibration time must be consistent with the electrode's response time.

Calibrating a pO_2 Electrode

1. Equilibrate the pO_2 electrode with gas or liquid having a pO_2 of zero.
2. Adjust the pO_2 meter to zero with the pO_2 calibration or balance control. This permits cancellation of the effect of the small residual current present even in the absence of oxygen.
3. Calculate the pO_2 value for the slope gas (as was done for the pCO_2 example).
4. Equilibrate the electrode chamber with the slope gas. Adjust the pO_2 meter to the correct value with the pO_2 slope control. The electrode is now calibrated and ready to determine unknowns.

Figure 9-6. Schematic diagram of sample chamber. The reference electrode of the *p*H system contacts the sample by a salt bridge (not shown).

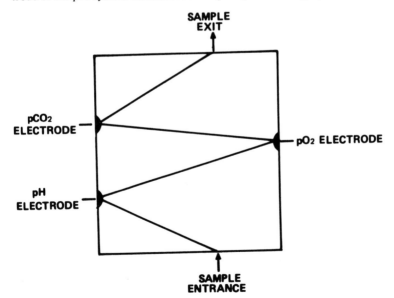

Semiautomated/Automated Instruments

Multipurpose instruments have been developed that will provide greater instrument stability, faster throughput, and additional calculated data important to the physician. A variety of them exist, varying in sophistication and cost. These instruments have part or all of the following configurational characteristics.

Sample Size.   Whole blood samples of from 70 to 500 μl are required. In most instruments, the sample chamber is located to permit visual inspection and identification of bubbles, clots, dirt, and so forth which could invalidate the results (Fig. 9-6). Some instruments have a sample error detector, an electronic sensor in the postelectrode sample line, to ensure that the electrode chamber is completely filled.

Measurement.   These instruments use standard electrode systems (*i.e.*, *p*H-sensitive glass, Clark-type polarographic pO_2, and Severinghouse pCO_2) with configurational changes to facilitate automatic calibration, sample introduction, and flush. The *p*H electrode is connected to the calomel reference electrode by a flowing open KCl liquid junction. Some instruments measure total hemoglobin, using a spectrophotometric system following lysis of the erythrocytes.

Additional Data Input.   Instrumental requirements are quite varied. The whole blood hemoglobin level can be entered electronically if it is not measured by the system. The patient's current body temperature may be required if "corrected" values are to be automatically determined. The barometric pressure is entered, if not automatically measured, so that the current values of the calibrating gases may be established.

Derived Data.   A wide variety of data helpful to the physician is often provided automatically, including standard bicarbonate, bicarbonate content, total CO_2 content, base excess, oxygen saturation, *p*H, pCO_2, and pO_2 corrected from 37°C to the patient's body temperature. The derivations are computed using programs that have been developed from equations containing constants that are empirically established. One should be familiar with the instrument's instruction manual to know the nature of the equations and constants used.

Calibration.   Calibration is performed manually or on a predetermined periodic cycle. Humidified gases or buffers equilibrated with CO_2, oxygen, and nitrogen are introduced into the chamber, usually with a peristaltic pump; *p*H calibration is performed with a pair of standard buffers. These usually have values of 7.384 for the zero calibration and 6.840 for the slope calibration. The calibration standards (and samples as well) are usually automatically preheated to 37°C prior to introduction into the electrode chamber.

Microprocessor-controlled blood gas instruments perform the calibration sequence automatically at fixed intervals. The instruments are programmed for the composition (in volume percent) of the calibration gases. Most instruments can also measure barometric pressure and will calculate the partial pressures of oxygen and CO_2 themselves. The results for patient samples are then calculated based on the responses of the electrodes and factors are derived from the calibration sequence. The instruments are capable of performing one-point and two-point calibrations. Generally, the one-point calibration is performed twice as frequently as the two-point. Instrument stability is required before patient samples are introduced. Most microprocessor-controlled instruments have diagnostics packages that monitor for faults such as electrode drift, out-of-range sensitivity, and unstable readings.

Flushing. The electrodes are automatically flushed following each use as well as periodically when not in use, using humidified "low" calibrating gas, buffer, or wash solutions such as polyethylene glycoloctylphenyl ether. This process automatically cleans the sample lines and keeps the electrodes humidified and equilibrated to some degree as well. Most instruments flush the sample out in the reverse direction from which it was introduced. This prevents the pump tubing from being contaminated with sample.

Maintenance. Daily maintenance involves injecting a cleaning solution through the system and checking the levels of the solution reservoirs and gas tanks. Weekly maintenance involves injecting a dilute bleach solution to remove protein build-up. Electrode membranes and electrolytes must be replaced approximately monthly.

QUALITY CONTROL

Standard systems for quality control in the clinical chemistry laboratory are generally applicable to pH and blood gas analysis. The periodicity of assay of the "control materials" should be varied to meet the individual instrumental needs, depending upon the instrument's stability, volume of use, time of day, number of persons performing the tests, and so on.

Control materials should be available and used. Some can be prepared by the laboratory whereas others are commercially available. Preparation in the laboratory involves equilibrating a series of buffers or whole blood with gas of known O_2, CO_2, and/or N_2 concentration in a tonometer and then making measurements before the values change. Preparation and stability are major problems that have to be overcome.[11,12,20] In addition, the potential for hepatitis transmission must be considered when whole blood is used.

Commercially prepared quality control materials are often more desirable. These are prepared in sealed glass ampules or aerosol cans at levels specified by the manufacturer. Usually, a trilevel control is used, with parameters designed to simulate acidemic, normal, and alkalemic conditions. They consist of aqueous buffers[13] or perfluorocarbon synthetic oxygen carriers equilibrated with gas to produce the desired pH, pCO_2, and pO_2 values. These materials should be opened and used immediately because of the small but significant rise in pH and pO_2 that occurs rather rapidly after exposure to room air. Microprocessor-controlled instruments have quality control routines that store the data, calculate means and data limits, identify outliers, and provide Levy-Jennings charts.

TRANSCUTANEOUS BLOOD GAS MEASUREMENT

Noninvasive techniques to estimate the partial pressure of arterial blood gas are becoming more popular because they seem to offer the opportunity for continuous monitoring without expenditures of large volumes of whole blood. This technique has been applied most frequently to neonates, especially those receiving oxygen therapy. Their stability and accuracy appear satisfactory at the level of calibration and for the purposes suggested. The results should be confirmed by standard whole blood measurements before definitive therapeutic decisions are made.

Skin is resistant to the diffusion of gas out of the vascular walls. Infants' skin is much less resistant than adults'. If the skin is heated externally to 43°C, skin capillary blood temperature is raised to 41°C and transcutaneous pO_2 closely approximates the arterial pO_2. Transcutaneous pCO_2 values tend to be higher than arterial pCO_2 values.

The transcutaneous electrode system[8] is held closely to the depilated skin surface by an airtight bond. A polypropylene membrane separates the heated skin surface from the electrode assembly, which consists of a polarized platinum mono-cathode surrounded by a silver ring-type anode held at a constant temperature, usually 43°C. Oxygen in the blood can diffuse from the capillary through the skin and electrode membrane and actuate the Clark-type electrode to produce the reading.

Chloride Coulometry

Coulometric methods of analysis measure the quantity of electricity (coulombs) required to carry out a specific chemical reaction. In this case, chloride ions are titrated with silver ions generated at the silver anode. This is accomplished by applying a direct current (dc) voltage across a pair of silver electrodes. When the coulometric circuit is activated so that silver ions are generated, an automatic timer is also initiated. Chloride ions present in the sample combine with the silver ions to form insoluble silver chloride. As in any titration, an indicator of some type must be used to signal the end of titration. In the Chloridometer,* amperometry is used as the indicator system. The amperometric system consists of a second pair of silver electrodes which are placed in the solution and are charged with a small, constantly applied potential. When sufficient silver ions have been generated to react with the chloride ions present, any additional generation of silver ion will result in a sharp increase in the silver ion concentration and consequently the conductivity of the titration solution. The current across the pair of amperometric electrodes increases owing to the silver ions being reduced. A relay is activated by this increase in current, and this in turn will stop the automatic timer and the additional generation of silver ions.

The constant rate systems[3,9,23] produce silver ions at a steady rate because a constant current is applied across the generating electrodes. When this is accomplished, chloride ions are titrated at a set rate, and concentration is directly proportional to the time of reaction. By analyzing standard and unknown solutions in a like manner, the time needed to reach the titration endpoint can be equated to the chloride concentration.

In the proportional systems,[22] the electrode potential and, consequently, the silver ions generated are regulated by a proportional control circuit. When a sample

*Trademark of Haake/Buchler Instruments Inc.

containing chloride is added, a difference of potential is detected by the silver detector electrodes, and the coulometric generator is started. As the endpoint of the reaction is approached, the proportion control circuit reduces the generation rate of silver ions, lessening the chances of overtitration. In this system, the total current that flows in the anode-to-cathode circuit of the coulometric generator is integrated electronically and displayed digitally in a direct conversion to chloride concentration in the sample.

PRINCIPLES

Coulometry is one form of titration. In this, like all titration methods, the basic principle is that equivalents of titrant react with equivalents of sample to produce equivalent amounts of product. In order to derive the number of equivalents of unknown, one must know the number of equivalents of titrant produced. In coulometry one can calculate the number of equivalent weights of titrant produced by application of the formula stated in Faraday's Law. Faraday showed that 96,487 C of electricity always liberated one equivalent weight of a compound or ions at each electrode. This law is stated in the formula

$$X = Q/F \tag{1}$$

where X is the number of equivalent weights of titrant generated at the electrode, Q is the number of coulombs of electricity used to generate the titrant, and F is Faraday's constant (96,487 C/equivalent weight).

Q can also be derived by a second equation,

$$Q = iT \tag{2}$$

where i is the electrical current (in amperes) that flows through the cell and T is the time (in seconds) during which the current flowed.

By combining equations (1) and (2), it is possible to relate the equivalents of titrant to current and time.

$$X = iT/F$$

Using this formula, one can calculate the number of equivalent weights of titrant generated. If the current is kept constant while titrating standard solutions and unknowns, one can derive a relationship between the equivalents of titrants in each case.

$$X_{unknown} = \frac{iT_{unknown}}{F}$$

$$X_{standard} = \frac{iT_{standard}}{F}$$

Because i and F are constants,

$$\frac{X_{unknown}}{T_{unknown}} = \frac{X_{standard}}{T_{standard}} \text{ or } X_{unknown} = \frac{T_{unknown}}{T_{standard}} \times X_{standard}$$

In practice, the timer is graduated in units of mEq Cl^-/l and the generator current is adjusted so the rate of silver ion production matches the register rate in concentration units of the timer. The value of a blank titration is automatically subtracted from the final result.

By using the basic principle of titrimetry, one can calculate the number of equivalents of the compound titrated in the unknown solution. In the Chloridometer, the coulometric circuit consists of a pair of silver electrodes immersed in a solution. The titration solution provides the medium for conduction between the anode and cathode of the generating electrodes. It consists of nitric acid, acetic acid, gelatin, and the sample to be titrated. The reaction at the anode is

$$Ag^0 \rightarrow Ag^+ + e^-$$

If the solution contains chloride ions, these will react immediately with the silver ions formed to produce insoluble silver chloride. This is shown in the following reaction:

$$Ag^+ + Cl^- \rightarrow AgCl \downarrow$$

The nitric acid present in the titration solution provides good electrolytic conductivity by providing protons for the cathode of the coulometric electrodes. The cathodic reaction is

$$2H^+ + 2e^- \rightarrow H_2$$

Generator Circuit

The coulometric circuit consists of a stable dc-voltage supply, an electrode pair to supply reagent ions, and a means of determining the amount of current flow (coulombs) through the electrode pair. The voltage supply may be a simple battery-powered unit capable of producing a constant set current, or a more sophisticated electronic supply that can furnish either a constant or a proportional current to the generator electrodes.

In the constant current system, the current is preset to give titration times of a specific range when the concentrations are within certain limits. When these criteria are met, only an accurate timing system is needed to complete the circuit.

In the proportional system, a more sophisticated means of current integration is used. This system employs direct electronic current integration that is related to the silver ions generated and is not dependent on the time rate principle of calculating ions generated.

Indicator Circuit

As in all titrations, some means must be provided for detecting the point in the titration at which the desired reaction is completed. This point in the titration is designated as the *equivalence point*. In practice, the equivalence point of the titration is detected by the appearance of excess titrant. In the Chloridometer, this is done amperometrically by placing a second pair of silver electrodes in the solution and applying a low potential across them. When the endpoint of the titration is reached, the current across the amperometric electrodes increases owing to the excess free silver ion being reduced. This increase in current activates a relay that stops an automatic timer and also the generation of additional silver ions.

In the Radiometer CMT 10 Chloride Titrator, a potentiometric detection method is used. This consists of a chloride-sensitive indicator electrode and a mercury/mercurous sulfate reference electrode. A calomel reference electrode cannot be used because the chloride in the calomel would interfere with the titration. Upon introduction of the sample into the titration vessel, the potential of the indicator circuit rises in response to the added chloride and the titration is automatically started. When the chloride is consumed by the titration reaction, the potential falls and the timer is stopped. This design has the advantages of starting automatically and not requiring as extensive maintenance as the amperometric method (see below).

INSTRUMENTAL PERFORMANCE

Titration Solution

The titration solution for the Buchler Chloridometer contains nitric acid, acetic acid, and gelatin. The acid solution helps to prevent the reduction of the precipitated silver chloride at the amperometric cathode. The nitric acid provides protons, which are reduced in the other half-reaction that occurs in the generator cathode.

Acetic acid reduces the polarity of the solution, making the silver chloride less soluble and thereby providing a sharper endpoint.

The gelatin is added to improve the reproducibility of the indicator circuit. Without the gelatin, silver reduction tends to take place preferentially at the high spots on the surface of the silver cathode. The gelatin inhibits this by adsorbing to the high spots and equalizing the reduction reaction over the surface of the electrode.

The other chloride titrators generally use a solution of sulfuric acid as the supporting electrolyte.

Accuracy

The Chloridometer is one of the most accurate means of determining chlorides used in the clinical laboratory. In a comparison with isotope dilution analysis, the coulometric-amperometric titration was shown to have an absolute accuracy within $\pm 0.5\%$. For greatest accuracy, the time of titration should be adjusted so that it is between 70 and 160 seconds for the CMT titrater; the working range is 5 to 999 mEq/l. The proportional systems are somewhat more versatile than the constant current units in that they can be used over a wider range of sample concentrations, and the endpoints are more precise. The working range of this system is 10 to 300 mEq/l with a readability of 1.0 mEq/l.

Precision

The precision of the constant rate system has been reported to be within $\pm 0.3\%$[3]; however, the between-run precision is about 2.6%[7] when using the high titration rate under normal operating conditions. The day to day precision of the proportional system is 2.0%[22] when operating at the 100 mEq/l level. As in most semiautomated procedures, the degree of precision is dependent upon the manual steps of analysis. This precision is also contingent upon good daily preventive maintenance. The generating electrodes in the constant rate systems must be kept clean, or the rate of silver ion production will not be constant. If the amperometric electrodes are not clean, the endpoints on all systems may not be sharp and therefore will cause overtitration.

Maintenance

The electrodes should be polished before each day's titrations. They should not be allowed to dry out because oxide forms on the surface. The generator anode should be periodically checked. As the Chloridometer is used, the terminal portion of this electrode will become thin. This thin portion should be cut off and the electrode length readjusted so that it extends down to the level of the other electrodes. The silver ion generating plate of the proportional units must be cleaned and inspected periodically, and it is recommended that this plate be replaced every 1000 determinations.

Daily maintenance:

1. Check reagents.
2. Check heater.
3. Check stirrer.
4. Check pumps and reaction cup for leaks.
5. Check indicator lamps.

Weekly maintenance:

1. Remove and clean reaction cup, magnetic stirrer, and all electrodes.

Monthly maintenance:

1. Remove and clean reaction cup, magnetic stirrer, and electrodes.
2. Replace generating electrode.
3. Remove and clean drain funnel.
4. Lubricate reagent and drain syringes.

Sources of Error

Other halogens (as well as cyanate, thiocyanate, and sulfhydryl ions) interfere. These ions combine with the silver ions generated; this leads to erroneously high results. Sulfhydryl groups can be a problem if one employs rubber stoppers or tubing. The aqueous solutions, especially if alkaline, extract sulfhydryl groups from the rubber. This interference can be avoided if glass polyethylene stoppers, Parafilm covering, and plastic tubes are used. Bacterial and mold growth in biologic fluids produces free sulfhydryl groups. Therefore, samples should be titrated promptly or stored at refrigerator temperature with a bacteriostatic agent such as Thymol crystals. Freezing the sample will also prevent this problem. Various anticoagulant problems[7] have been mentioned. A change in blood pH and loss of

CO_2 from blood sample before serum and cell separation will cause a shift of chloride from serum to cell,[7] thereby causing a lowered serum chloride. One should not work in direct sunlight because the silver chloride formed in the titration will decompose in the presence of light (chloride ion will reform). Analysis should be performed rapidly and in successive order so that electrode oxidation does not occur. This will also prevent drying of the electrode, which is a cause of uneven reaction rates.

Anodic Stripping Voltammetry

Anodic stripping voltammetry (ASV) is an electrochemical technique that offers an alternative to atomic absorption spectrophotometry for the determination of heavy metals. Anodic stripping voltammetry is related to polarography, which was the principle of the Clark pO_2 electrode, except that in ASV the applied potential is varied over time. Anodic stripping voltammetry is most often applied to the analysis of lead in biologic samples.

PRINCIPLES

The apparatus for performing an ASV experiment consists of a working electrode, a reference electrode, a sample chamber, a variable dc voltage source, a voltmeter, and a microammeter. In ASV, a large, negative (cathodic) potential is first applied to the working electrode. This causes the metal ions in solution to be reduced onto the surface of the working electrode. (The current is not recorded in this step). The purpose of this step is to concentrate and purify the metals from the solution. The metals are concentrated from a volume of several milliliters down to the volume that covers the surface of the electrode, perhaps 10^{-3} to 10^{-4} cm^3. Then the potential is increased in the positive direction (anodic) in a linear fashion (sweep). The metals are reoxidized (stripped) in order of their characteristic potentials (Fig. 9-7) and currents flow owing to the oxidation reactions of the metals that were plated onto the surface of the electrode. The heights (or areas) of the current-vs-voltage peaks are directly proportional to the amounts of the metals originally present in the solution.

The working electrode consists of mercury plated onto a wax-impregnated carbon rod. A silver–silver chloride reference electrode is used. The sample, either blood or urine, is first treated with an exchange reagent that lyses the red blood cells and releases the metals from any complexes. The exchange reagent contains chromium (III) and is an acidic, oxidative medium. Even small amounts of EDTA can be used as an anticoagulant. Only 100 μl of blood sample is required.

PERFORMANCE

The Environmental Science Associates Model 3010A Trace Metal Analyzer can determine lead, arsenic, cadmium, copper, or zinc.[14] A typical reaction requires 90 seconds per sample. Standards are run both to determine the oxidation potential and the standard curve relationship for each metal. The potentials for some metals can lie close to one another, so large amounts of copper, for example,

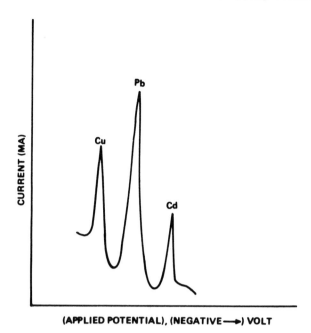

Figure 9-7. Recorder tracing for anodic stripping analysis of blood.

in a sample can interfere with the determination of lead if the peaks are not carefully identified. The starting and stopping points and the rate of the voltage sweep are selected and the current peaks are recorded on a strip chart recorder. Because the voltage sweep rate is known, the chart speed can be related to voltage.

Anodic stripping voltammetry has a linear range for whole blood lead of 5 to 700 μg/dl. Centers for Disease Control proficiency surveys for lead[2] have shown that the accuracy and precision for ASV are similar to atomic absorption, as shown in Table 9-1. Method comparison with atomic absorption gives a correlation coefficient of 0.87.[16] The mercury plating on the carbon working electrode must be periodically replaced by plating a new surface on the electrode.

Table 9-1
CDC Blood Lead Proficiency Testing Summary of Results
by Method, Shipment 1985-II

Method	CV*	% Satisfactory*
Atomic absorption		
Delves cup	7.0	96
Extraction	12.0	85
Graphite furnace	14.0	84
Anodic stripping voltammetry	10.0	87
All methods	13.0	85

*Average of three samples.

References

1. Beckman Instruments: Chloride/Carbon Dioxide Analyzer Operating Instructions. Fullerton, CA, Beckman Clinical Instrument Division, 1977
2. Centers for Disease Control: Proficiency Testing for Blood Lead (Toxicology). Shipment 1985-II. Atlanta, 1985
3. Cotlove E, Trantham HV, Bowman RL: An instrument and method for automatic, rapid, accurate, and sensitive titration of chloride in biological samples. J Lab Clin Med 51:461, 1958
4. Clark LC: Monitor and control of blood and tissue oxygen tensions. Trans Am Soc Artif Intern Organs 2:41, 1956
5. Clark LC, Lyons C: Electrode systems for continuous monitoring in cardiovascular surgery. Ann NY Acad Sci 102:29, 1962
6. Ganong WF: Review of Medical Physiology, 12th ed. Los Altos, CA, Lange Medical Publications, 1985
7. Henry RJ: Clinical Chemistry: Principles and Technics, 2nd ed. Hagerstown, Harper & Row, 1974
8. Huch R, Huch A, Rooth G: An Atlas of Oxygen-Cardiorespirograms in Newborn Infants. London, Wolfe Medical Publications, 1983
9. Instruction Manual, Corning 920 Direct-Reading Digital Chloride Meter, Corning, 1972
10. Ladenson JH, Apple FS, Koch DD: Misleading hyponatremia due to hyperlipidemia: A method-dependent error. Ann Intern Med 95:707, 1981
11. Leary ET, Delaney CJ, Kenny MA: Use of equilibrated blood for internal blood-gas quality control. Clin Chem 23:493, 1977
12. Mass AHJ et al: Evaluation of ampouled tonometered buffer solutions as a quality-control system for pH, pCO_2 and pO_2 measurement. Clin Chem 23:1718, 1977
13. Noonan DC, Komjathy ZL: Long-term reproducibility of a new pH/blood gas quality control system compared to two other procedures. Clin Chem 22:1817, 1976
14. Oakes B: Personal communication. Environmental Science Associates, December 6, 1985
15. Orion Research: Handbook of Electrode Technology. Cambridge, MA, Orion Research, 1982
16. Searle B, Chan W, Davidow B: Determination of lead in blood and urine by anodic stripping voltammetry. Clin Chem 19:76, 1973
17. Severinghaus JW: Electrodes for blood and gas pCO_2, pO_2 and blood pH. Acta Anaesthesiol Scand (Suppl) 11:207, 1962
18. Severinghaus JW, Bradley AF: Electrodes for blood pO_2 and pCO_2 determination. J Appl Physiol 13:515, 1958
19. Siggard-Andersen O: Factors affecting the liquid-junction potential in electrometric blood pH measurement. Scand J Clin Lab Invest 13:205, 1961
20. Steiner MC et al: A stable blood product for pH-blood-gas quality control. Clin Chem 24:793, 1978
21. Trenchard D, Noble MIM, Goz A: Serum carbonic acid pK: Abnormalities in patients with acid-base disturbances. Clin Sci 32:189, 1967
22. Underwood T: Chloride/Carbon Dioxide Analyzer, Operating Instructions. Beckman Instruments, 1976
23. User's Handbook, Radiometer CMT 10 Chloride Titrator. Radiometer Copenhagen, 1978
24. Wenger WC, Lott JA: Current controversy in acid-base chemistry: The inconstant constants in the Henderson-Hasselbalch equation. J Med Technology 1:109, 1984
25. Winstead M: Instrument Check Systems. Philadelphia, Lea & Febiger, 1967

Suggested Reading

Bates RG: Determination of pH: Theory and Practice. New York, John Wiley & Sons, 1973
Bauer HH, Christian GD, O'Reilly JE (eds): Instrumental Analysis. Boston, Allyn and Bacon, 1978
Bender GT: Chemical Instrumentation: A Laboratory Manual Based on Clinical Chemistry. Philadelphia, WB Saunders, 1972

Cotlove E: Determination of chloride in biological materials. Methods Biochem Anal 12:277, 1964

Cotlove E: In Meites S (ed): Standard Methods of Clinical Chemistry, Vol III. New York, Academic Press, 1961

Fischer RB: Ion-selective electrodes. J Chem Educ 51:387, 1974

Fisher JE: Measurement of pH. Am Lab 16 (June): 54, 1984

Fleischer WR, Gambino SR: Blood pH, pO_2, and oxygen saturation. Chicago, American Society of Clinical Pathology, 1972

Hicks JM: In situ monitoring. Clin Chem 31:1931, 1985

Rothstein F, Fisher JE: pH Measurement: The meter. Am Clin Products Rev 4 (August): 26, 1985

Siggard-Andersen O: The Acid-Base Status of the Blood, 4th ed. Baltimore, Williams & Wilkins, 1974

Westcott CC: pH Measurements. Orlando, FL, Academic Press, 1978

Willard HH, Merritt LL Jr, Dean JA, Settle FA Jr: Instrumental Methods of Analysis, 6th ed. Princeton, NJ, Van Nostrand, 1981

10

OSMOMETRY
Mary Ann Steinrauf

Definitions

Colligative Properties: Any property that depends only on the number of particles in solution and not on the nature of these particles. These properties are boiling point, freezing point, osmotic pressure, and vapor pressure.

Colloid: A particle (*e.g.,* protein) that, instead of dissolving, is held in a state of suspension and does not pass through a cell membrane.

Colloid Osmotic Pressure (Oncotic Pressure): The osmotic pressure due to the presence of colloids in a solution.

Dew: Moisture from the air that condenses and collects in small drops on cool surfaces.

Dew Point: The temperature of the air at which dew begins to form.

Freezing Point: The temperature at which a solution will turn from liquid to solid. More precisely, it is the temperature at which an infinitesimal amount of the solid phase will exist in equilibrium with the liquid phase.

Heat of Fusion: The heat that is released when a supercooled liquid crystallizes. The process of crystallization considerably reduces the random molecular motion of the liquid state. This loss of molecular energy is released in the form of heat. This heat of "putting together" actually warms the solution, causing the paradox of sample warming during freezing.

Milliosmole (mOsm): 1/1000 of an osmole.

Molal: A solution of one gram-molecular weight of solute dissolved in one kilogram of solvent.

Molar: A solution of one gram-molecular weight of solute per liter of solution.

Newton's Law of Cooling: The rate of cooling is proportional to the difference in temperature between the sample and its environment.

Osmolality: A measure of the concentration of free particles in solution. These particles may be ions or un-ionized molecules.

Osmole: The number of particles (6.0224×10^{23}) that will lower the freezing point of a solution 1.858°C, irrespective of whether the particles are ionic or molecular. A solution containing 1 osmole of solute per kilogram of solvent has a concentration of 1 osmolal and is equal to the gram-molecular weight divided by the number of particles or ions into which the substance dissociates in solution.

Osmotic Coefficient: A factor for correction of the observed osmolality to the ''ideal'' behavior of a solute.

Osmotic Pressure: The pressure that must be put upon a solution to keep it in equilibrium with the pure solvent when the two are separated by a semipermeable membrane.

Solution: A homogeneous single-phase mixture of solute (solid component) and solvent (liquid component).

Specific Gravity: The ratio of the mass of a solution to the mass of an equal volume of water at a specified temperature.

Supercooling: The tendency of any solvent or solution to cool below the freezing point in a liquid state. The greater the amount of supercooling, the less stable the liquid and the more likely it is to crystallize spontaneously. (It corresponds, in a sense, to supersaturation of a solute in a solvent.)

Thermistor: Electronic semiconductors of fused metal oxides whose electrical resistance varies with, and is extremely sensitive to relatively minute changes in, temperature.

Thermocouple: Two conductors of different metals joined at their ends and producing a thermoelectric current when there is a difference in temperature between the ends.

Thermodynamics: The study of heat transfer.

Transducer: A device that changes one form of energy to another (*e.g.*, pressure to electrical signal).

Vapor Pressure: Expresses the relative ease with which the molecules may escape from the surface of a pure liquid or a pure solid at a given temperature.

Wheatstone Bridge: A circuit for measuring an unknown resistance by comparing it with known resistance.

Introduction

The *osmometer* is an instrument capable of determining the osmolality of a solution by measuring an activity of that solution called a *colligative property.* There are three types of instruments in clinical use. These are the freezing point, vapor pressure, and colloid osmometers. Because of the various detection systems used, how they are applied in measuring the specific colligative property, and the kinds of interfering substances encountered, it is imperative that the clinician be informed as to the methodology employed.

The freezing point osmometer[10] is a very sensitive instrument incorporating a thermistor, a modified Wheatstone bridge, a galvanometer, and digital display in a detection and measuring system. This instrument is capable of measuring very small changes in temperature but requires the largest sample volume of the three. It can accurately measure the freezing point of a solution and can indicate the corresponding osmolality within 1% of the scale reading.

In the vapor pressure osmometer, measurement is based upon vapor pressure depression instead of freezing point depression. Using a vapor pressure osmometer, a microsample is placed into a small closed chamber. The dew point temperature depression is measured inside the closed chamber. It is an explicit function of the vapor pressure in the chamber. When the vapor pressure has reached equilibrium, the dew point temperature depression is measured by means of a sensitive thermocouple junction inside the chamber. A Wheatstone bridge and digital readout complete the measuring system. Calibration of vapor pressure at room temperature is performed using a single NaCl standard.

Colloid osmometry utilizes an electronic pressure transducer and two chambers of fluid separated by a semipermeable membrane (permeable to small molecules but impermeable to large molecules). The colloid osmotic pressure (COP) created at the membrane is measured by the transducer.

Principles

When a solute is dissolved in a solvent, the colligative properties of the solution change in a linear relationship as the molal concentration (number of particles) increases: the freezing point is lowered, the boiling point is raised, the vapor pressure is lowered, and the osmotic pressure is increased.

A 1-osmolal solution consists of 1 mole of solute dissolved in 1 kg of solvent and contains 6.02×10^{23} particles (Avogadro's number) per kilogram of water. The freezing point of this solution will be lowered by 1.86°C and the vapor pressure will be lowered by 0.3 mm Hg, as compared to pure water. In solution, a molecule of a nonelectrolyte such as glucose does not ionize and, therefore, produces one particle. In addition, sodium chloride dissociates into two particles and calcium chloride dissociates into three particles, provided that complete ionization occurs. Therefore, if one gram-molecular weight of these compounds is dissolved in one kilogram of water, the resulting solutions would be 1, 2, and 3 osmolal, respectively. Thus, it is evident that the colligative properties of a solution will change in proportion to the number of dissociated ions or particles found per molecule.

Although the concentration of these particles in solution can be determined by measuring the variation of any of the colligative properties, the most common procedure is to monitor either the freezing point or the vapor pressure reduction compared to pure solvents and to known solutions.

Freezing Point Osmometer

COOLING MODULE

An insulated tank contains the thermostatically controlled cooling bath. The bath is usually filled with a solution of ethylene glycol mixed with water. It is maintained at approximately −7°C (Fig. 10-1).

OPERATING HEAD

The operating head (Fig. 10-1) controls the vibrator coil, stirring rod, and temperature probe, which are inserted into the sample tube when it is placed on the mandrel. This operating head is mounted on a movable arm supported on a vertical rod so it can be raised or lowered. In some instruments, it is rotated to the side.

The stirring rod is a small wire next to the probe. It vibrates back and forth in order to stir the sample and to ensure that the cooling process is uniform. When

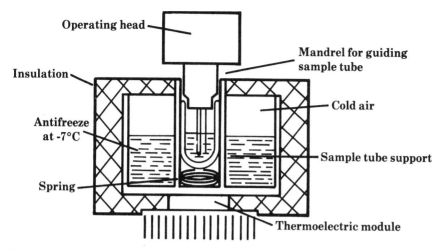

Figure 10-1. Cooling bath with sample and probes in place.

the sample is supercooled, the wire is made to vibrate violently, causing the initiation of the seeding process in which ice crystals are formed.

The thermistor (Fig. 10-2) is the temperature-sensing device of this system. It is an electronic component of metal oxides, encapsulated in glass, whose electrical resistance varies with temperature. This device makes it possible to determine the temperature of a solution by varying its resistance.[8]

MEASURING SYSTEM

A *galvanometer* (Fig. 10-3) is a system for measuring small increments of current. It is used to show the direction of current flow in the Wheatstone bridge. In the galvanometer, the current flows through a fine gold wire and a coil suspended between two magnets. Because the coil is in a magnetic field, it will tend to twist

Figure 10-2. Thermistor probe.

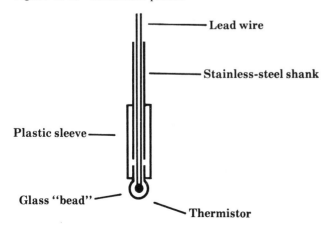

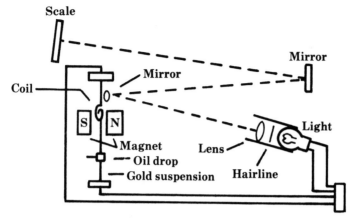

Figure 10-3.   Optical galvanometer diagram.

in proportion to the amount of current. The hairline image is focused on the galvanometer scale by reflecting it with a mirror attached to the coil. A galvanometer reading of zero indicates that no current is flowing through the balance leg of the Wheatstone bridge. When current does flow, movement of the hairline image indicates the direction of flow and its magnitude (Fig. 10-4).

In the Wheatstone bridge circuit (Fig. 10-5) a battery provides direct current in the direction of the arrows. When the resistance ratio of the Q → R divided by R → S equals one, there will be no flow of current through the galvanometer.

Figure 10-4.   Instrument freezing curve. (Osmometry and Cryoscopy School Outline. Needham Heights, MA, Advanced Instruments)

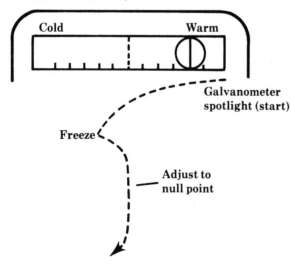

There are four points in the circuit where the resistance may be varied and, therefore, cause a flow of current through the galvanometer. These are the thermistor, two variable resistors (potentiometers labeled A and B), and another variable resistor (M) that is calibrated in definite divisions representing milliosmoles (mOsm). To calibrate the instrument so that the measuring control (M) is calibrated directly in milliosmoles, two standards of known concentration (100 and 1000 mOsm/kg) are taken through the operating procedure and frozen with the milliosmole dial (M) set at the appropriate concentration. The variable resistors at A or B are used to bring the current flow, registered by the galvanometer, back to the null point. These controls are used for vertical and slope adjustments during calibration. These potentiometers are then locked so that they cannot be moved. This procedure calibrates the instrument so that the resistance change of the thermistor can be set to coincide with the change in osmolality, thereby making it possible to read this change directly in milliosmoles. Instruments using automated measuring systems carry out these steps automatically and the values are displayed digitally.

PROCEDURE

When measuring the osmolality of a pure solvent, heat is removed and the solvent cools according to Newton's Law until its freezing temperature is reached. Then, provided crystallization occurs, the temperature stays constant until the

Figure 10-5. Osmometer schematic showing Wheatstone bridge circuit. (Osmometry and Cryoscopy School Outline. Needham Heights, MA, Advanced Instruments)

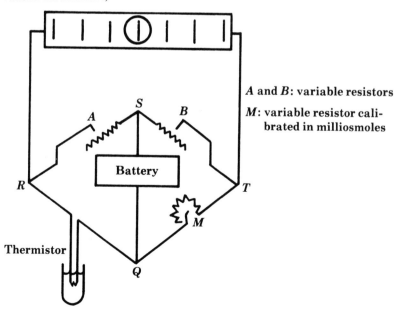

A and *B*: variable resistors

M: variable resistor calibrated in milliosmoles

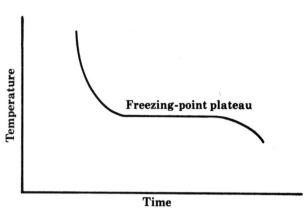

Figure 10-6. Solvent freezing curve. (Osmometry and Cryoscopy School Outline. Needham Heights, MA, Advanced Instruments)

transition from liquid to solid phase is complete. After that, the crystal mass cools to the bath temperature (Fig. 10-6).

When a solute is added to a solvent and the mixture is cooled through the freezing cycle, the time-temperature curve proceeds differently. The same initial pattern is observed until the freezing temperature is reached. However, the temperature will not "plateau" but will abruptly decrease its rate of descent (Fig. 10-7). As the solvent crystallizes out, the ratio of solute to the remaining liquid solvent increases continuously, and the freezing point is thereby gradually lowered. This lack of exactness of the freezing point results in a hyperbolic curve (Fig. 10-7). Most biologic solutions contain more than one solute, which tend to interact with one another to make measurement of the freezing point of such a solution more difficult than that of a pure solvent. For this reason, a solution is supercooled so that its temperature is maintained below the freezing point; the

Figure 10-7. Solution freezing curve. (Osmometry and Cryoscopy School Outline. Needham Heights, MA, Advanced Instruments)

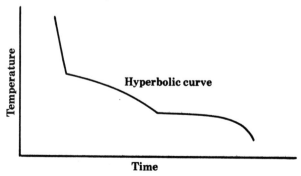

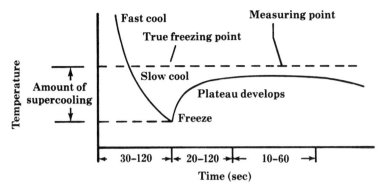

Figure 10-8. Uniform freezing curve. (Osmometry and Cryoscopy School Outline. Needham Heights, MA, Advanced Instruments)

solvent molecules aggregate in a subcrystalline form but will not crystallize spontaneously. Crystals will form only after the solution is "seeded." The seeding used is the violent agitation of the stirring rod.

With the supercooling technique, the time-temperature curve descends to a point well below the normal freezing point, at which time seeding is induced by violently agitating the probe. As the heat of fusion is released, the temperature rises to a plateau and this is a convenient time to determine the reading (Fig. 10-8).

The specimen, with thermistor probe and stirring wire inserted, is lowered into the cooling bath and the sample is supercooled. The sample must be stirred gently during the cooling step. When the galvanometer reading indicates that sufficient cooling has occurred, the stirrer is violently agitated to initiate crystallization (Fig. 10-9). The galvanometer movement changes direction as the heat of fusion is released. There follows an equilibration period of 2 to 3 minutes when

Figure 10-9. Sample immediately after freezing.

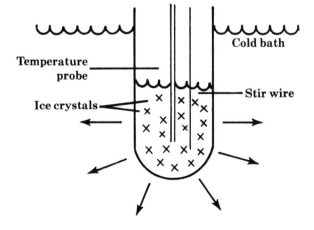

the temperature at the sample probe remains relatively constant (Fig. 10-8). This temperature is the freezing point of the solution. During this time, the Wheatstone bridge is balanced with the measuring potentiometer as indicated by the galvanometer.

The readings are usually in milliosmoles. If the instrument reads in degrees Centrigrade of freezing point depression, the milliosmoles can be calculated using the following formula:

$$\text{mOsm/kg } H_2O = \frac{\text{observed freezing point}}{1.86} \times 1000$$

The molal freezing point constant of $-1.86°C$ was determined by experimentation using 1 mole of a nonelectrolyte dissolved in 1 kg of water. Calibration of the osmometer must be done daily with the desired standards (100–1000 mOsm/kg) to ensure accurate results.[4]

Vapor Pressure Osmometer

The vapor pressure osmometer operates upon the principle that, as solute is added to solvent, the vapor pressure is reduced. This instrument actually measures the dewpoint temperature of a solution, which is a linear function of the vapor pressure.[4] The dewpoint measurement is made by a thermocouple set up to exhibit the Peltier effect. Using this system, current is passed through the thermocouple loop to cool one section of the detector below the dewpoint. Moisture will condense from the chamber onto the loop until the dewpoint is reached. At this time, the rate of condensation and evaporation within the chamber is at an equilibrium (dewpoint) and the temperature is measured.

The operation of the instrument is usually automatic once the sample is introduced into the chamber. Because of the small sample size, careful measurement and consistent sampling are required (the routine 8 μl sample may be increased to 10 μl for pipetting convenience, but sample size must be the same for standardization and sample measurement). The specimen as standard is placed on a filter paper disk and inserted into the sample chamber by means of a sample slide. The sample and chamber are allowed to equilibrate, and the temperature is measured. This is the reference temperature. The thermocouple sensor is cooled below dewpoint temperature to produce condensation. At the equilibrium point (plateau), the temperature is again measured. This is the dewpoint temperature. The difference between the measured dewpoint temperature and the reference temperature is directly proportional to the vapor pressure and, therefore, to osmolality. The standardization of this system is best performed by running samples of pure solutions so the sensitivity (slope) can be set and calibration can be made directly in milliosmol units.

Barlow[1-3] claims four main advantages of vapor pressure osmometry over other methods: microsampling capability, low maintenance, high reliability, and lower cost. Varied physiological specimens of differing viscosities, particle content, and even tissue may be analyzed by this system.

Colloid Osmometer

Colloid osmometry[9] employs a two-chamber pressure system with the chambers separated by a semipermeable membrane. The membrane selected must be freely permeable to small molecules but impermeable to large molecules. The lower chamber is filled with isotonic saline solution and is connected to the pressure transducer. The upper chamber is filled with the specimen to be measured. If isotonic saline is placed in the upper sample chamber, a zero reference value is obtained. The colloid osmotic force created at the membrane causes fluid to move from the lower chamber to the sample chamber, creating a negative pressure in the transducer chamber. This pressure equals the colloid osmotic pressure of the unknown solution. The output from the transducer is amplified and converted to give the concentration in mm Hg on a digital display. The instrument is calibrated using a known concentration of albumin in the unknown chamber. The major use for the measurement of the colloid osmotic pressure is to monitor water/plasma-protein balance in detecting and treating conditions leading to pulmonary edema.[4,7]

Calculated Osmolality

Serum osmolality is determined by a relative small fraction of the serum constituents. Many equations for the estimation of serum or plasma osmolality are reported in the literature. One equation[11] uses the concentrations for serum sodium, glucose, and urea nitrogen to approximate the osmolality:

$$\text{mOsm/kg } H_2O = 1.86 \, (Na^+) + \frac{\text{glucose}}{18} + \frac{BUN}{2.8}$$

where

$$1.86 = \text{osmotic coefficient of sodium chloride}$$
$$Na = \text{mmol/liter}$$
$$\text{Glucose} = \text{mg/dl of measured glucose}$$
$$18 = \text{molecular weight of glucose and conversion from mg/dl to}$$
mmol/liter
$$BUN = \text{mg/dl of measured BUN}$$
$$2.8 = \text{molecular weight of BUN and conversion from mg/dl to}$$
mmol/liter

This estimation is useful when there is no osmometer available or when one wishes to check for the presence of volatile substances such as ethanol in the serum.[7]

Specimen

Blood should be collected with a minimum of stasis. Evacuated tubes containing a gel for serum separation are acceptable. The serum should be separated by centrifugation as rapidly as possible and stored in a sealed container.[5] If carbon dioxide is lost, low values may result. If the test cannot be performed immediately, the specimen should be frozen. Serum and urine samples are stable for several days when stored in sealed vials at 5°C or for several months when stored at or below −20°C. Before analysis, specimens must be warmed to room temperature. Hemolysis should be avoided; however, lysed red blood cells (RBCs) have nearly the same osmolality as serum. Therefore, the error introduced by slight hemolysis is not great. The serum should be free of particulate matter that could act as a seeding agent (*e.g.*, chylomicrons or fibrin threads). Volatiles such as ethanol present in serum will not be detected by the vapor pressure instrument but will be measured by the freezing point instruments.

Urine specimens should be centrifuged until clear. The determination should be performed promptly. If the sample has been refrigerated and contains precipitate, warm the sample before centrifugation. It is best to freeze specimens unless the osmolality can be determined immediately after collection.

Normal serum osmolality is between 285 and 310 mOsm/kg. Urine osmolality depends upon the state of hydration of the patient; values can vary between 50 and 1400 mOsm/kg H_2O.[6]

Standards

The following formulas show the relationship of the various standards to their respective osmotic pressure and osmolality:

$$O = \text{osmole/kg } H_2O$$
$$O = \phi \, nc$$

where

ϕ = osmotic coefficient
n = number of particles into which the molecule dissociates
c = concentration in moles/kg H_2O

The dissociation of a molecule in solution can be characterized by n = 1 for nonelectrolytes, and n = 2 and n = 3 for salts that ionize into two and three ions respectively. The osmotic coefficient, ϕ, may be determined by dividing the actual freezing point depression by the theoretical freezing point depression.

$$\phi = \frac{\Delta a}{\Delta t}$$

where

Δa = actual freezing point depression
Δt = theoretical freezing point depression

The osmolality of serum or urine is determined by comparing the freezing point of the unknown specimen with that of a sodium chloride standard of known osmolality. Molal solutions must be used when measuring changes in the physical properties of a solution. Changes in temperature will alter the weight/volume relations of molar solutions but will not alter the weight/weight relationship of a molal solution. Therefore, standards must be prepared as *molal* rather than *molar* solutions. Because of the nature of molal solutions (weight/weight), working standards cannot be made by diluting a stock solution; each standard must be prepared individually.

Standards should be stored in stoppered borosilicate glass or polyethylene bottles. These standards should be checked frequently for contamination because shelf life is limited after containers have been opened. It is a general rule that no standard bottle should be entered by a pipette; therefore, standards should be poured into clean tubes for the day's use. Sampling of standards in this fashion will prevent errors caused by dissolved gases in these solutions.

Sources of Error

1. The bath
   a. Temperature—It must be controlled ($-5°$ to $-9°C$).
   b. Composition—Concentrated antifreeze leads to erratic cooling. The cooling bath must be filled with a 1 to 2 dilution of antifreeze and water.
   c. Level—It must be within the tolerances set by manufacturer.
   d. Age—As the fluid in the bath ages, viscosity increases, heat conductivity decreases, cooling is slowed down, and the reproducibility of the results decreases.
2. A defective thermistor probe will cause erratic results.
3. Insufficient stirring will cause the sample to cool slowly and erratically. Results will not be reproducible. Too much stirring may cause premature freezing of the sample.
4. Plastic tubes cannot be used because of their low thermal conductivity.
5. The probe must be positioned in the center of the sample.
6. The probe should be wiped between samples to minimize carry-over.
7. The unknown sample and the standards must receive identical treatment in performance of the test.
8. Samples should be at room temperature when analyzed.
9. The general problems in changes of temperature, humidity, and vapor pressure must be considered in vapor pressure osmometry. This may require recalibration immediately prior to analysis.

References

1. Barlow WK: Vapor pressure osmometery. Med Electron Data 6:64, 1975
2. Barlow WK: Volatiles and osmometry. Clin Chem 22:1230, 1976
3. Barlow WK, Schneider PG: Colloid osmometry. Logan, UT, Wescor, 1978
4. Ferris CD: Guide to Medical Laboratory Instruments. Boston, Little, Brown & Co, 1980
5. Foreback CC, King RC: Osmolality: Selected methods. Clin Chem 9:282–292, 1982
6. Henry JB: Clinical Diagnosis and Management, 17th ed. Philadelphia, WB Saunders, 1984
7. Kaplan LA, Pesce AJ: Clinical Chemistry Theory, Analysis, and Correlation. St Louis, CV Mosby, 1984
8. Lee LW, Schmidt LM: Elementary Principles of Laboratory Instruments, 5th ed. St Louis, CV Mosby, 1983

9. Morissette MP: Colloid osmotic pressure: Its measure and clinical value. Can Med Assoc J 116:897, 1977
10. Osmometry and Cryoscopy School Outline. Needham Heights, MA, Advanced Instruments, 1967
11. Weisberg HF: Osmolality: Calculated, "delta," and more formulas. Clin Chem 21:1182, 1975

Suggested Reading

Cockayne MS, Anderson SC: Minute mystery. Journal of Medical Technology 1:7, July 1984

Draviam EJ, Custer EM, Schoen I: Vapor pressure and freezing point osmolality measurements applied to a volatile screen. Am J Clin Pathol 82:706–709, 1984

Fligner CL, Jack R, Twiggs GA, Raisys VA: Hyperosmolality induced by propylene glycol: A complication of silver sulfadiazine therapy. JAMA 253:1606, 1985

Henry RJ, Cannon DC, Winkelmann JW: Clinical Chemistry: Principles, and Techniques, 2nd ed. Hagerstown, Harper & Row, 1974

Loeb JN: The hyperosmolar state. N Engl J Med 290:1184–1187, 1974

Osmometry and Cryoscopy School Outline. Needham Heights, MA, Advanced Instruments, 1967

Tietz NW: Fundamentals of Clinical Chemistry, 2nd ed. Philadelphia, WB Saunders, 1976

Weisberg HF: Osmolality. ASCP Commission on Continuing Education Critique cc-71, 1971

11

REFRACTOMETRY

Richard D. Juel
Mary Ann Steinrauf

Definitions

Critical Angle: When light passes from a medium, such as air, into a more dense medium, like glass or water, the angle of refraction is always less than the angle of incidence. As a result of this decrease in angle, there exists a range of angles for which no refracted light is possible. Consider the diagram for which several angles of incidence and their corresponding angles of refraction are shown (Fig. 11-1). In this diagram, angle 4 is the critical angle.

One should note that in the limiting case where the incident rays approach the angle of 90° (*i.e.,* where they graze along the surfaces), the refracted rays approach a certain angle *c*, beyond which no refracted light is possible. This limiting angle is called the critical angle. In any medium, the value for the critical angle depends upon the index of refraction. One can calculate the critical angle of refraction by using Snell's Law.

$$\frac{\sin i}{\sin r} = n$$

In determining the critical angle, angle *i* equals 90° (sine of 90° angle = 1), and angle *r* equals angle *c*. Therefore, solving for the critical angle:

$$\frac{1}{\sin c} = n$$

$$\sin c = \frac{1}{n}$$

The rays formed by the refraction of the grazing rays are termed *critical rays*.

Dispersion: The angular spread of all the various wavelengths (colors) produced by sending white light through a prism is called the dispersion. The band of colors so produced is called a spectrum. A prismatic spectrum is characteristically nonlinear.

Index of Refraction: If a medium *A* is a vacuum (or, for practical purposes, air), the

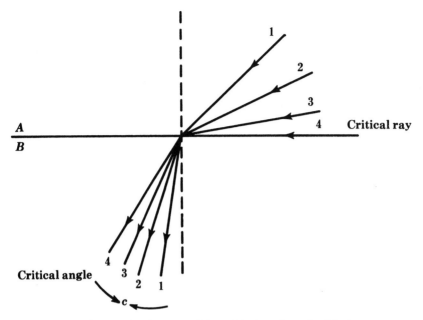

Figure 11-1.   Schematic diagram of the critical angle and critical ray.

value of the constant in the above equation is called the index of refraction, *n*, of medium *B*. By experimental measurements of the angles *i* and *r*, one can determine the values of *n* for various transparent substances.

Law of Reflection: The angle at which a ray of light strikes the reflecting surface is equal to the angle the reflected ray makes with the same surface. These angles are customarily measured from a line perpendicular to the plane of the reflective surface. This line is called the normal.

Law of Refraction: The sine of the angle of refraction (*r*) bears a constant ratio to the sine of the angle of incidence (*i*). This constant is the same for all angles of incidence. Again, these angles are measured in relation to the normal. This law is also referred to as Snell's Law.

$$\frac{\sin i}{\sin r} = \text{constant}$$

Reflection and Refraction: When a ray of light (incident ray) strikes any boundary between two transparent substances (*A* and *B*) in which the velocity of light is appreciably different, part is reflected (reflected ray), and the rest is refracted (refracted ray). The bending is due to a change in the velocity of the light upon entering the second medium. The angle of incidence (*i*) is the same for the incident ray and the reflected ray (Fig. 11-2).

Principles

The refractive index, like the melting point and the boiling point, is a characteristic constant for each substance. It is related to the number, charge, and mass of the vibrating particles in the materials through which the radiation is

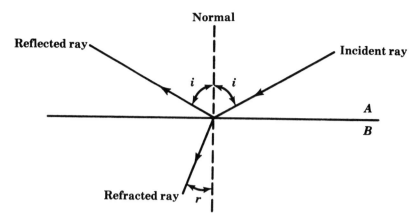

Figure 11-2. Reflection and refraction of radiation.

transmitted. It can be used in confirming the identity of substances, analyzing mixtures, and estimating properties of polymers, such as molecular weight, size, and shape.

Because a determination of the refractive index requires only the measurement of angles, the refractive index can be precisely determined by the use of an optical instrument called the *refractometer*. Most refractometers utilize a principle based on the measurement of the critical angle; these include the Abbe, Pulfrich, and immersion (dipping) types. These instruments differ mainly in the ranges covered and the type of light sources used.

In these instruments, a convergent beam of light strikes the surface between the unknown sample of refractive index n and a prism of known refractive index n'. This ray of light passes from a rarer to a denser medium (Fig. 11-3).

The beam is so oriented that some of its rays just graze the surface; thus, there is a sharp boundary between the light and dark portions. Measurement of the angle at which this boundary occurs allows one to compute the value of c, and hence the value of n. All nongrazing rays are refracted at angles smaller than the critical angle. Because the grazing rays may enter the prism (refractive index n') anywhere along the interface, an endless set of critical rays and not just one

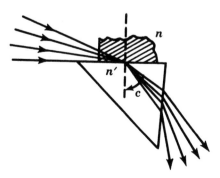

Figure 11-3. Schematic diagram of refraction in the prism of a critical angle refractometer (Jenkins FA, White HE: Fundamentals of Optics, 3rd ed. New York, McGraw-Hill, 1957)

critical ray will be formed. By the use of a condensing or focusing lens, these rays can be coalesced into a single light–dark boundary as viewed through the telescope of the instrument.

The refractometer has the following positive features: the instruments are of simple design; the measurements can be made very simply and rapidly; the analysis is nondestructive; most instruments require only small samples; and it has a wide range of application.

Components

LIGHT SOURCES

For operating convenience, refractive indexes are commonly obtained in the visible range. In this range, most substances are nonabsorbing. The latter is an advantage, because detection would be a problem if there is significant loss of light intensity. For a precise determination of refractive index, monochromatic

Figure 11-4. Amici prism. (Meloan CE, Kiser RW: Problems and Experiments in Instrumental Analysis. Columbus, Ohio, Merrill, 1963)

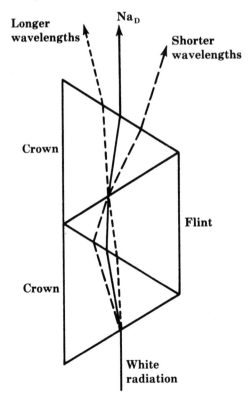

light must be used. A variety of electrical discharge lamps are able to produce either a suitable single spectral line or a closely spaced pair of lines. The most widely used is the intense sodium doublet (the "D line") at 589.0 and 589.6 nm, although a mercury or hydrogen lamp can also be used. The advantage of a sodium lamp is that a filter is seldom necessary; even though other emission lines are present, their intensity is less than 1% that of the D lines. On occasion, a determination of the dispersion of the refractive index (*i.e.*, its variation with wavelength) is helpful. For this, a mercury lamp with different filters yields four intense line spectra at 579.0 (yellow), 546.1 (green), 435.8 (blue), and 404.7 (violet) nm. A still more versatile unit is a mercury lamp to which cadmium is added so that there is also a bright red cadmium line at 643.8 nm.

White light can be used for precise refractometry. However, dispersion is the deterent to its use in critical-angle refractometry. It is imperative that there is compensation for the dispersion. Critical-angle instruments using daylight or tungsten sources utilize Amici prisms for this compensation. These prisms are small, direct-vision spectroscopes. They are constructed of different varieties of glass and are designed so that the light is dispersed without deviating the wavelengths at the D line. This combination of prisms is termed an *Amici compensator* (Fig. 11-4).

With the Amici compensator, the boundary appears sharp; however, the accuracy of the measurement of *n*, regardless of the type of refractometer, only approaches 0.0001. A disadvantage when using the Amici prisms is that the index of refraction cannot be measured at wavelengths other than the D line without making an elaborate reading correction.

TEMPERATURE CONTROL

The refractive index is dependent on temperature and wavelength as is shown by the data for water (Table 11-1). Most liquids show a change in the refractive index of approximately 0.00045 unit/°C. Solids, although less sensitive, do show changes of approximately 0.00001 unit/°C. This decrease in *n* is a direct result of

Table 11-1
Influence of Wavelength and Temperature on Refractive Index of Water

Color	Fraun-hofer Symbol or Line	Source Element	Wavelength (nm)	n_D^{20}	Temperature (°C)	n_D
Red	C	H	656.3	1.3312	10	1.3337
Yellow	D	Na	589.3	1.3330	20	1.3330
Blue	F	H	486.1	1.3371	30	1.3320
Violet	G	Hg	435.8	1.3403	40	1.3306
	G'	H	434.0	1.3404	50	1.3290

(Strobel HA: Chemical Instrumentation: A Systematic Approach to Instrumental Analysis. Reading, MA, Addison-Wesley, 1973)

the thermal expansion of the substances. For a reading to be reliable to the fourth decimal place, liquid samples must be thermoregulated to ±0.2°C. If better precision is desired, temperature control must be improved. At high levels of precision, the entire refractometer must be thermoregulated. This is usually accomplished by circulating fluid from a constant-temperature bath through a "jacket" surrounding the sample. Maintaining the uniformity of the liquid sample temperature can also be a problem unless evaporation is minimized.

Instruments

ABBE REFRACTOMETER

The Abbe refractometer (Fig. 11-5) utilizes the principle of the measurement of the critical angle. A few drops of the liquid being examined are placed between the illuminating prism P_1 and the refracting prism P_2. The prisms are partially hollowed to allow the circulation of thermostated water. Light is reflected from a mirror and passed through the prism P_1, which has a rough ground upper surface. The rough surface acts as a source of an infinite number of rays. These rays pass through the thin layer of liquid in all directions and strike the polished surface of the refracting prism P_2, where they are refracted. The critical angle (c) is formed

Figure 11-5.   Abbe refractometer. (Meloan CE, Kiser RW: Problems and Experiments in Instrumental Analysis. Columbus, Ohio, Merrill, 1963)

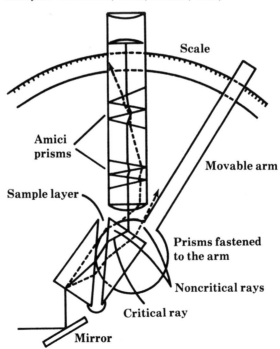

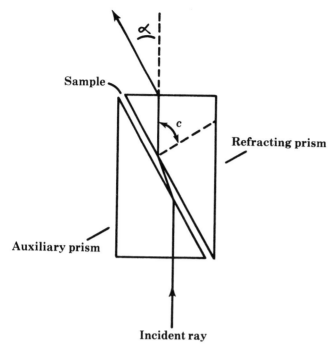

Figure 11-6. Schematic diagram of double prisms of the Abbe refractometer and the angle of emergence.

in prism P_2 and cannot be measured. What is measured is the angle of emergence (α) of the critical ray (Fig. 11-6).

The critical ray forms the border between the light and dark portions of the field when viewed with the telescope, which is attached to the scale. The sharp edge of the light-dark boundary is aligned with the cross hairs in the telescope ocular, and the reading is taken from the ruled scale. The scale is graduated in refractive indexes based on the D lines, and can be read to the nearest 0.001 unit. An attached magnifier allows the next decimal to be estimated, providing a readability of ±0.0001. The indexes may be determined over the range of 1.30 to 1.70.

White light in the form of a tungsten lamp is usually used as a light source. Two Amici prisms are placed, one above the other, in front of the objective of the telescope. These prisms prevent a colored indistinct boundary between the light and dark fields due to differences in refractive indexes for light of different wavelengths.

PULFRICH REFRACTOMETER

In this instrument, the refracting prism is always under the sample (Fig. 11-7). A horizontal beam of monochromatic light is directed along the surface of a refracting prism at the grazing angle. The sample reservoir is mounted on the horizontal surface of the prism. There is a right-angle prism that reflects the rays

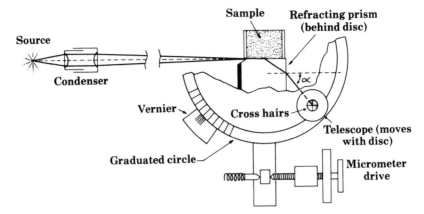

Figure 11-7. Pulfrich refractometer. (Strobel HA: Chemical Instrumentation: A Systematic Approach to Instrumental Analysis. Reading, MA, Addison-Wesley, 1973)

emerging from the refracting prism and allows the identification of the angle of emergence (α). A telescope is mounted at the side on a rotatable scale, which is ruled in degrees. The scale is also fitted with a vernier, which allows estimation to the nearest minute (1/60 of a degree). The telescope is moved until the light–dark boundary is focused on the cross hairs of the eyepiece, and the scale reading is then taken. Tables are furnished that allow one to obtain the value for n for different wavelengths of illumination. The accuracy and precision of this instrument is approximately 0.0001 unit for direct measurements. The usual range of measurement is from 1.33 to 1.60. However, this may be extended to 1.84 by inserting other refracting prisms furnished as interchangeable parts. The accuracy of the instrument can be increased to 0.00005 by the use of a micrometer drive to position the telescope cross hairs.

IMMERSION (DIPPING) REFRACTOMETER

This type of refractometer (Fig. 11-8) is the simplest to use but requires a large sample of approximately 10 to 15 ml. It is similar to the Abbe refractometer but differs in that it has no auxiliary prism. The refracting prism is mounted rigidly in the telescope, which contains the compensating prisms and the eyepiece. An accurately ruled scale is mounted below the eyepiece inside the tube. White or artificial light is used as a light source. The refracting prism is immersed in a small beaker containing the sample. A mirror is mounted below to reflect light up through the liquid. Again, the critical ray projects as a light–dark boundary on the scale. The exact position of this line is determined by moving the scale with a micrometer screw until the nearest division falls on the boundary. Both the scale and micrometer are read and, using a table as a reference, the readings are converted to refractive indexes. The micrometer drum shows the decimal to be added. A change of 0.01 division corresponds to 0.000037 in refractive index at the sodium doublet line (n_D). Thus, this instrument can give greater precision in its readings than either the Abbe or the Pulfrich refractometer.

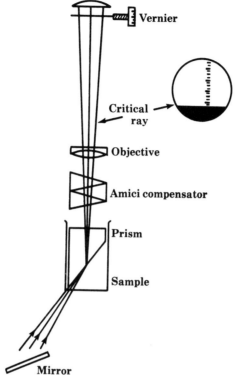

Micrometer eyepiece

Vernier

Critical ray

Objective

Amici compensator

Prism

Sample

Mirror

Figure 11-8. Immersion refractometer. (Courtesy of Bausch and Lomb Optical Co., Rochester, NY)

Total Solids (TS) Meter

The TS meter is the refractometer most commonly used in the clinical laboratory. Like the other refractometers discussed, it employs the principle of critical-angle measurement. Although the property that is measured is the refractive index, certain models are calibrated in other quantities such as protein concentration, solids concentration, or specific gravity. Numerous studies have established the relationship between the refractive index and these other quantities.

The instrument, as ordinarily used, requires only a drop of sample. It can also be used as a dipping refractometer. When employing a small sample, a drop of fluid is drawn by capillary action into the space between the cover plate and the prism cover glass (Fig. 11-9). The instrument is then exposed to a light source, which can be either natural or artificial illumination. The light–dark boundary is brought into focus by rotating the eyepiece. The variation in the critical angle will determine the location of the light–dark boundary on the calibrating scale, indicating the refractive index of the solution under examination.

The TS meter eliminates significant temperature errors by incorporating a

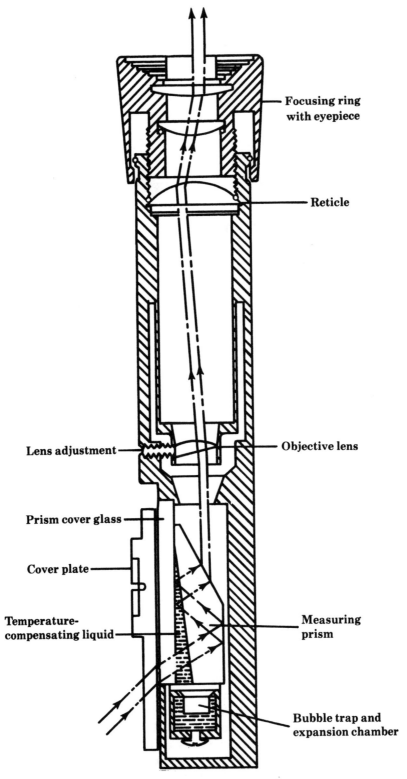

Labels in figure:
- Focusing ring with eyepiece
- Reticle
- Objective lens
- Lens adjustment
- Prism cover glass
- Cover plate
- Temperature-compensating liquid
- Measuring prism
- Bubble trap and expansion chamber

Figure 11-9. Schematic diagram of the total solids meter. (Courtesy of American Optical Co., Buffalo, NY)

temperature-compensating liquid in a sealed chamber located in the optical path. This chamber is situated in front of the measuring prism. This provides compensation for aqueous solutions at temperatures ranging from 15° to 37°C. The refractive index of this liquid varies with the temperature so that, as the temperature of the liquid varies, there is a change in the deflection of the light rays passing through it, thereby compensating for changes in the refractive index of the sample. Because an increase in the temperature of the sample or the environment results in thermal expansion of the liquid, an air bubble is placed in the liquid, which allows accommodation for this expansion. The air bubble is kept out of the optical path by a bubble trap located at the end of the chamber.

When a small sample is used, temperature equilibration between the sample and the instrument occurs almost instantaneously. However, when using the instrument as a dipping refractometer, several minutes must be allowed for this equilibration to be reached.

The zero setting of the instrument should be checked regularly; however, it should need readjustment rarely, if ever. This can be checked by taking a reading with distilled water when the temperature of the instrument is between 20° and 30°C. This adjustment should be made when the reading departs from zero by more than 0.05% (one-half division). The correction is made by means of a small screw that is a fine adjustment of the objective lens in the path of light. This in turn changes the location of the light–dark boundary on the reticle on which the scale is located. Readings at other points on the scale can be checked with various materials, depending on the quantity being measured.

The instrument has an accuracy of 0.0001 refractive index unit. It lends itself well to the clinical laboratory in that, in addition to being relatively inexpensive, it is durable, precise, accurate, and simple to operate.

Suggested Reading

American Optical Bull 10400–101, 1972

Jenkins FA, White HE: Fundamentals of Optics, 3rd ed. New York, McGraw-Hill, 1957

Meloan CE: Instrumental Analysis Using Physical Properties. Philadelphia, Lea & Febiger, 1968

Pickering WF: Modern Analytical Chemistry. New York, Dekker, 1971

Strobel HA: Chemical Instrumentation: A Systematic Approach to Instrumental Analysis. Reading, MA, Addison-Wesley, 1960

Willard HH, Merritt LL, Jr, Dean JA, Settle FA Jr: Instrumental Methods of Analysis, 6th ed. Princeton, Van Nostrand, 1981

12

ELECTROPHORESIS

Carl R. Jolliff

Definitions

Ampholyte: A preparation that contains a heterogeneous mixture of aliphatic polyaminopolycarboxylic acids of a given range of isoelectric points.

Amphoteric: A substance that possesses the capability of having a net positive, negative, or zero charge dependent upon its acidic or alkaline environment.

Boundary: The edge of a zone such as between interfaces of a discontinuous buffer and gel matrix, pH gradients, molecular size gradients, or voltage gradients.

Conductivity: The ability of a conductor to carry a current as determined by the overall contribution of each dissolved ionic species.

Convection: The movement of molecules concentrated in one area to another area, generally related to density differences.

Discontinuous Buffer System: A system in which the chamber buffer is different than the buffer within the support medium. A continuous buffer system would be the same for both chamber and medium-entrapped buffer. Improved separation may be obtained in a discontinuous system depending on the differing ionic compositions of the buffers.

Electro-osmosis (Endosmosis): The flow of one phase relative to another stationary phase with the application of an external voltage. The amount of flow will depend upon the charge contributed by the support medium and the type of buffer used. This is usually seen as a net flow of the solvent in one direction.

Electropherogram: The pattern of proteins distributed on a separation medium as the result of electrophoresis.

Electrophoresis: The movement of charged particles in an electric field.

Gel: Any solid medium composed of a network of interstices of pores that are capable of entrapment of solvent.

Ionic Strength: In a buffer system, the sum of the concentration of each ion, which is multiplied by the square of its effective charge.

Isoelectric Point, pI: The pH at which a substance exhibits a zero net charge.

154

Mobility: The migratory capacity of a substance as expressed by the distance traveled during an electrophoretic separation. This ability depends upon many variables (see text).

Molecular Sieving: Separation of molecules relative to their molecular sizes.

Resolving Power: The ability of a system to separate one molecule from others in a mixture of molecules.

SDS: Sodium dodecyl sulfate. A highly effective detergent used to denature proteins.

Tailing: Due to adsorptive properties observed in certain media, molecules of an individual species of protein may not migrate at the same rate, thereby producing a so-called "tail." This is particularly true of albumin during paper electrophoresis.

Zone: The area within a larger area distinguished by the presence of a particular feature or character such as protein bands within an electropherogram.

Principles

Electrophoresis, as performed in the clinical laboratory, involves the separation of proteins, isotypes, or degradation products of proteins. In all forms of electrophoresis, an electric field must be established within the boundaries of buffer interfaces. A potential applied results in a directional migration of the components toward either the anode or the cathode. The rate and direction in which migration occurs depends on numerous factors.

Factors Influencing Electrophoretic Migration

PARTICLE CHARGE

Proteins are generally large molecules composed of amino acids (polypeptides). Amino acids consist of polar amino (NH_3) and carboxyl (COOH) groups, each capable of carrying an ionic charge. The charge depends upon the pH of the medium in which the molecule occurs. If the medium is acidic, the amino acid becomes positively charged. If the medium is alkaline, the amino acid becomes negatively charged. Due to this property, amino acids are termed *amphoteric*. Polypeptides behave in the same manner. The isoelectric point (pI) of a polypeptide occurs at a particular pH when a balanced state exists between positive and negative charges. If the pH of the buffer supporting the molecule is below its pI, the molecule will migrate toward the cathodic electrode. A higher pH will result in anodic attraction. Most plasma proteins are electrophoresed in pH 8.6 buffer systems, thereby resulting in migration toward the anode.

NET CHARGE

Net charge will depend upon the total charges contributed by the molecules' amino and carboxyl groups, the pI of the protein, and the pH of the buffer system. As net charge increases, mobility increases.

IONIC STRENGTH

The choice of a particular ionic strength buffer will depend upon the ionic species contributed by the migrant. Ionic strength is defined by the formula

$$\mu = \tfrac{1}{2}(i \times n^2)$$

where

μ = ionic strength (current-carrying capacity of the dissolved buffer electrolyte)

i = molal concentration of a particular ion

n = valence of the ion

Factors such as solubility of the migrant and the ability of the buffer to maintain a constant *p*H at varying ionic strengths are extremely important. Lower ionic strength buffers permit faster migration rates, thereby lessening heat development. (In general, for agarose electrophoresis, barbital buffers are used with ionicity of 0.025 to 0.075.)

TEMPERATURE

The support medium offers resistance to the current flow, thereby causing a concentration of ions and increased migration, all of which result in increased temperature. Heat-dissipating devices such as water-cooled cells, submersible medium chambers, and refrigerated units have been developed to reduce temperature. The use of thin-layer agarose systems has circumvented the need for most of these systems due to the short running times involved.

POTENTIAL

Potential or power of driving the migrant in the electric field is provided by a power supply that may offer constant voltage, current (amps), or both. Migration will increase as amperage or voltage increases. If temperature and buffer concentration remain constant, resistance will remain constant. If temperature increases, resistance decreases and current increases for any given voltage setting. If temperature is a problem and cannot be controlled, constant current should be used.

TIME

Increased separation results from increased time of electrophoresis. As the distance of migration increases, so does the diffusion of the molecule into the medium, which results in patterns of poor definition.

DIFFUSION

Low molecular size of the migrant, increased thickness of the support medium, and increased time of electrophoresis will increase diffusion of the migrant. Increased temperature and concentration of the migrant will also result in greater diffusion (Fig. 12-1).

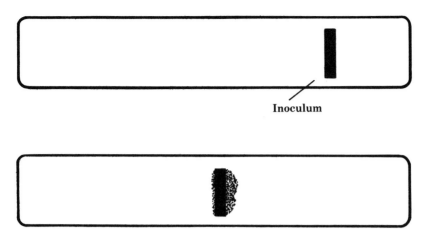

Figure 12-1.   Diffusion of initial inoculum.

MOLECULAR SIZE AND SHAPE

Larger molecular weight, irregular-shaped molecules will migrate at a slower rate. Small pore size of the support medium also inhibits the migration of such molecules (Fig. 12-2).

CONCENTRATION OF BUFFER

Ionic strength varies directly with electrolyte concentration and with the square of the valence of the electrolyte. Therefore, the electrolyte concentration appears to have less effect on ionic strength than does its valence (see formula for ionic strength, above).

Figure 12-2.   Pore size versus particle size and shape.

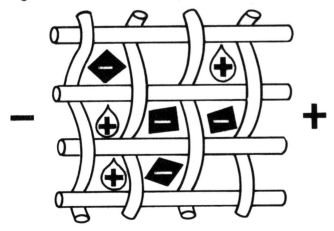

The media employed for electrophoretic separation depends upon the analyte under examination. A summary of the media available and their applications is presented in Table 12-1.

Support Media

PAPER

Paper as a support medium is seldom used today. Paper has the advantages of being self-supporting, easy to use, and capable of being heat resistant during protein fixation. Smaller molecular weight substances (*i.e.,* amino acids and peptides) are easily separated with the use of paper. The main disadvantages are the length of time required for separation, the nonuniformity, and the adsorption, which tends to produce "tailing."

GELS

Agarose

The most common support medium used today in clinical laboratories is agarose gel.[6] Unlike agar, agarose has no agaropectin, thereby allowing little or no adsorption and less endosmosis. With improved buffer systems, increased resolution for serum proteins is obtained, thereby allowing greater clinically related interpretative capabilities.

Commercially available thin-layer gels on plastic backing ready for immediate use have increased the demand for this procedure. The method provides for rapid separation time and decreased hands-on time. Thin-layer gels (99% water) can be fixed, stained, cleared, and dried with final patterns on a transparent background capable of being scanned densitometrically. Immunologic procedures combined with electrophoresis such as immunoelectrophoresis, immunofixation, and electroimmunodiffusion are best performed on this medium because the agarose can be poured at around 50°C, which will not denature most antibody molecules. Agarose also allows for maximum diffusibility of both separated antigens and antibody to occur. Low background fluorescence makes this medium preferred for isoenzyme studies utilizing fluorescence visualization and densitometric quantitation.

Disadvantages of the thin-layer agarose gels are temperature variations experienced in shipping and the necessity of storing the gels in a horizontal position. Freezing as well as extreme heat will affect gel performance. Gels tend to pool if not stored in a horizontal position.

Starch Gel

Although not widely used in routine clinical laboratories, starch gel offers excellent separation of plasma proteins and hemoglobins.[8] It has the disadvantage of being a time-consuming procedure combined with technical difficulty. Starch must be heated to boiling and degassed before pouring. The molecular sieving phenomenon due to gel porosity is an advantage in the separation of certain

Table 12-1
Migrants Separated by Electrophoresis

Migrant	Stain	Support Medium
Serum and body fluid proteins	Amido black 10-B	Agarose
	Ponceau S	Cellulose acetate, HR*
	Coomassie blue	Polyacrylamide
	Nigrosin	Isoelectric focusing
	Silver	Isotachophoresis
Amino acids	Ninhydrin	Paper
		Cellulose acetate
		Polyacrylamide
Lipoproteins	Oil red O	Agarose
		Paper
		Cellulose acetate, HR
Glycoproteins	Periodic acid-Schiff	Agarose
Hemoglobins	Amido black 10B	Starch gel
	o-Dianisidine	Agarose
	Peroxide	Cellulose acetate, HR
	Silver	Isoelectric focusing
	Ferricyanide	
Isoenzymes		
Lactate dehydrogenase	NADH (fluorescent) or tetrazolium	Agarose
Creatine kinase	NADH (fluorescent) or tetrazolium	Agarose
Alkaline phosphatase	1-napthylphosphate plus fast blue B or 5-bromo-4-chloroindolyl phosphate	Agarose Cellulose acetate Polyacrylamide
Immunoglobulins		
Oligoclonal CSF	Coomassie blue	Agarose
	Silver	Cellulose acetate, HR
	Immunofixation with specific antisera followed by stain— Amido black 10-B	
Serum and body fluid proteins by specific techniques	Amido-black 10-B	Agarose
	Coomassie blue	Cellulose acetate, HR
Immunoelectrophoresis		
Immunofixation		
Electroimmunodiffusion		
Crossed electroimmunodiffusion		
Counter immunoelectrophoresis		

*High resolution

proteins. Thicker gels may be used to isolate electrophoretically separated proteins by the process of gel elution, thereby enhancing its research uses.

Polyacrylamide Gels

Separations requiring high resolution are best performed on polyacrylamide gels. This medium is prepared by the polymerization of polyacrylamide with bifunctional N, N'-methylene bisacrylamide resulting in crosslinking of the acrylamide polymers. Such gels possess considerable strength, have low endosmosis, and are capable of being used in gradient procedures by varying the concentration of the polyacrylamide. Because separation of molecules utilizing this procedure is based upon both molecular size and charge, some 100 proteins may be visualized. The material also possesses the attributes of being clear, chemically inert, electrically neutral, and free from endosmosis.

Cellulose Acetate

Cellulose acetate as a separation medium largely replaced paper some years ago. An advantage of this medium is that it is a homogeneous, uniform, foam-like structure consisting of multiple interlocking chambers. Each chamber consists of walls of cellulose acetate polymer prepared by the action of acetic anhydride on cellulose. The chamber-like structure results in approximately 80% void space, which is capable of holding the electrolyte. Manufacturing control over the strips maintains constant pore size, chemical content, and thickness, all of which could not be said for paper. The strips may be made transparent with the use of chemical solvents and oils.

In recent years, further refinements in the cellulose acetate strips and buffer systems have resulted in methods for higher resolution of separated proteins and the capability for combining immunodiffusion procedures and electrophoresis.[10] Some of the disadvantages of the media are the necessity for clearing in organic solvents, difficulty in handling the thin films, and their storage. The gelatinized strips must also be kept in solvent until use.

Sucrose

The Tiselius technique of moving-boundary electrophoresis utilizes fluid in a U-shaped tube. One of its greatest technical problems involves convection currents, due either to heat or to differences in the concentration of migrants. Convection can be minimized if a chemically and electrically inert substance, such as sucrose, is added to the solution to produce a concentration gradient throughout the length of the tube. The sucrose is more concentrated at the dependent portion of the tube and becomes gradually less concentrated near the upper end. This concentration gradient is stable and counteracts convection. This technique is commonly used in column electrophoresis.

Types of Electrophoresis

ZONE

Zone electrophoresis involves separation on a stabilized medium. Paper, cellulose acetate, starch gel, agarose, and polyacrylamide gels are of this type.

Application of the analyte may be invasive (cutting or slotting of the media) or noninvasive (template or applicator applied).

Once the analyte is applied, the medium is placed in a chamber (Fig. 12-3) so that one end is in contact with the anode and the other is in contact with the cathode. The media itself may dip into the buffer chambers or wicks may conduct the buffer to the medium. The cell is covered to prevent drying of the medium and a potential is applied through the use of constant voltage, current, or both by a power supply. After a given time for separation, the medium is removed and the protein is fixed, stained, destained, and visualized. Proteins will be separated into bands if the sample was placed on the medium in that manner, as is usually the case for serum proteins. Hence, the term *zone electrophoresis*.

The "disk" electrophoresis procedure incorporates the use of polyacrylamide-containing tubes. The material to be electrophoresed is placed in one end of the tube. A potential is applied through the tube and separation occurs as a series of disk-like bands. This system is commercially available with prepoured tubes ready for use.

Precast polyacrylamide gels are available allowing for the availability of a technique that was, at one time, only used in research facilities. Ampholytes with varying *p*H ranges and SDS gels also are commercially available.

MOVING BOUNDARY

The moving-boundary electrophoresis technique of Tiselius utilizes a U-shaped tube having a rectangular cross section (Fig. 12-4). The volume of the tube varies

Figure 12-3.   Zone electrophoresis, agarose, thin layer, support medium.

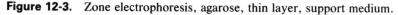
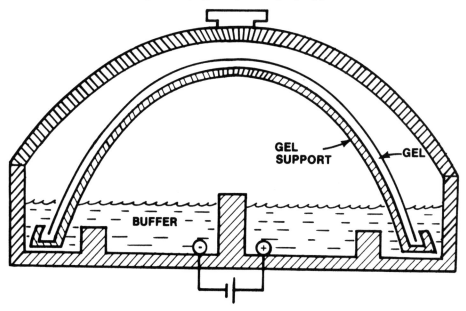

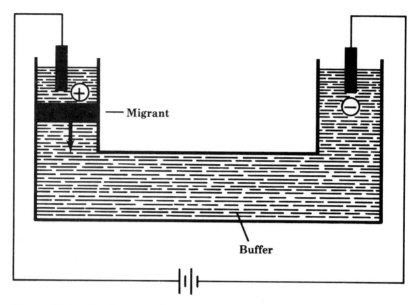

Figure 12-4. Moving boundary electrophoresis.

from 2 to 80 ml, depending on the purpose. The U-shaped tube or cell is filled with buffer and a discrete layer of liquid containing the substance to be migrated is added. The tube is placed in a constant-temperature water bath to minimize thermal convection currents. A stable electrical current is applied to the tube. Migration may take several hours, and the movement of migrant can be monitored during electrophoresis. A system of Schlieren optics is used to determine the boundaries of the migrant. In this way, the concentration of migrant at different levels of the U-shaped tube can be determined. Moving-boundary electrophoresis requires relatively large amounts of migrant, a large and cumbersome apparatus, relatively purified solutions of migrant, and a relatively long time of migration. Also, the zones of migration are indistinct because of convection currents. One of its advantages is that the movement of the migrant may be observed continuously during migration. An additional advantage is that interference of migration by the support medium is not a consideration as it is in other types of support media.

CURTAIN ELECTROPHORESIS

In curtain electrophoresis, a square of special filter paper is hung vertically (Fig. 12-5) and buffer is added to the upper margin. A single spot along the upper margin is inoculated with the migrant. Except for a moderate amount of diffusion, the migrant will form a straight line as it is carried by gravity down the strip of filter paper until it drips off at the bottom edge. If an electrical current is passed horizontally through the filter paper, the migrant will form a fan-shaped series of bands depending upon the mobility of the fractions in the migrant. These different

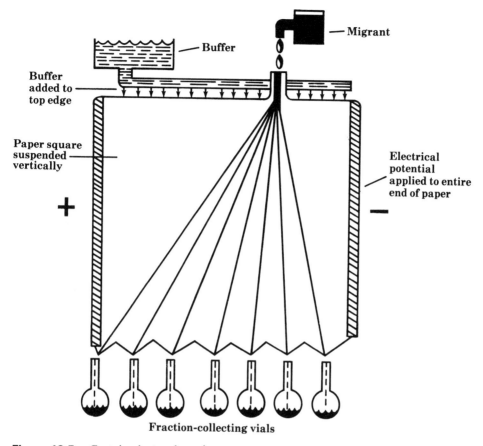

Figure 12-5.   Curtain electrophoresis.

fractions will reach the bottom of the filter paper at different points and can be collected by a test tube along the lower margin of the filter paper. The migrant can be continuously added at the top. This technique allows electrophoretic separation of large volumes of material and is especially applicable to purification of large volumes of solution.

ISOELECTRIC FOCUSING

Isoelectric focusing accomplishes the separation and focusing of proteins according to their isoelectric points with a continuous stable and linear pH gradient (Fig. 12-6).[12] The buffer substance for this technique is a carrier ampholyte, which is an aliphatic polyamino-polycarboxylic acid. These ampholytes are synthesized from acrylic acid and a number of polyethylene-polyamines in an aqueous solution. Numerous aliphatic polyamino-polycarboxylic acids exhibiting various isoelectric points over a wide range are thus available within the support medium, polyacrylamide, and will selectively orient themselves in the gel during electropho-

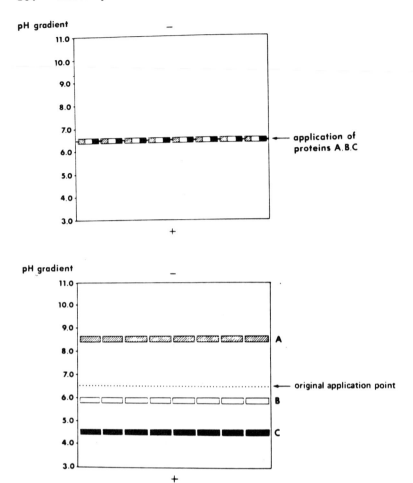

Figure 12-6.   Isoelectric focusing with flat-bed polyacrylamide gel electrophoresis. Isoelectric point of protein A = 8.5, B = 6.0, and C = 4.5. The net charge of proteins A, B, and C at their respective pH gradient focus will be zero.

resis, as will the proteins according to the pI. Polyacrylamide gels offer a support medium that can be used as a flat bed or a thin layer allowing for the separation of numerous samples on one flat bed plate.

Hemoglobins, specific protein genetic variants such as α_1-antitrypsin protease inhibitor (Pi) types, and isoenzymes have been separated by this method. The method has also been used in combination with immunodiffusion techniques to identify specific proteins utilizing antibody-charged agarose. The advantages of isoelectric focusing are as follows:

1. Diffusion of protein during electrophoresis is eliminated.
2. Separation of more components is possible due to selectivity of 0.02 pH units between separated proteins.

3. Proteins are separated solely with respect to the *p*I and are not dependent on molecular size and shape.

HIGH-RESOLUTION TWO-DIMENSIONAL GEL ELECTROPHORESIS

With this powerful new research tool,[5,9] proteins are separated according to their isoelectric points by isoelectric focusing in the first dimension. The second dimension is accomplished by electrophoresing the separated proteins into an SDS gel, which separates the proteins according to molecular weight. The completed electropherogram will result in the visualization of over some 1000 proteins. Computer systems have been designed for the analysis of these patterns and it is postulated that this procedure may pinpoint disease-related changes of serum and body fluid protein with more clarity.

Identification of Migrants

Methods used for the visualization of separated migrants depend on the support media used. Some media such as paper and forms of cellulose acetate allow for the fixation of proteins by heating, whereas others require chemical or immunologic fixation. Fixation must be performed or diffusion of the separated proteins will occur. Once fixed, the proteins may then be visualized in the following ways:

DYE ADSORPTION

A wide variety of dyes may be utilized to stain the electrophoretically separated substances. Proteins are usually stained with Amido black, Ponceau S, or Coomassie blue. In instances of low concentration, nigrosin or a silver stain may be employed. Lipoproteins are stained with lipid-soluble dyes such as Sudan black B and oil red O. Glycoproteins are best stained with periodic acid-Schiff (PAS) stain.

It is necessary for the investigator to be aware of the fact that serum proteins, after separation, do not equally adsorb stain in an amount proportional to their fraction by weight. Even though the same stain is used, dye lots may vary in their propensity to stain a particular protein. It is with these facts in mind that one must treat serum protein electrophoresis as a semiquantitative procedure.

ELUTION

The migrant bands that are identified by one of the methods above can be cut apart and eluted from the support medium. They can then be quantitated by spectrophotometric analysis of the eluent. This method is generally considered too tedious for routine use, but it is one of the most accurate methods of quantitation.

DENSITOMETER

If the support medium is transparent, the migrant bands will stand out as more or less dense zones, depending upon their concentrations and affinities for dye. Specially designed densitometers or "strip scanners" are used to measure the densities of the bands. This technique utilizes a light source of a specific wavelength and a photoelectric cell. The strip is moved in front of the light source at a constant, known rate. The optical densities of the bands are recorded on graph paper. The amount of migrant in a given band depends upon the length of the band and the optical density of the band. Quantitation can be obtained by integrating the area under the curve. Because of multiple variables previously discussed, this method is considered to be semiquantitative. Additional variables that need to be considered in quantitation of proteins by densitometry are the following:

1. There are problems related to specific staining of the protein bands by the various dyes. Therefore, the amount of light of a given wavelength that is absorbed is not directly proportional to the concentration. Thus, the technique does not follow Beer's Law.
2. The albumin fraction migrates farthest from the point of application. Some media, especially paper, will absorb a small amount of the first protein with which it comes in contact. In the case of albumin, this may amount to 5% to 10% of the total quantity when paper is used. This albumin "tailing" produces a false elevation of the globulins that subsequently come to rest on the tail and also produces a false depression in the quantity of albumin.

In spite of these theoretical problems and the semiquantitative results, medically useful and reliable information can be obtained from densitometry of proteins. Its value lies especially in the determination of percentage values attributed to each separated fraction. These percentage values help the individual responsible for interpreting the pattern to not rely on visual inspection alone. Both visual and densitometric values are required for adequate classification and interpretation of serum protein patterns.

CHEMICAL REACTIONS

Migrants can be identified in some cases on the basis of a biochemical reaction. An example is the catalytic action of lactic dehydrogenase isoenzymes on the oxidation of lactate to pyruvate, with the concomitant reduction of the coenzyme nicotinamide-adenine dinucleotide (NAD). The reduced coenzyme, NADH, then reacts with phenazine methosulfate, which reduces nitro-blue tetrazolium chloride yielding a blue formazan pigment.

ULTRAVIOLET LIGHT ABSORPTION

Some compounds do not absorb light in the visible spectrum but do absorb ultraviolet light. Techniques for spectral identification and quantitation are available utilizing this characteristic.

FLUORESCENCE

Some compounds will fluoresce when excited by exposure to light (usually ultraviolet light) and, as a result, will emit visible light. Techniques for identification and quantitation utilize these characteristics.

RADIOAUTOGRAPHY

Substances labeled with a radioisotope may be identified after electrophoresis by exposing the bands to sensitive radiographic film.

Techniques Employing Electrophoresis and Immunodiffusion

IMMUNOELECTROPHORESIS

Immunoelectrophoretic (IEP) patterns are based upon the electrophoretic separation of serum, cerebrospinal fluid, urine, or other body-fluid proteins, followed by the diffusion of those proteins into that separation medium which also supports the diffusion of antibody to those proteins (Fig. 12-7). As the protein antigen and precipitating antibody combine, a precipitation arc will form over a prescribed period of time, thereby resulting in an IEP pattern (Fig. 12-8). At the end of development of this pattern, the arcs may be photographed with the use of a camera viewing box.

The IEP pattern may also be washed in cold saline until excess antigen and antibody are removed and then stained with numerous protein stains, dried, destained, and kept for a permanent record, as well as visualized for interpretation. The advantage of agar gel and agarose over cellulose acetate is that the resulting pattern may be visualized prior to staining.

The use of polyvalent antiserum with serum, urine, cerebrospinal fluid, or other body fluids provides for the development of numerous arcs, 30 or more in number, providing the protein is present in amounts above 5 mg/dl. The use of monovalent antiserum to a specific protein will delineate that protein in relation to the other proteins as previously developed with the polyvalent antiserum. Monovalent antiserum specificity, therefore, becomes very critical in the interpretation of the IEP pattern, and each laboratory intending to utilize the procedure should perform a series of monovalent antiserum patterns in relation to the polyvalent patterns to establish arc identification. Variability between laboratories and electrophoretic procedures, separation media, protein genetic polymorphism, and antiserum lots all have a distinct bearing on the appearance of the IEP patterns. The use of patterns as developed by other laboratories should serve only as a guide to the interpretation of patterns from individual laboratories.

Figure 12-7.   First stage of immunoelectrophoresis.

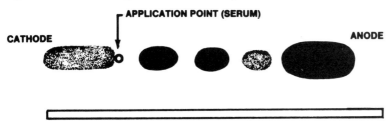

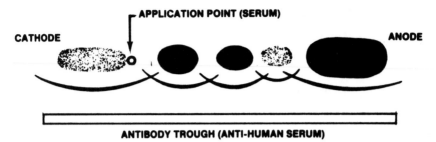

Figure 12-8.   Second stage of immunoelectrophoresis.

In the interpretation of immunoelectrophoretic patterns, the quality and quantity of the separate protein may be distinguished by six important observations (Figs. 12-9 and 12-10):

1. The distance of the arc to the antibody trough. The closer the arc to the trough, the greater the concentration of protein.
2. Size of the arc. The denser and greater the length of the arc, the greater the concentration of protein in the arc.
3. Shape of the arc. Abnormal arc configuration indicates the possible presence of monoclonality.
4. Arcs of identity. Proteins in both arcs have common antigenic determinants.
5. Arcs of partial identity. Proteins share some but not all antigenic determinants.
6. Arcs of nonidentity. The two proteins do not share common antigenic determinants.

Immunoelectrophoresis kits are available from commercial sources and are very reliable. Today, antiserums are excellent compared to earlier efforts of com-

Figure 12-9. Distinguishing features of antigen arcs in immunoelectrophoresis.

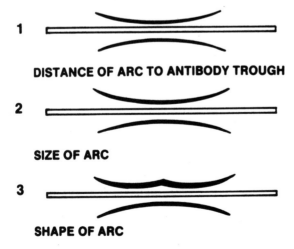

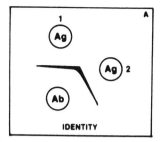 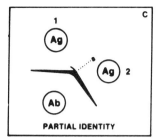 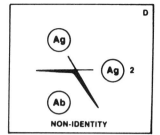

Figure 12-10. Comparison of arcs between antigens of identity, partial identity, and nonidentity.

mercial sources. One is referred to excellent monographs on the procedure and interpretation of patterns.

ELECTROIMMUNODIFFUSION

In electroimmunodiffusion (EID) (electroimmunoquantitation [EIQ], rocket electrophoresis, one-dimension single electroimmunodiffusion), serum is placed in an antigen well and is electrophoretically migrated through a field of agarose containing antiserum to a specific protein (Fig. 12-11).[7] In the classic quantitative procedure, a single "rocket" is developed as the antigen is electrophoresed into the gel. The height of the rocket from the leading edge or the center of the antigen well to the tip of the precipitated Ag/Ab rocket is directly related to the amount of antigen present in the serum sample placed in the well.

Several elements must be provided in the test system:

1. The gel must contain a low concentration of antibody that is specific for the antigen.

Figure 12-11. Rocketlike precipitin pattern of Ag/Ab complex. Note narrowing and confluence of precipitate as antigen travels toward the anodic end of gel.

**ONE DIMENSION
SINGLE ELECTROIMMUNODIFFUSION
UTILIZING MONOVALENT ANTISERUM**

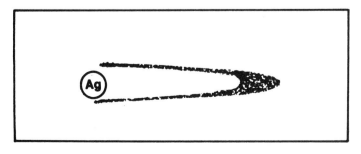

2. The gel must be adjusted so that very little migration of antibody occurs during the electrophoresis (*p*H 8.2–8.6).
3. The sample wells should be formed in the gel media where the electrophoretic field is uniform (parallel to the electrodes).

As electrophoresis begins, the antigen leaves the sample well and at once encounters antiserum antibody. Due to the fact that a high concentration of antigen is present initially as it enters the antibody-containing medium, antigen excess prevails; thereby, a soluble Ag/Ab complex exists. The Ag/Ab complex has a slower mobility than the antigen alone, resulting in the antigen passing through the medium and leaving behind a trail of the slower migrating Ag/Ab complexes lateral to the path of migration. Because the antigen concentration on these peripheries is at equivalence to the antibody in the gel, an insoluble precipitin line forms. As antigen diminishes in concentration due to the combination of fresh antibody, the rocket narrows toward a line drawn from the center of the antigen well to the anodic end of the gel. At complete depletion of the antigen, the two lateral precipitin lines converge into a loop or tip of precipitate.

By the incorporation of known antigen standards in each run, a standard curve can be constructed and an unknown specific protein antigen concentration can be determined. The slides may be stained or the precipitin lines may be intensified with the use of 2% tannic acid before measurement. All such measurements must be compared with known protein standards and such values must be plotted against concentration.

TWO-DIMENSIONAL SINGLE ELECTROIMMUNODIFFUSION

In two-dimensional EID (crossed electroimmunodiffusion), popularized by Laurell,[4] electrophoresis of serum proteins proceeds in agarose allowing for the first separation of the protein components. The agarose is then charged with a polyvalent antihuman serum and the pattern is then electrophoresed into the antibody-charged agarose at a right angle to the first separation. Like in EID, Ag/Ab peaks develop, thereby allowing for the detection of two or more isomers of a given protein as well as the elucidation of all the plasma proteins due to their differences in electrophoretic mobilities (Fig. 12-12).

Quantitation may also be accomplished by this methodology if standardized antigens for comparison are included in each run. This method of quantitation requires considerable experience in the identification and interpretation of the various separated antigen rockets. The immunoglobulins in this system as well as in EID would behave as cathodically migrating proteins and would have to be treated by carbamylation for their migration to be anodic.

ONE-DIMENSIONAL DOUBLE ELECTROIMMUNODIFFUSION

One-dimensional double electroimmunodiffusion (counterimmunoelectrophoresis, electroosmophoresis, immunorheophoresis) for the identification of either antigen or antibody relies on the ability of antibody to migrate cathodically and antigen to migrate anodically in the conventional electrophoretic system (Fig.

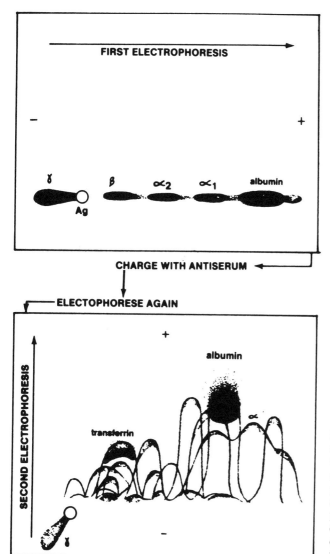

Figure 12-12. Two-dimensional single electroimmunodiffusion (Laurell). Example of crossed immunoelectrophoresis into gel containing antihuman serum. Note the position of γ-globulin peaks developed by the application of antihuman serum cathodic to serum (antigen) well.

12-13). The antigen and antiserum wells must be placed in a suitable separation medium under controlled *p*H conditions. It is also necessary that the ratio of antigen to antibody be near equivalence because equal proportions are involved in the identical wells; therefore, the two reactants meet in the same proportion as in the original wells.

The advantages of this method are as follows:

1. It is fast.
2. It is economical.
3. It is extremely sensitive.

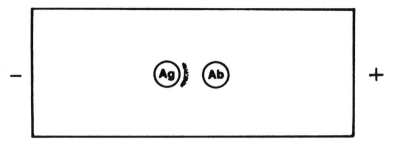

Figure 12-13.   One-dimension double electroimmunodiffusion; example of counterimmunoelectrophoresis. Note curvature of precipitin band due to configuration of round wells. Slit wells allow for straight line precipitin band.

4. It can concentrate the reaction into a small area.
5. It can utilize antigen molecules too large to diffuse through conventional media (as in strict immunodiffusion methodology).
6. It may be used when small samples for identification are available.

By the adjustment of voltage and ionic strength parameters, a lower rate of migration of the reactants can be obtained, which will enhance the size and intensity of the final precipitin reaction. Intensity of the resultant precipitin band may be enhanced by the use of tannic acid (2%) or by staining after the removal by washing of the unreacted protein.

IMMUNOFIXATION

Immunofixation utilizes the separation of serum proteins by electrophoresis in a stabilized medium followed by the fixation of those separated proteins by specific protein antiserum. Unlike immunoelectrophoresis, the separated protein is not allowed to diffuse to any great extent; therefore, the precipitation of the Ag/Ab complex allows for better resolution of the separated components and, at the same time, when compared with a stained electrophoretic pattern, it identifies the area of the protein in question.

The method, as defined by Alper and Johnson[1] and later elaborated upon by Ritchie and Smith and Cawley and associates,[3] allows for monospecific protein antiserums to detect separated serum proteins in numerous types of stabilized media (*i.e.,* starch gel, polyacrylamide, and agarose). These aforementioned systems allow for greater separation and therefore clearer definition of the specific proteins, such as complement split products, antibody classes in cerebrospinal fluid, and, in circulating immune complexes, α_1 antitrypsin Pi types and group-specific components (Gc) types.

Immunofixation is undoubtedly best used in the clinical laboratory for the identification of the monoclonal and/or multiple clonal gammopathies and can be used in conjunction with IEP for this purpose. The procedure (Fig. 12-14) consists of the application of specific antiserum to the separated protein pattern with the

IMMUNOFIXATION

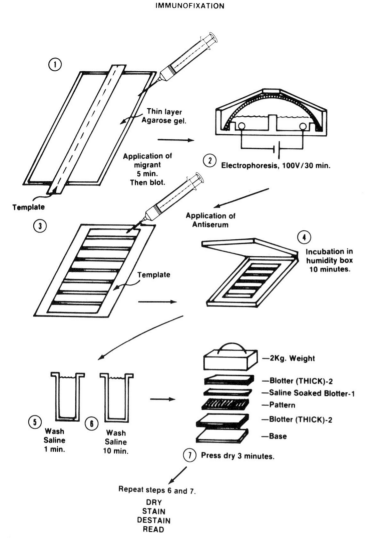

Figure 12-14. Immunofixation electrophoresis.

use of a template or with antiserum-soaked filter paper or cellulose acetate strips. The fixation of the antigen by the antibody is allowed to occur in a moist environment for approximately 30 minutes. After the development of the precipitin band, a visual inspection may be made or the pattern may be subjected to a process to remove unreacted antigen and antibody and then stained.

The method offers speed, allows for the use of small amounts of antiserum, and, depending on antiserum specificity, is quite comparable to IEP without the loss of resolution that is sometimes evident in IEP. A disadvantage is that there must be an equivalence of Ag/Ab, or, at most, a slight excess of antibody, or dissolution of the complex will occur. In this event, no banding, visible or stained, will be evident; consequently, the investigator may report an antigen as not being present. Excellent commercial kits are now available.

References

1. Alper CH, Johnson AM: Immunofixation electrophoresis: A technique for the study of protein polymorphism. Vox Sang 17:445, 1969
2. Bon WF, Swanborn PL: Electro-osmophoresis. Anal Biochem 11:16, 1965
3. Cawley LP, Minnard BJ, Tourtettotte WW et al: Immunofixation electrophorectic techniques applied to identification of proteins in serum and cerebrospinal fluid. Clin Chem 22:1262, 1976
4. Clarke HGM: Two dimensional (Laurell) immunoelectrophoresis for estimation of antigens in relative units. In Williams CA, Chase MW (eds): Methods in Immunology and Immunochemistry. New York, Academic Press, 1971
5. Clinical Chemistry: Two dimensional gel electrophoresis (Special Issue) 28(4):, 1982
6. Jeppsson JO, Laurell CB, Franzen B: Agarose gel electrophoresis. Clin Chem 25:629, 1979
7. Laurell CB: Quantitative estimation of proteins by electrophoresis in agarose gel containing antibodies. Anal Biochem 15:45, 1966
8. Marsh CL, Jolliff CR, Payne LC: A rapid micromethod for starch-gel electrophoresis. Am J Clin Pathol 41:217, 1964
9. O'Farrell PH: High resolution two-dimensional electrophoresis of proteins. J Biol Chem 250:4007, 1975
10. Pesce MA, Covolo C, Imblum RL: Electrophoresis of serum proteins on cellulose acetate. In Faulkner ER, Meites S (eds): Selected Methods for the Small Clinical Chemistry Laboratory. Washington, DC, Am Assoc Clin Chem, 1982
11. Ritchie RF, Smith R: Immunofixation: General principles and application to agarose gel electrophoresis. Clin Chem 22:497, 1976
12. Righetti PG, Drysdale JW: Isoelectric Focusing. New York, Academic Press, 1976

Suggested Reading

Brewer JM: Electrophoresis. In Kaplan LA, Pesce AJ (eds): Clinical Chemistry, pp 152–165. St Louis, CV Mosby, 1984
Cawley LP: Electrophoresis and Immunoelectrophoresis. Boston, Little, Brown & Co, 1969
Wieme RJ: Agar Gel Electrophoresis. New York, Elsevier, 1965

13

GAS LIQUID CHROMATOGRAPHY

Jim Noffsinger
Arden E. Larsen
Arthur L. Larsen

Definitions

Efficiency: The narrowness of the peaks. This is related to the number of theoretical plates per foot of column packing length.

Leading: A term applied to a peak that manifests an elongated ascending limb with a straight descending arm. This phenomenon is due to overloading of the column.

Peak Broadening: This phenomenon refers to the longitudinal expansion of the vapor plug as it travels through the column. Therefore, compounds that are retained longer are broader when they are eluted from the column.

Relative Retention Time: The ratio of the retention time of an unknown compound to the retention time of a standard.

Resolution: A measure of the completeness of the separation of two peaks. A combined term incorporating both sensitivity and efficiency.

Retention Time: That period of time in which a compound remains within a column under given conditions of temperature, gas flow, column packing, length of column, and diameter of column.

Retention Volume: The retention time multiplied by the flow rate.

Selectivity: The distance between the maxima of two peaks.

Tailing: This phenomenon refers to peaks that are asymmetric on the descending side due to adsorption of solute on the active site of the solid support. This phenomenon is reduced by deactivating the support.

Temperature Programming: When compounds of markedly varying boiling points are analyzed, the speed with which they are eluted from the column may be increased by increasing the temperature of the column stepwise, so that those compounds with the lower boiling points will come off first; then, as the temperature is increased, the higher boiling substances will be eluted faster.

Principles

Gas liquid chromatography (GLC) is an analytical technique by which compounds of similar chemical structure and boiling points can be separated from one another on the basis of both chemical and physical properties. The technique is applicable to compounds with relatively high boiling points. The mixture to be analyzed is converted to a suitable form for separation, is volatilized by flash evaporation, and is carried as a gas through a column packed with an inert supporting phase covered with an active liquid separating phase. The size, structure, polarity, relative boiling point, and other features of the compounds in the mixture will cause some to be eluted from the column more rapidly than others. As each compound in the mixture is eluted, it is detected by one of several different detecting devices. The impulse created by the detector is converted to electrical energy and amplified. This electrical energy can be recorded as a graph on a recorder (Fig. 13-1).

Sample Preparation

Only in relatively few instances can a biologic sample be injected directly into a gas chromatograph. Ordinarily, some preliminary purification must be accomplished. The sample most frequently used is urine, although blood and gas samples from a patient may also be utilized. In the clinical laboratory, the components most frequently analyzed by gas chromatography are nonprotein hormones, therapeutic drugs, fatty acids, and alcohol. The technique is also of great value in toxicologic studies. Samples derived from blood, urine, and other body fluids may be used in this process. Depending upon the desired compound to be analyzed, the purification procedure may be simple or rigorous. Analysis of urinary hormones requires multiple extractions with solvents. On the other hand, some

Figure 13-1.   Diagram of principal components in a gas liquid chromatograph.

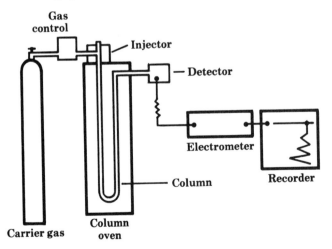

methods for the determination of blood alcohol allow direct injection of whole blood into the gas chromatograph. The sample preparation depends upon the number of compounds in the unknown, their concentration, the presence of interfering substances, and the column packing used.

After purification, this sample may require further manipulation before injection into the gas chromatograph. Some substances in a family of compounds are so similar that they cannot be well separated from one another unless they are first converted into derivatives. Examples of commonly used derivatives are silyl ethers, methyl esters, and acetate esters. By converting the compounds in a mixture to derivatives, more efficient separation of the components may be achieved. The formation of derivatives may provide additional advantages such as increasing the volatility or thermal stability of the compound. As soon as the sample has been purified and derivatives have been made, a suitable solvent must be used for sample injection. The solvents most frequently used in gas chromatography are acetone, alcohol, chloroform, hexane, and other volatile organic solvents. Aqueous solutions are very rarely used in gas chromatographic analysis.

The sample is introduced by means of a *microsyringe,* which is a finely calibrated, rather expensive piece of equipment. The size of the sample to be injected may range from less than 1 μl to as many as 5 μl for analytical gas chromatography. In some very large gas chromatographs, which are used for preliminary separation of industrial compounds, much larger samples are used. This type of chromatography is referred to as *preparative chromatography.*

Using the microsyringe requires good technique. One must be sure to avoid the inclusion of bubbles in the syringe. The barrel of the syringe should be handled as little as possible in order to avoid warming it with the fingers, thereby causing expansion of the glass and consequently an inaccurate volume.

Injection

The sample is introduced into the gas chromatograph through an injection port sealed with a rubber septum. The injection port is surrounded by a metal block which is heated by an independent heating unit to a temperature considerably higher than the column. The setting for the temperature of the injection block is determined by the boiling point of the least volatile compound in the mixture. In general, the injection port is maintained at a temperature approximately 50° to 100°C above the column temperature. However, it is important to avoid temperatures that will result in pyrolysis or isomerization of the material. The purpose of this injection block is to *flash evaporate* the solvent and the compound when they are injected. The evaporated sample is converted into a discrete "plug" of gas which is pushed through the column by an inert carrier gas (such as argon or nitrogen). The speed with which the plug of gas moves through the column is directly proportional to the carrier gas flow rate and the temperature of the column.

The time required for an individual component to emerge from the column is referred to as that compound's retention time under the specific conditions of column temperature, carrier gas flow rate, injection block temperature, column length, and column packing stated. Because these precise conditions are difficult to duplicate exactly from one laboratory to another, the term *relative retention time* has been employed. This term describes the retention time of a particular compound in comparison to the retention time of a reference compound. Each compound has its own characteristic retention time, forming the basis for gas chromatographic separation.

Types of Columns

Columns may be constructed of metal, glass, or nylon capillaries. Metal and glass columns may be straight, coiled, or U-shaped and may range in length from a few feet to as long as 300 feet. Capillary columns, on the other hand, are usually of very fine dimension and extremely long. Nylon capillary columns may be up to 1 mile in length.

Column packing consists of two essential ingredients: the *inert supporting phase* and the *stationary liquid phase*. The solid supporting phase is usually an inert material of uniform particle size. Diatomaceous earth is a frequently used solid support, although celite, firebrick, and glass beads are also used. The particle size is important in achieving the maximum efficiency from the columns. Usually, the smaller the particle, the greater the column efficiency will be. However, smaller particles inhibit the flow rate of gas owing to increased resistance of the denser medium.

The analysis of many types of samples requires that the solid support be treated to minimize decomposition or irreversible adsorption of the sample. For example, the diatomaceous earths contain hydroxyl groups, which can be treated with dimethyldichlorosilane to prevent interaction of these polar groups with polar components in the sample. Metal impurities will, in some instances, cause decomposition of the sample under heat. Acid washing is often used to remove mineral impurities from the surface of the solid support.

The liquid phase of the column packing is that chemical actually responsible for separating the various compounds in the mixture. The stationary phase should not react irreversibly with the sample and should not "bleed" excessively at the temperature required for the analysis. The sample should be soluble in the stationary phase. The liquid used will be chosen to effect separation of the compounds to be analyzed. The principal characteristics of the compounds to be considered are their polarity and their volatility. The melting point should ensure that the coating becomes liquid at the optimum temperature of analysis. Frequently, these coatings are not liquid at room temperature and appear to be a sticky solid.

Nonpolar column coatings include squalane, silicone oil, esters of high molecular weight alcohols, and dibasic acids. Polar compounds are polyethylene glycol, polyesters, ethers, carbohydrate esters, and derivatives of ethylene diamines.

The selection of the proper column packing is essential to good analytical performance. The choice of the stationary (liquid) phase is particularly critical. The choice must be made with regard to the chemical nature of the compounds to be analyzed and must take into consideration their physical properties as well. A wide variety of liquid phases are available both as pure products and coated onto solid supports. The selection of a desirable liquid phase has been simplified somewhat by the studies of W.O. McReynolds. These studies include the behavior of selected substances of widely different chemical composition, using a very large number of different liquid phases. This work has been summarized in table form and relates the polarity of each liquid phase toward each of the chemicals chosen for comparison.

For separations within a chemical class of compounds, a liquid phase of similar polarity usually provides the best choice. The separation of materials of differing chemical classes may be obtained by selecting a liquid phase capable of eluting either compound first.

Consideration also must be given to the relative amounts of liquid phase and solid support. Low concentrations of liquid phase are favored because of increased efficiency and rapidity of analysis. There is, however, the risk that, at low concentrations, active sites on the support will be exposed, resulting in adsorption of the sample. The use of 3% weight/weight liquid phase as a column packing is common.

Column packing material may be purchased already prepared. In fact, columns can be purchased that are already packed with the desired inert and liquid phases. In preparing columns, however, a few points should be observed.

1. The ratio of liquid to support phase is important. An increase in the percentage of liquid phase will decrease the efficiency of the columns.
2. The length, diameter, and material of the column are important. For instance, a long narrow column may not be suitable for use with a very fine mesh packing. Also, a metal column may react with certain packing materials or with the samples to be analyzed.
3. The coating of the inert support phase should be uniform in order to achieve maximum column efficiency.
4. Packing should not be so dense that flow rate is impeded.
5. Many liquid phases require conditioning prior to injection through the column. Conditioning refers to heating the column at a temperature slightly higher than optimal operating temperature for a period of 6 to 12 hours prior to introducing a sample into the column. This conditioning will "bleed off" any excess coating in the column.

The ability of a given column packing to separate two compounds is described by the term *resolution*. This term is described by the following equation:

$$R = 2\left(\frac{t_{R2} - t_{R1}}{W_1 + W_2}\right)$$

where t_{R1} and t_{R2} are the retention times for peaks 1 and 2 respectively, and W_1 and W_2 are the peak widths at baseline for peaks 1 and 2. Complete separation occurs when the resolution (R) is 1.5 or greater. Resolution is the combined effect of selectivity (the retention time between the two peaks) and column efficiency (the narrowness of the peaks). The efficiency of a column is affected by the following factors:

1. Turbulence due to eddy diffusion; this may occur when there are gaps in the column packing
2. Molecular diffusion within the gas phase

3. Mass transfer of the sample between the carrier gas and the liquid phase
4. Flow rate of carrier gas

Peak Analysis

The signal recognized by the detector is converted into electrical energy in the electrometer. This small signal is amplified greatly and is registered on the recorder as a peak.

Qualitative identification of an unknown substance is obtained from the relative retention time or by comparing the retention time compared to known materials analyzed under identical conditions on the same column. Because several substances may have nearly the same retention time, a second column with a widely different polarity should be used to confirm the identity of the unknown.

Quantitation is obtained by comparing the area under the peak with that of a known standard. Sampling errors are common, due to the normally small volumes injected (often less than 10 μl). To overcome these errors, an "internal standard" is often used in quantitative work. The internal standard is a substance that elutes in the near vicinity of the substance to be measured but is clearly resolved from it. A known quantity of internal standard is added both to the sample to be analyzed and to a pure standard solution of known concentration. Quantitation is achieved by comparing ratios (either peak height or area) of sample to internal standard versus standard to internal standard.

Detectors

The function of the detector is to sense and quantitate the various components that have been separated within the column and that are carried into and through the detector by the effluent carrier gas. Although there are many different types of detectors used in gas chromatography, only a few are used in biomedical applications. All of these produce a very small electrical current, which varies proportionately to the quantity of the compound in the effluent carrier gas. This small electrical current is then amplified by the electrometer to a level sufficient to drive the recorder. Because very small amounts of solute (in the range of 10^{-10} moles) are present, all of the detectors used must be extremely sensitive and stable.

THERMAL CONDUCTIVITY DETECTORS

The thermal conductivity detector is one of the first detectors used successfully in biomedical applications. It is a rugged detector, responds to all types of compounds, and has a sensitivity of approximately 10^{-8} moles of solute. However, it is quite sensitive to temperature changes as well as to changes in the flow rate of the carrier gas. In this type of detector, a thin filament of wire is placed at the end of the column and is heated by passing a current through it. When the effluent gas passes over this wire, a temperature change occurs, thereby changing the resistance in the wire. When the carrier gas contains various solutes, a greater temperature change is caused than with the carrier gas alone, thus producing a greater change in resistance in the wire and a greater change in the flow of current through the wire. In actual practice, two detectors are used (Fig. 13-2). One detector, D_2, is the reference cell through which only carrier gas passes; and the other, D_1, is the cell through which the carrier gas plus the vaporized solutes pass. These two detectors are placed in a balanced electrical circuit that is adjusted by the variable resistors, R_1 and R_2, with only carrier gas flowing through both detectors so that no flow of electricity occurs across points A and B. When solute is in the carrier gas passing through detector D_1, there is a change in resistance, and current now flows between points A and B through the electrometer E, and the amplified impulse is then recorded as a peak on the chart.

FLAME IONIZATION DETECTORS

Organic compounds yield ions when burned in a hydrogen-air flame; and if two electrodes at a potential difference of approximately 150 V are inserted into this flame, differences in conductivity of the flame can be measured as the solutes elute from the column and are burned (Fig. 13-3). This is the principle upon which the flame ionization detector is based. In the usual flame detector, the column effluent is mixed with hydrogen. This mixture is fed into the flame jet of the detector. The jet is a thin-walled stainless-steel tube which also acts as one elec- trode. The other electrode is a fine platinum wire held above the jet. The com- bustion chamber is supplied with filtered air because dust particles create distur- bances in the flame. The response of this detector is practically instantaneous. It is not affected as much as the thermal detector by changes in temperature and carrier gas flow rate. It is very sensitive and can detect approximately 10^{-10} to 10^{-15} moles of solute. For hydrocarbons, the response of the detector is roughly a function of the carbon number; however, large deviations are encountered with low molecular weight compounds. The detector is not sensitive to air, carbon dioxide, or water, but care must be taken to keep it clean.

It is obvious that the use of such a detector leads to burning of the solute. Therefore, if samples are to be collected for other types of analyses, stream splitters must be used. In this way, only part of the effluent passes through the flame, and the remainder can be collected and further analyzed.

Figure 13-2. Diagram of a thermal conduc- tivity detector.

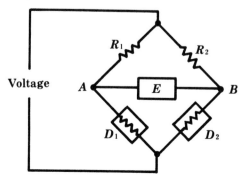

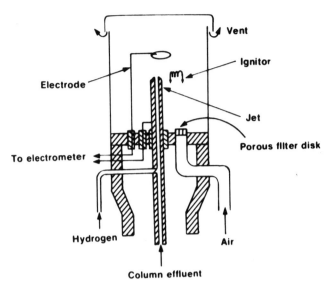

Figure 13-3. Diagram of a flame ionization detector. (After Chattoraj SC: Gas Chromatography. In Tietz NW (ed): Textbook of Clinical Chemistry. Philadelphia, WB Saunders, 1986)

ALKALI FLAME IONIZATION DETECTOR (NITROGEN PHOSPHORUS DETECTOR)

Alkali flame ionization detectors (AFID) are very similar to flame ionization detectors (FID). The former make use of an alkali source within the flame. The presence of the alkali metal produces an increase in ionization current for compounds containing selected elements. Nitrogen, phosphorus, halogens, sulfur, arsenic, tin, silicon, and lead are all known to produce this effect. Although sodium hydroxide was used in early AFID detectors, the less volatile rubidium salts are more commonly used in more recent detectors.

One mode of operation of the AFID detector is illustrated in Figure 13-4A. An air flow of approximately 100 to 120 ml/minute is supplied to the flame compared to the usual 200 to 300 ml/minute used in the FID detector. The cool flame minimizes the ionization of carbon-containing materials. The presence of a hot alkali source within the flame allows for the ionization of both nitrogen- and phosphorus-containing compounds. The alkali source may be heated externally to produce the desired temperature. Very large increases in sensitivity have been reported for both nitrogen- and phosphorus-containing compounds using this detector. The exact mechanism for increased ionization in the presence of alkali sources is not presently known. In the proposed mechanism given below, ionization is presumed to take place on the surface of the alkali source.

$$C \longrightarrow minimal\ ionization$$
$$N \longrightarrow CN\cdot \xrightarrow{Rb^*} CN^-$$
$$P \longrightarrow OP\cdot = O\ (or\ \cdot P = O) \xrightarrow{Rb^*} P = O^-$$

(Rb* represents an excited form)

An alternate mode shown in Figure 13-4*B* allows for a more specific detection of phosphorus-containing materials. In this system, a higher flow rate of air is used in order to produce a hot flame. No external heat supply is required for the alkali source. Ionization of carbon- and nitrogen-containing compounds takes place in the hot flame, but these ions are conducted to ground. Ionization of phosphorus, on the other hand, occurs on the surface of the bead.

Figure 13-4.   Alkaline flame ionization detector in the nitrogen phosphorus (NP[*A*]) mode and phosphorus (P[*B*]) mode. (After Kolb B, Bischoff J: A New Design of a Thermionic Nitrogen and Phosphorus Detector for GC. J Chromatogr Sci 12:625, 1974)

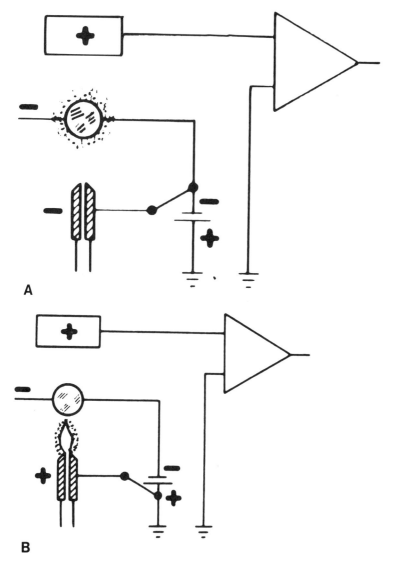

ELECTRON CAPTURE DETECTORS

In this type of detector (Fig. 13-5), the chamber has a source of ionizing radiation. The electrons that strike the solute molecules have just enough energy to penetrate the electrical field of the molecule and be captured but not enough energy to break the molecule into ions. The original electrical signal is now decreased because of the electrons being captured. Compounds containing halogen atoms and certain polar functional groups are most easily identified by electron capture, the decrease in current being virtually independent of the size and shape of the hydrocarbon moiety of the solute. If the compounds to be analyzed do not contain halogen atoms, they must be halogenated prior to chromatography. The detector is somewhat more sensitive to temperature fluctuations than the argon ionization detector, but is relatively insensitive to changes in carrier gas flow rate. This detector is extremely sensitive and, in certain types of analysis, can detect 10^{-15} to 10^{-20} moles of solute.

Despite the indisputable importance of detectors in gas liquid chromatography and their theoretical complexity, this topic has been condensed because all of the useful types of detectors are readily available commercially and detailed instructions of their theory, operation, and maintenance are obtainable from the manufacturers.

Advantages of Gas Chromatography

1. *Speed.* Once the sample is prepared for injection into the gas chromatograph, most analyses require between 5 and 60 minutes to determine 8 to 10 compounds. There are a few uncommon procedures that require up to 24 hours for final elution of the last component; but for the most part, gas chromatography is a rapid technique after the lengthy purification process is completed.

Figure 13-5. Diagram of an electron capture detector. (After Chattoraj SC: Gas chromatography. In Tietz NW (ed): Textbook of Clinical Chemistry. Philadelphia, WB Saunders, 1986)

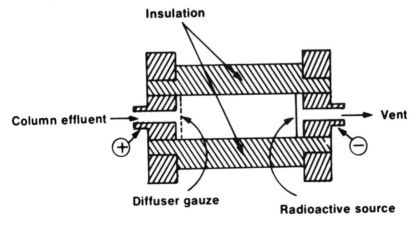

2. *Wide temperature range.* Substances may be measured in a temperature range from $-200°C$ to $+1000°C$ because freezing- and boiling-point problems are eliminated when using gases.

3. *Recovery of sample.* It is possible to insert a device called a splitter into the system so that only a portion of the sample is detected by the detector; the remaining material is vented to the outside, where it may be collected for further analyses.

4. *Sensitivity.* The gas chromatograph is an extremely sensitive analytical tool capable of determining substances in the nanogram range.

5. *Small sample sizes required.* Less than 1 μl of material may be injected into the gas chromatograph.

6. *Automation.* It is possible to obtain gas chromatographs with automatic setting devices so that the recording will be accomplished automatically and the analyst need not be in attendance at the instrument for the entire run.

Disadvantages of Gas Chromatography

1. Lengthy preparation time for samples
2. Contamination of detectors in the case of impure samples
3. Time-consuming column preparation

Suggested Reading

dal Nogare SD, Juvet RS: Gas Liquid Chromatography Theory and Practice. New York, John Wiley & Sons, 1962

Kolb B, Bischoff J: A new design of a thermionic nitrogen and phosphorus detector for Gc. J Chromatogr Sci 12:627, 1974

McReynolds WO: Characterization of some liquid phases. J Chromatogr Sci 8:685, 1970

Meloan CE: Instrumental Analysis Using Physical Properties. Philadelphia, Lea & Febiger, 1968

Supina WS: The Packed Column in Gas Chromatography. Bellefonte, PA, Supelco, 1974

Tietz NW: Textbook of Clinical Chemistry. Philadelphia, WB Saunders, 1986

Walker JQ, Jackson MT, Maynard JB: Chromatographic Systems Maintenance and Troubleshooting. New York, Academic Press, 1977

Willard HH, Merritt LL Jr, Dean JA, Settle FA Jr: Instrumental Methods of Analysis, 6th ed. Princeton, Van Nostrand, 1981

14

LIQUID CHROMATOGRAPHY

Marilyn K. Hiatt
Ernest J. Kiser

Definitions

Chromatography: A process that permits the resolution of a mixture as a consequence of differences in rates at which the individual components migrate through a stationary medium under the influence of a mobile phase.

Mobile Phase: The solvent that flows through a chromatographic column.

Stationary Phase: The separating material that remains in a fixed position in a chromatographic column.

Support: The material to which the stationary phase is attached in a chromatographic column.

Introduction

Liquid chromatography (LC) is a chromatographic technique that utilizes a liquid mobile phase to separate mixtures of compounds. Recent advances in pump technology have increased liquid chromatography's utility in the clinical laboratory. The separations that were once performed on long columns requiring hours of elution time are now feasible in minutes with the use of high-pressure pumps and small particle-size columns. This chapter discusses the basic principles, the various types, the important parameters, and the common equipment used in liquid chromatography.

Principles

The chromatography of the components of a mixture is based on simple principles. Separation of the components of a mixture may be accomplished because each component interacts with its environment differently from the other compounds under the same conditions. The solubility and miscibility of compounds are the primary factors affecting their interactions.

The polarity of individual molecules determines their solubility and miscibility. The simplest organic compounds, alkanes and alkenes, are nonpolar. A good example of a nonpolar compound is hexane.

$$
\begin{array}{ccccccc}
 & H & H & H & H & H & H \\
 & | & | & | & | & | & | \\
H- & C & -C & -C & -C & -C & -C-H \\
 & | & | & | & | & | & | \\
 & H & H & H & H & H & H
\end{array}
$$

Factors affecting polarity are the presence or absence of electron donating or withdrawing groups, conjugation, and molecular symmetry. Examples of electron withdrawing groups and molecular symmetry affecting polarity are hexanol (*left*, below) and hexanoic acid (*right*, below), the latter being the more polar.

$$
\begin{array}{ccccccc}
 & H & H & H & H & H & H \\
 & | & | & | & | & | & | \\
H- & C & -C & -C & -C & -C & -C-OH \\
 & | & | & | & | & | & | \\
 & H & H & H & H & H & H
\end{array}
\qquad
\begin{array}{ccccccc}
 & H & H & H & H & H & O \\
 & | & | & | & | & | & \parallel \\
H- & C & -C & -C & -C & -C & -C-OH \\
 & | & | & | & | & | & \\
 & H & H & H & H & H &
\end{array}
$$

Most biologic molecules vary from slightly polar to polar. Water is a very polar molecule because of its molecular structure, which results in a permanent dipole.

The polarity of molecules is predictive of their general solubility: the rule "like dissolves like" may be applied in liquid chromatography for selection of appropriate mobile and stationary phases.

The components of a liquid chromatography column may be itemized as follows:

1. Stationary phase—may be a solid or a liquid
2. Mobile phase—is a liquid
3. Support—is most often a solid

Separation of solutes may be achieved if the stationary and mobile phases are selected so that separation of the solutes occurs due to either differences in solubility of the solutes between the stationary and mobile phases or differences in adsorption on the stationary phase.

As a discrete band of sample-containing solution is forced through the column, the portion of solution high in concentration of a specific component is equilibrated with the stationary phase and the mobile phase; the next increment of mobile phase containing less of this component will extract a portion of the adsorbed component into the mobile phase. If every specific component enters into this "back and forth" exchange to different degrees and at different speeds from all other components, separation is achieved.

Types of Liquid Chromatography

There are four basic types of liquid chromatography: liquid-solid (adsorption), liquid-liquid (partition), ion-exchange, and gel permeation (molecular sieving).

ADSORPTION

Adsorption chromatography is performed with a liquid mobile phase and a solid stationary phase, which reversibly adsorbs solutes. Common examples of stationary phases are silica gel, porous glass beads, and alumina. The mobile phase is usually a relatively nonpolar solvent mixture. This technique is applicable when sample components vary widely in polarity (*e.g.*, lipids).

PARTITION

Partition chromatography is performed with a liquid-coated stationary phase, which is immiscible with the mobile phase. The relative distribution of the sample components between the mobile phase and the stationary phase determines the relative separation. Usually, stationary liquid phases are polar whereas the mobile phase is nonpolar (normal phase). Water and polyethylene glycol are typical normal-phase stationary phases. Hexane and chloroform are common normal-phase mobile phases. It is possible to damage a column by removing the polar coating if a polar mobile phase is used. As shown in Figure 14-1, a very nonpolar molecule would move rapidly through a normal-phase column if the mobile phase were hexane. The nonpolar molecule would have a greater attraction for the nonpolar hexane than for the polar groups of the stationary phase.

Another form of partition chromatography, reverse phase, consists of a nonpolar stationary phase and a polar mobile phase. Typical mobile phases in this form of chromatography are water, acetonitrile, and methanol. Common station-

Figure 14-1. Normal phase liquid chromatography.

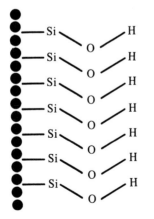

Non-polar mobile phase

Polar Stationary Phase

ary phases are hydrocarbon chains chemically bonded to the support. Partition chromatography is employed when sample components have known differences in solubility (*e.g.*, drugs). Figure 14-2 illustrates the molecular structures of typical stationary and mobile phases employed in reverse-phase partition chromatography.

ION-EXCHANGE

Ion-exchange chromatography is performed using an ion-exchange resin as the stationary phase and an aqueous solution as the mobile phase. The resins are highly polymerized crosslinked hydrocarbons that contain ionized functional groups. The resin may be thought of as having two distinct parts; one is a large, nondiffusible but permeable ion (basic resin structure), and the second part is a small, equally but oppositely charged ion that is free to migrate throughout the resin structure during the exchange. The ionic functional group attached to the structure of the resin determines the exchanger characteristics. Cation resins are produced when an acidic functional group, for example $(-SO_3H)$, is attached to the resin structure. The acidic hydrogen is available for exchange. Conversely, anion exchangers are produced when basic functional groups are attached to the resin structure. Figure 14-3 illustrates a typical structure for a cation-exchange resin.

The mechanism of the exchange is illustrated as follows:

$$X^- + R^+Y^- \quad Y^- + R^+X^- \quad \text{(anion exchange)}$$
$$X^+ + R^-Y^+ \quad Y^+ + R^-X^+ \quad \text{(cation exchange)}$$

where

$$X = \text{sample ion}$$
$$Y = \text{mobile-phase ion}$$
$$R = \text{ionic sites on exchanger}$$

Figure 14-2. Reverse phase chromatography.

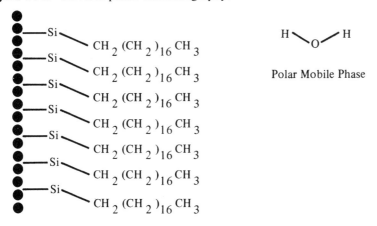

Polar Mobile Phase

Nonpolar stationary phase

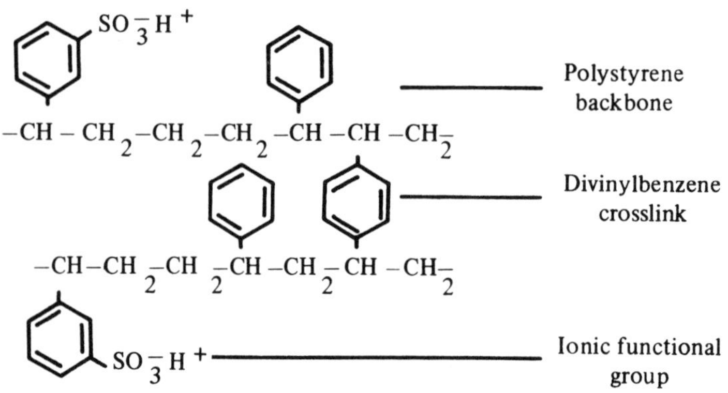

Figure 14-3. Cationic ion exchange resin.

In an anion-exchange system, the sample ion X^- is in competition with the mobile-phase ion, Y^-, for the ionic sites, R^+, on the ionic exchanger. In cationic-exchange chromatography, the sample cations, X^+, are competing with the mobile-phase ions, Y^+, for the ionic sites, R^-, on the ion exchanger. Solutes interacting weakly with the resin in the presence of the mobile-phase ions are eluted rapidly, whereas solutes that react strongly with the resin are retained much longer. *p*H and ionic strength of the mobile phase determine the solute ion-resin interaction. Clinically, this technique is used for separation of small ions, small hormones, heme-break-down products, and amino acids.

GEL PERMEATION

Gel permeation is a mechanical sorting of molecules based on molecular size. Size separation is accomplished with a porous packing gel through which the smallest components in the sample migrate into the smallest pores of the gel while the large molecules are excluded from the gel and elute from the column early in the separation. This technique is used for separation of high molecular weight enzymes and proteins from other serum constituents.

Chromatographic Parameters

Columns vary with their packing material, according to the type of liquid chromatography to be performed. It is important to choose the appropriate type of column for the compounds to be separated. A general rule to follow is: adsorption chromatography is most applicable for nonpolar compounds, whereas partition chromatography is the method of choice for slightly polar-to-polar compounds. Any ionized compounds are best separated utilizing ion-exchange chromatography.

An additional parameter that is useful for controlling separation is temperature. Increasing temperature may, in some instances, improve component separation and will reduce solvent viscosity, which results in reduced column back pressure.

There are two basic methods for solvent delivery. The first is isocratic solvent delivery, in which a mobile phase of fixed composition is delivered to the column at a set rate throughout the chromatogram. The second method is gradient solvent delivery, in which one component of the mobile phase is varied in concentration throughout the chromatogram.

Equipment for Liquid Chromatography

The basic components of a liquid chromatography system are illustrated in Figure 14-4.

The solvent delivery system may be one of three basic types. The first is a syringe pump, which is driven by a worm-screw drive. This mechanism yields a precise, pulseless flow. Another type is the single-piston reciprocating pump, which maintains constant pressure by a pressure-sensitive feedback circuit. The third type of delivery system is a dual-reciprocating pump, which has two pistons diametrically positioned and driven by the same cam. Both the single-piston and the dual-piston pump have a pulsed flow that is controlled by various damping mechanisms, resulting in low baseline noise. Table 14-1 illustrates the advantages and disadvantages of each solvent delivery system.

There are three basic types of sample injector systems for liquid chromatographs. The first is the on-column injection system, which consists of a siliconized

Figure 14-4.   Basic liquid chromatograph components.

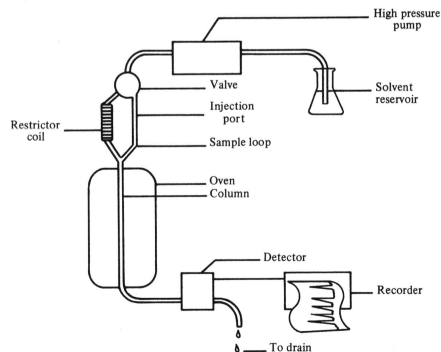

Table 14-1
Solvent Delivery Systems

Solvent Delivery System	Advantages	Disadvantages
Syringe pump	Even solvent flow rate Low flow rates precisely controlled	Unable to replenish solvent without shutting system down; high pressures not attainable
Reciprocating pump	Solvent reservoir easily refilled during operation; high pressures attainable; relative ease of operation	Pulsing solvent flow
Dual-headed reciprocating pump	Same as the reciprocating-pump system	Small amount of pulsing in the flow of solvent

rubber disk, and a septum through which the sample is loaded into the flowing mobile phase at a point just above the column bed using a micro high-pressure syringe. Upkeep of this system is difficult because of leaks and punctured septums which cannot be replaced unless the pumping mechanism is shut down. Small particles of septum material, dislodged by the syringe needle puncturing the septum, tend to collect at the head of the column, causing high back pressure and peak broadening.

The second type of injector is a fixed-loop injector in which the sample is loaded into the injector with a syringe to completely fill the injector sample loop. When the valve is turned to the "inject" position, the total volume of the sample loop is washed onto the column by the mobile phase.

The third type is the syringe-loop injector in which the sample, premeasured by microsyringe, is loaded into the sample loop which is partially filled with mobile phase. The sample is then flushed onto the column when the injector is placed in the "inject" position.

The advantage of the fixed-loop injector is that a reproducible volume is applied to the column; but this system lacks the flexibility of varying the injection volume. Both loop injector systems, however, allow ease of sample injection against high solvent pressure and are superior to the septum injector.

There are four basic detectors used for liquid chromatography: fixed wavelength adsorption, multiple wavelength adsorption, fluorescent, and electrochemical.

The fixed-wavelength ultraviolet-visible detector generally consists of a mercury lamp light source and utilizes filters to select the desired wavelength. The multiple-wavelength ultraviolet-visible detector utilizes a monochromater to obtain the wavelengths of choice. Both the fixed- and multiple-wavelength detectors are spectrophotometers utilizing a microflow cell as a cuvette. The fluorometric detector is a fluorometer adapted with a microflow cell to detect fluorescent compounds.

Table 14-2
Liquid Chromatograph Detectors

Detector	Advantages	Disadvantages
Fluorometric	High sensitivity for fluorescent compounds	Moderately specific
Electrochemical	Extremely sensitive Good specificity	Too sensitive Mobile phase must be an electrolyte
Fixed wavelength	Cheap Stable Relatively sensitive	Poor specificity
Multiple wavelength	Good specificity	Moderately sensitive

Electrochemical detectors are employed to detect compounds that can be oxidized or reduced, thus changing the conductivity of the compounds as compared to the solvent flowing through the flow cell.

The advantages and disadvantages of each detector are listed in Table 14-2.

Advantages and Disadvantages of Liquid Chromatography

The first advantage of liquid chromatography, as compared to other types of chromatography, is the simple sample preparation. A single extraction is usually sufficient, and derivatives are usually not required; therefore, a step is removed in which experimental error is likely to be introduced. This technique may be used at ambient or slightly above-ambient temperatures. Because of the relatively low temperatures involved in liquid chromatography, sample stability is of little concern. Finally, the instrumentation for liquid chromatography is reliable, and routine maintenance is simple compared to gas chromatography.

Two major disadvantages of liquid chromatography are the lack of sensitivity to some compounds and the requirement of moderately expensive equipment to perform analyses.

Suggested Reading

Berg E: Physical and Chemical Methods of Separation. New York, McGraw-Hill, 1963

Parris NA: Instrumental Liquid Chromatography. Journal of Chromatography Library, Vol. 5. New York, Elsevier, 1976

Johnson EL, Stevenson R: Basic Liquid Chromatography. Palo Alto, Varian, 1978

Snyder LR, Kirkland JJ: Introduction to Modern Liquid Chromatography. New York, John Wiley & Sons, 1979

Water's Guide to Therapeutic Drug Monitoring by Liquid Chromatography. Milford, MA, Water's Associates, August, 1978

Willard HH, Merritt LL Jr, Dean JA, Settle FA Jr: Instrumental Methods of Analysis, 6th ed. Princeton, Van Nostrand, 1981

Yost RW, Ettre LS, Conlon RD: Practical Liquid Chromatography: An Introduction. Norwalk, CT, Perkin-Elmer, 1980

15

SCINTILLATION COUNTERS

Mary C. Haven
Guy T. Haven

Definitions

Alpha (α) Particle: A helium nucleus ejected from the nucleus during radioactive decay that contains two protons and two neutrons and is positively charged, $^4_2He^{2+}$.

Annihilation Radiation: The production of two 0.51-MeV γ rays resulting from the combination and subsequent annihilation of an electron-positron pair.

Beta (β) Particle: An electron ejected from the nucleus during radioactive decay.

Cocktail: In this context, an undrinkable mixture of organic solvent (usually toluene) and a fluor.

Compton Effect: The interaction of a γ ray with an atom resulting in ejection of a weakly bound electron with incident energy being divided between the ejected electron and a photon (γ ray) of less energy.

Crossover: The detection of γ rays in crystals adjacent or near an isotopic source in another well in a multiwell system.

Excitation: Orbital electrons in the atoms are raised to a higher energy state.

Fluor: A substance that emits light when exposed to energetic electrons.

Gamma (γ) Rays: In electromagnetic radiation, a unit of energy emitted by a radioactive atom.

Half-Life: The time required for the disintegration of one-half of the radioactive atoms.

Ionization: The formation of an ion pair, an electron, and a positively charged ion from an atom.

Isotopes: Nuclides of the same atomic number (Z) but different atomic mass (A); number of protons = Z = atomic number, number of neutrons + protons = A = atomic mass.

keV: 10^3 eV.

MeV: 10^6 eV.

Normalization: The process by which the efficiencies of multiple crystals in a multiwell counter are matched.

Pair Production: γ ray interaction with the field surrounding the atomic nucleus resulting in the formation of an electron-positron pair.

Photoelectric Effect: The interaction of a γ ray with an atom resulting in the ejection of a tightly bound electron with all incident energy transferred to the electron.

Positron: A positively charged β particle with the same mass as an electron.

Radioactive Decay: A nuclear reaction that occurs spontaneously in unstable nuclei as the nuclide approaches stability.

Radioactivity: A spontaneous reaction of unstable nuclei as they approach stability.

Resolution: A measure of the energy width of the actual counted spectrum in a particular crystal.

Spilldown: Counts from a higher energy isotope that overlap into the window of a lower energy isotope when more than one isotope are being counted.

Introduction

All instruments for the detection and measurement of radiation require a sensing element, which converts the energy of radiation to electrical energy. The most common means of detecting radiation is via its production of light flashes (scintillation). This chapter will be limited to that instrumentation called scintillation counters. Scintillation counters are used to detect both β and γ emissions. A brief discussion of radioactivity will form a basis for understanding how radiation is measured.

NUCLEAR DECAY

Radioactive isotopes undergo spontaneous radioactive decay, releasing both nuclear particles and energy. The rate of nuclear decay and the character of the emissions identify specific isotopes. The radiation emitted from a radioisotope can be α, β, or γ rays.

Beta particles represent electrons derived from nuclear events, and their energy spectrum depends on the speed with which the electron leaves the nucleus. Beta particles are emitted from a given radioisotope over a continuous range of energy up to a maximum value (E_{max}), which is characteristic of each radioisotope. Commonly used isotopes such as ^3H and ^{14}C emit β particles of relatively low energy (Figs. 15-1 and 15-2). Beta particles, both because of their mass and charge,

Figure 15-1. Beta spectrum of ^3H.

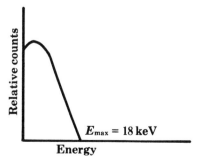

$E_{max} = 18\,keV$

Figure 15-2. Beta spectrum of ^{14}C.

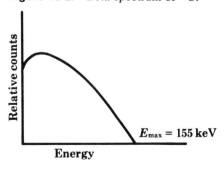

$E_{max} = 155\,keV$

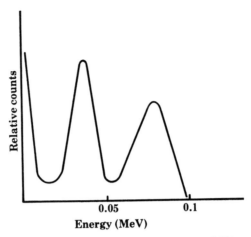

Figure 15-3. Gamma-ray spectrum of [125]I.

readily interact with matter and travel only short distances. As the β particle traverses material, it causes ionization and excitation of orbital electrons.

Gamma rays represent pure energy emissions that are analogous to x-rays, except for their origin. Gamma rays are derived from events in the nucleus of an atom, whereas x-rays are caused by the excitation of electrons outside the nucleus. Gamma rays are emitted from specific radioisotopes at characteristic energies generally ranging from 10 keV to 6 MeV.[9] The spectrum of each γ-emitting isotope is unique and can be used to identify the isotope (Figs. 15-3 and 15-4). Because γ rays have neither mass nor charge, they are capable of traveling great distances through matter (*e.g.*, cosmic rays represent high-energy γ rays).

Figure 15-4. Gamma-ray spectrum of [131]I.

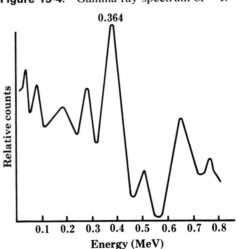

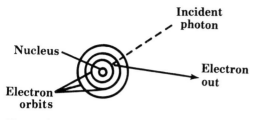

Figure 15-5. Photoelectric effect.

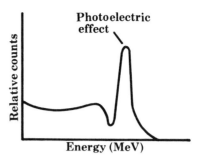

Figure 15-6. Spectrum showing photoelectric effect.

INTERACTION OF GAMMA RAYS WITH MATTER

Gamma rays characteristically interact with matter in three unique ways, producing energetic electrons:

Photoelectric effect refers to the total transfer of the γ ray's energy to an orbital electron; the energy is therefore transformed to the kinetic energy of the electron. This process is especially prevalent with low-energy (<0.5 MeV) γ rays (Figs. 15-5 and 15-6).

The *Compton effect* occurs most commonly with γ rays of medium energy (0.5–1.0 MeV). Here, only a portion of the γ ray's energy is imparted to the electron, the result of Compton effect being the production from the incident γ ray of an energetic electron and a γ ray of lesser energy. These Compton electrons may possess any amount of energy up to a defined maximum. Compton recoil electrons thus have a wide energy spread even when they result from mono-energetic γ rays (Figs. 15-7 and 15-8).

Pair production is a unique process in which high-energy γ rays are transformed into matter. It occurs only with γ rays having energy in excess of 1.02 MeV. The energy of the incident γ ray becomes mass in the formation of an electron–positron pair. The resulting positron reacts with surrounding matter by colliding with an electron. The mass of both positron and electron are annihilated

Figure 15-8. Spectrum showing Compton effect.

Figure 15-7. Compton effect.

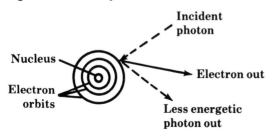

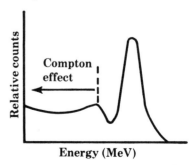

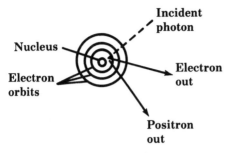

Figure 15-9. Pair production.

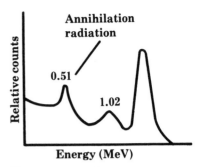

Figure 15-10. Spectrum showing annihilation effect.

to become two 0.51 MeV photons. This represents annihilation radiation, which always accompanies pair production (Figs. 15-9 and 15-10).

Both β and γ emissions are referred to as ionizing radiation, since during their interaction with matter they produce ions. Several devices for the detection of radioactivity are based on the measurement of this ionization in gas-filled chambers. Gas ionization detectors such as ion chambers, proportional counters, and Geiger-Mueller counters, however, are now only rarely used in clinical laboratories.

Solid Scintillation Counters

BASIC COMPONENTS

The three effects—photoelectric, Compton, and pair production—all ultimately yield energized electrons which, in solid scintillation systems, can interact with the fluor.[8] When these electrons pass near the orbital electron of the fluor, part of the energy is imparted to the orbital electron, raising the electron to a higher energy level. On return of this electron to the ground state, a characteristic photon is emitted. The number of photons released by the fluor is dependent upon the kinetic energy of the electrons and therefore on the total energy of the incident γ ray.

The fluor generally used for solid scintillation counting is a single large crystal of sodium iodide containing thallium. This crystal, usually well-shaped, virtually surrounds the sample to increase counting efficiency. The thallium-activated sodium iodide crystal characteristically emits photons at a visible wavelength suitable for detection by photomultiplier tubes. The sodium iodide crystals are hygroscopic (absorb water) and are therefore completely enclosed. The crystal is sealed in light-reflecting aluminum, except where attached to the photocathode through a transparent window. Through this window, photons may pass from crystal to the photocathode. This arrangement both protects the crystal from moisture and maximizes the light reaching the photomultiplier tubes.

By the use of photomultiplier tubes, the photons arising from the interaction of a single γ ray with the crystal are transformed to an electrical pulse; the magnitude of this pulse is increased by more than a million times. If this multiplication is to be useful, it must be reproducible so that a γ ray of 1 MeV might always result in the production of 1×10^8 electrons at the photomultiplier anode, whereas a γ ray of 2 MeV would result in the production of 2×10^8 electrons. Reproducible multiplication within the photomultiplier tube requires extreme stability of the high-voltage power supply. Ideally, the output of these power supplies, which provide overall gradients of up to 3000 V, should vary 0.01 V or less with a line voltage change of 1 V. The line voltage should be monitored before installing scintillation counters, and auxiliary voltage-regulation devices should be installed if necessary.

Closely coupled to the photomultiplier tube is a preamplifier, which further amplifies or multiplies the photomultiplier output. Thus, the amplifier, upon receiving 1×10^8 electrons from the photomultiplier tube, might generate a pulse of 0.6 V, whereas, upon receipt of 2×10^8 electrons, a pulse of 1.2 V would result. The duration required from the impingement of a γ ray on the crystal to the generation of a measurable voltage pulse is measured in nanoseconds. This allows high counting rates to be achieved using scintillation counting.

The combination of crystal, photomultiplier tube, and preamplifier produce discrete voltage pulses proportional in magnitude to the energy of incident γ rays. The addition of a pulse-height analyzer to this system results in a spectrometer which will discriminate among energies of the incident γ rays. This analyzer classifies the pulses according to their height or amplitude.

A single-channel pulse-height analyzer consists of two variable discriminators, which allow selection of lower and upper levels of detection. The lower discriminator setting is termed the *base*. The upper discriminator setting is selected by adding a voltage increment (a window) to the base. These two discriminators, in conjunction with an anticoincidence circuit, allow only those energies between the two discriminator levels to pass to the scaler.

Discriminator I, the base, establishes the lower limit of detection. Pulses with an amplitude less than the base are rejected and do not appear as analyzer output. Discriminator II rejects all pulses with an amplitude less than the base plus the window. The anticoincidence circuit is designed to block all pulses arriving simultaneously (*i.e.*, all pulses with amplitudes greater than both discriminators). Only those pulses passed by discriminator I and rejected by discriminator II will reach the scaler.

Figure 15-11 represents an example of a single-channel pulse-height analyzer with the base set at 1 V and the window at 0.5 V. In this case, a pulse of 0.5 V will be rejected by both discriminators. A pulse of 1.2 V will be passed by discriminator I and rejected by discriminator II, and will reach the scaler. A pulse of 2.0 V will be passed by both discriminators I and II, arrive simultaneously at the coincidence counter, and therefore be rejected. Only those pulses greater than 1 V and less than 1.5 V will reach the scaler.

To illustrate how a pulse-height analyzer can isolate and count only the principal photopeak of a spectrum, the example of ^{137}Cs will be used. The principal photopeak has an energy of 0.661 MeV. The assumption (this will be explained in differential counting) will be made that the base setting can be varied between 0 and 1000 keV; that is, 0 and 1 MeV. The base sets the lower discriminator and

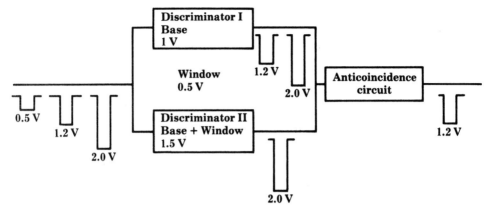

Figure 15-11.   Single-channel pulse-height analyzer.

the window sets the increment increase above the base which will serve as the upper discriminator. If the base can vary between 0 and 1 MeV and a 10% window is employed, this window is 10% of 1 MeV, or 0.1 MeV. The Poisson distribution peaks at 0.661 MeV, but there are a significant number of counts on each side of 0.661 MeV. To center this peak in a 10% window, or, in this case, a 0.1-MeV window, half of this 0.1 MeV should be on either side of 0.661 MeV. Therefore, the base should be set 0.05 MeV lower than the 0.661-MeV peak. The base should then be set at 0.611 MeV; the 10% window would set the upper discriminator 0.1 MeV higher than the base, or 0.711 MeV. At these settings, most of the counts resulting from the photopeak of ^{137}Cs will reach the scaler (Fig. 15-12).

The counts derived from the scintillation process and isolated according to amplitude are recorded and displayed on a scaler which displays the counts accumulated during the counting period selected.

A single-channel γ-ray spectrometer (Fig. 15-13) then includes a NaI (Tl)

Figure 15-12.   Isolation of ^{137}Cs photopeak.

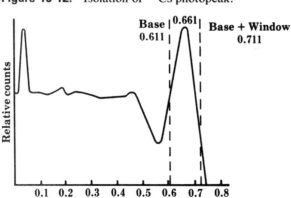

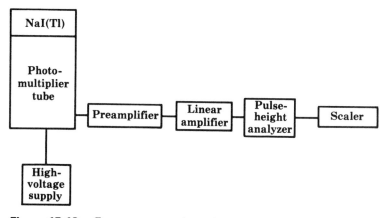

Figure 15-13. Gamma-ray spectrometer.

crystal attached to a photomultiplier tube. A high-voltage supply is necessary for the photomultiplier tube. The signal is transmitted by a preamplifier to a linear amplifier, where further amplification occurs. A pulse-height analyzer then classifies the pulses according to their height or amplitude, and a scaler registers the number of pulses received.

TYPES OF COUNTING

A scintillation counter can be used for two types of counting, integral and differential. In integral counting, a rejection of low pulses can be set, but no limit is set on higher-energy pulsing. In Figure 15-14, which shows a ^{131}I emission spectrum, pulses below 0.314 MeV are rejected (0.314 MeV is the base), but all

Figure 15-14. Integral count of ^{131}I spectrum.

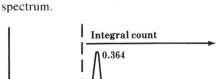

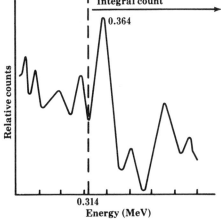

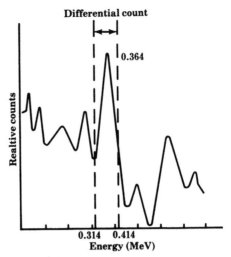

Figure 15-15. Differential count of ^{131}I spectrum.

higher pulses are counted. Differential counting employs the pulse-height analyzer. It not only rejects pulses lower than the base but also sets a limit on high-energy pulses. The same ^{131}I sample, set to count differentially with a 10% window, would count only the principal photopeak (Fig. 15-15).

DIFFERENTIAL COUNTERS

In the discussion of pulse-height analyzers, the assumption was made that the base could be varied between 0 and 1000 keV (0 and 1 MeV). In order that the pulse can be calibrated in γ ray energy, the optimum high voltage to be applied to the photomultiplier tube must be determined experimentally.

By adjusting the voltage to the photomultiplier tube and the amplification of the linear amplifier (called attenuation or gain), the pulse height can become a multiple of the incident γ ray energy. To accomplish this calibration, a mono-energetic source, usually [137]Cs (Fig. 15-16), with a photopeak at 0.661 MeV is used, and an attenuation to correspond to a maximum amplified pulse of 10 V is selected. The 0.661 MeV peak can be perfectly centered between 0.611 and 0.711 MeV by a base setting at 0.611 and a window of 10% or 1 V (Fig. 15-12). The voltage to the photomultiplier tube is then varied in small increments until a maximum count rate is obtained. As the voltage is increased, the pulse height produced by the γ ray will be increased until the pulses fall within the area set by the base and window (Fig. 15-17). When the applied voltage causes some of the pulses to exceed the upper discriminator level, the count rate begins to decrease. When the maximum count rate is achieved, the high voltage is fixed, placing the instrument in calibration. Now a 0.661-MeV γ ray will give a pulse of 6.61 V at this attenuation and high-voltage setting. The high-voltage setting is not changed after this calibration regardless of the γ-emitting isotope counted.

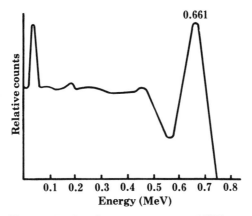

Figure 15-16. Gamma spectrum of ^{137}Cs.

An amplified pulse of 10 V now corresponds to a 1 MeV γ ray. If the attenuation is changed, the amplification is changed proportionately (*e.g.,* one-half of the 10 V setting would make the maximum detectable pulse 5 V [corresponding to 0–0.5 MeV] and a ^{137}Cs γ ray would not be detected). Lower attenuations are used for the lower-energy γ emissions from ^{125}I, ^{57}Co, and ^{51}Cr.

In many differential counters found in the clinical laboratory, the instrument manufacturers have selected the base and window for the two commonly used isotopes, ^{125}I and ^{57}Co. Adjustment of gain and high voltage to the photomultiplier may also have been done at the factory. In these instruments, the technologist does not adjust high voltage but relies on regular quality control measures to signal changes in instrument performance.

Integral Counters

A simpler scintillation counter without a pulse-height analyzer, only a lower-level discriminator (base), is used for integral counting. If a detector is to be used

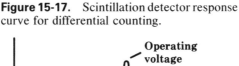

Figure 15-17. Scintillation detector response curve for differential counting.

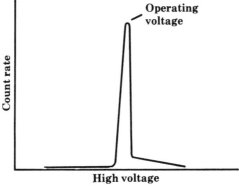

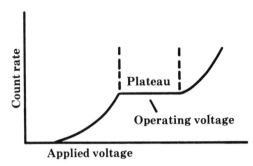

Figure 15-18. Scintillation detector response curve for integral counting.

for integral counting, adjustment of the voltage applied to the photomultiplier tube is needed, and the optimum voltage again is determined experimentally.

While counting an isotope, the applied voltage is varied, and a graph of count rate versus voltage is prepared. A typical response curve is shown in Figure 15-18. An applied voltage midpoint of the resulting plateau will ensure a count rate relatively independent of small voltage changes, thereby increasing instrument stability. This operating voltage should be determined for each isotope to be counted in the instrument.

Multiwell Counters

Speed in reporting results was the impetus for the introduction of multiwell γ counters into the clinical laboratory. With these counters, multiple samples (usually 10 to 24) can be counted simultaneously in closely matched scintillation crystals. These crystals are usually smaller (1 to 1.5 inches) than the more standard crystals (2 to 3 inches) used in the single-well counters. They are not as efficient for counting high-energy γ rays, but are suitable for the low-energy isotopes usually used in clinical diagnostics, ^{125}I and ^{57}Co. Most multiwell instruments have dual pulse-height analyzers so that these two isotopes can be counted simultaneously. High voltage to the photomultiplier is adjusted at the factory; the individual laboratory matches the various detectors through a normalization process. Each detector is surrounded by lead to decrease the amount of radiation detected in wells adjacent to the sample being counted; these unwanted counts are usually called *crosstalk* or *crossover*. The multiwell counters frequently include software for normalization, crosstalk correction, spilldown (counts from a higher-energy isotope that overlap into the window of the lower-energy isotope), as well as data reduction of standard curves and calculation of unknown samples.

Liquid Scintillation Counting

BASIC COMPONENTS

The measurement of β emissions of the widely used isotopes ^3H and ^{14}C cannot be performed by solid scintillation counting, in part because these weak-energy emissions cannot traverse the aluminum envelope of the scintillation crystals. The low energy and slight penetration ability of β particles necessitate an intimate admixture of sample and fluor for efficient counting. Liquid scintillation derives its name from the liquid mixture composed of sample, solvent, and the fluor. With luck, both sample and fluor are soluble in the solvent, although emulsions of sample in the solvent may sometimes be satisfactory. Toluene is the most common solvent used, and reagent grade is satisfactory. For samples containing water, dioxane is often the solvent of choice. However, dioxane must be specially purified. The addition of a solubilizing agent often aids in obtaining homogeneous solutions of organic and aqueous mixture.[4]

A wide variety of fluors is available for liquid scintillation counting. The fluors are generally complex heterocyclic, organic compounds that, when excited, emit photons in the near ultraviolet and visible regions. The fluors typically comprise less than 1% of the solvent-fluor mixture (cocktail).

The β emissions from the sample interact with the material surrounding them and cause excitation first of the solvent molecules. This excitation energy of the solvent is transferred to the solute, the fluor, causing excitation of fluor electrons. The excited electrons in the fluor emit photons of light as they fall back to the ground state. These photons of light are detected by the photomultiplier tube and result in electrical pulses as in solid scintillation counters. Power supplies for the provision of a high-voltage dc potential to the photomultiplier tube are similar to those used in γ ray spectrometry, except that, in the former, two potentials are supplied for paired photomultiplier tubes. Because the low-energy ranges of β emission result in photomultiplier output of the same order of magnitude as thermionic emission (noise), coincidence circuitry has been employed. The use of paired photomultiplier tubes and coincidence circuitry ensures that only pulses seen simultaneously (usually within less than 20 nsec) are passed on to the spectrometer. Pulses simultaneously observed are most often due to β emission. By contrast, the thermionic emission arising in each photomultiplier tube is random, and this background noise is unlikely to be detected simultaneously. Thermionic emission is also often decreased by refrigeration of the entire detector unit. However, refrigeration is of relatively less importance when newer photomultiplier tubes are used. Many current instruments can be operated at ambient temperature. Two preamplifiers are often attached to the photomultiplier tube to provide initial amplification. Pulses from the two detection circuits are passed through a coincidence circuit and are electronically summed. Pulses then pass to two or more channels, each consisting of a linear amplifier, pulse-height analyzer, and scaler, much like in γ scintillation counting (Fig. 15-19). Because of the multiplicity of instrument types available for liquid scintillation counting, it would be impractical to describe instrument setting for counting a specific β-emitting isotope. The directions provided by each manufacturer should be carefully followed.

QUENCHING

The admixture of sample and fluor in liquid scintillation can lead to the problem of quenching. This is especially true of biologic samples that may contain a great variety of chemical compounds. Even the oxygen in air, as well as any number of chemicals in the sample, may result in quenching. As noted previously, β

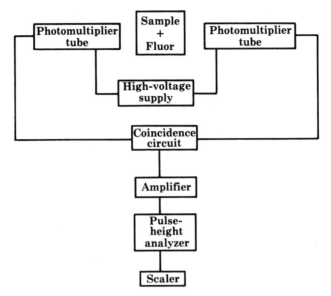

Figure 15-19. Block diagram of a liquid scintillation counter.

particles are emitted at a continuous spectrum of energies, the characteristic feature of each isotope being the maximum energy of β emission, the E_{max}. Quenching shifts this β emission curve to the left, lowers the energy of the E_{max}, increases the number of counts in the lower-energy range, and decreases the total detectable count (Fig. 15-20). Quenching may be of three types: chemical, chromatic, and optical.

Chemical quenching is caused by a variety of polar organic compounds that can absorb energy from the excited solvent molecules, preventing, in part, excitation of the fluor. Color quenching can be expected whenever the scintillant solution does not have its usual light blue color due to colored impurities in the sample. Yellow and red solutions especially may absorb the blue light that is

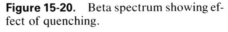

Figure 15-20. Beta spectrum showing effect of quenching.

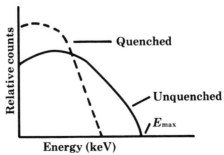

emitted by the fluors. Finally, optical quenching results when the mixture of scintillation cocktail and sample result not in true solutions but suspensions. Because quenching decreases the detectable energy of β-emitting isotopes, it should be minimized whenever possible. Quenching is sometimes unavoidable, however, and the degree of quenching unpredictable; therefore, it must be recognized and corrected.

Compared to most γ emissions, the β emissions of ^{14}C and especially ^{3}H are of very low energy. Even in the absence of quenching, only approximately 90% of the ^{14}C emissions and 60% of the ^{3}H emissions will be detected. These percentages are referred to as counting efficiency, and they equal detected counts per minute divided by disintegrations per minute × 100 [% E = (cpm/dpm) × 100]. Disintegrations per minute (dpm) is an absolute number proportional to the isotopic content of the sample, whereas counts per minute (cpm) refers only to the observed count. By correcting for quenching (*i.e.*, determining efficiency), an estimation of the dpm of each sample and consequently of the isotopic content is obtained. Chemical and color quenching both result in a decrease in cpm and a shift of the energy spectrum to a lower range, but the shapes of the resulting curves are different (Fig. 15-21).

QUENCH CORRECTION

Internal Standard Method

The internal standard method for determining counting efficiency is considered by some to be the most reliable method.[10] The sample is counted once, and then a sample aliquot of radioactive standard with known dpm is added, and the sample is again counted.

$$\% E = \frac{\text{cpm due to added standard}}{\text{dpm of added standard}} \times 100$$

The drawbacks of this method include a small pipetting error, the inability to recount unaltered sample since it has become contaminated with standard, and the necessity for counting the sample twice. However, the internal standard method corrects equally well for all types of quenching.

Figure 15-21. Beta spectrum shifts due to quenching.

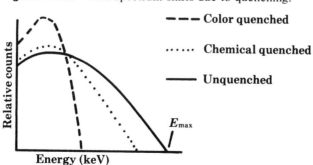

Channels Ratio Method

The channels ratio method[6] is based on the observation that the β spectrum is always displaced to the left when quenching occurs. Using a two-channel instrument to measure a single isotope, the first channel is set to encompass all energies of a given isotope. The second channel is set to encompass approximately 50% of the counts in an unquenched sample, usually in the lower-energy range. As the degree of quenching increases, the count rate in the first channel decreases proportionately more than in the second channel because of the spectral shift. The channels ratio method is standardized by counting multiple samples containing a standard amount of radioisotope with known dpm in the presence of varying quantities of chemical quenching agents. A curve relating the percent efficiency [% E = (cpm $\times$ 100)/dpm] to the ratio of counts in the two channels is constructed. When unknown samples are counted, the ratio between the two channel counts is determined and the percent efficiency is determined graphically. Channels ratio corrections are most applicable to chemically quenched samples; small errors are produced when mild optical quenching is present. Large errors may be introduced when quenching is due to color or precipitation of the sample. A major weakness in this method occurs when samples of low activity are counted, necessitating very long counting periods to accumulate statistically significant counts in each channel. Recognizing these disadvantages, the channels ratio method is less time consuming than the internal standard method, is not subject to pipetting errors, and does not result in contamination of the sample.

External Standard Method

In this method, the sample is irradiated by a γ source which produces Compton electrons. The assumption is made that the Compton electrons behave as β particles in solution and that quenching in the sample results in proportionate quenching of Compton electrons. After the sample is counted, the external standard is automatically positioned near the sample vial, and the sample is again counted for an additional minute. Depending on the γ-emitting isotope used as external standard, the energy range of the Compton electrons may or may not overlap with the energy range of the β-emitting isotope within the sample. Depending upon the instrument used, either the gross counts of the external standard or the channels ratio of the external standard counts in two separate channels can be plotted against percent efficiency to generate a curve. This curve is produced experimentally and used in the same manner as channels ratio curves. The major advantage of the use of the external standard is that it allows one to rapidly determine counting efficiency regardless of the amount of radioactivity in the sample. The reproducibility of the technique depends on a constant geometric relationship between γ source and sample. Thus, the γ source must be positioned automatically in the identical position for each count, and sample volume and vial characteristics must be constant. Because the Compton electrons produced are all of relatively high energy compared to the β emissions of tritium, it is possible that minor quenching of low-energy β emissions from tritium may go undetected.

Electronic Method

Electronic quench correction is currently available on several instruments. In general, the instrument monitors the external standard ratio of the sample and adjusts instrument performance to produce results proportional to dpm when subsequently counting the sample. Automatic instrumental adjustment consists of either varying amplifier gain or altering the efficiency of the photomultiplier tubes by varying a magnetic field surrounding the photomultiplier tubes. This technique is least efficient in correcting low-energy samples such as tritium or highly quenched samples from other β-emitters.

Quality Control of Scintillation Detectors

GAMMA COUNTERS

Peak resolution should be checked in the instrument at the time of installation, and occasionally thereafter, to ensure that the instrument meets specifications. The energy width of the actual counted photopeak is dependent upon the quality of the crystal. A perfect crystal would have a peak width of 1 pulse height. The lower the percent resolution, the sharper the photopeak, the better the signal-to-noise ratio for narrower windows may be set. Peak resolution is determined from the spectrum of a standard isotope. To determine this spectrum, a narrow window is selected, 1%; the base of the pulse-height analyzer is varied in small increments, 5 keV, across the entire photopeak; and the standard isotopic source is counted at each setting for the same time unit. A graph of counts versus energy will yield the isotope spectrum. The full width at half maximum (FWHM) of the photopeak expressed in energy divided by the energy of the γ ray times 100 equals the percent resolution (Fig. 15-22).

$$\frac{\Delta E}{E} \times 100 = \% \text{ resolution}$$

For ^{137}Cs, resolutions of 7% to 12% can be found in clinical laboratory instruments.[3] Counting efficiencies of ^{137}Cs and/or ^{125}I should also be determined at installation, occasionally thereafter, and when troubleshooting the instrument. A source of known activity (corrected for decay since calibration) is counted and percent efficiency is calculated from the following equation:

$$\frac{\text{cpm}}{\text{dpm}} \times 100 = \% \text{ efficiency}$$

The counting reproducibility of each crystal should be checked at regular intervals. The standard method for checking the assumed normal distribution (the Poisson distribution of radioactive decay approaches a normal Gaussian distribution as N, the number of observations, becomes larger[2]) is by using the chi-square test. An isotopic standard (count rate $\approx$ 100,000 cpm) is counted several times, usually between 15 and 30, but the same number of observations is checked each time. The mean of the multiple observations is considered the *expected count*

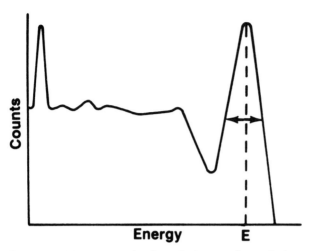

Figure 15-22. Determination of photopeak resolution: full width at half maximum (FWHM) of the photopeak divided by the energy of the γ ray.

rate; the individual count is considered the *observed count rate*. The chi-square is calculated from the following equation:[7]

$$\chi^2 = \Sigma \frac{(O - E)^2}{E}$$

where

O = observed count or each individual count
E = expected count or mean of all observations
χ^2 = chi-square
df = degrees of freedom or (N − 1)
N = number of observations

The calculated chi-square should fall between the two chi-square values found in standard chi-square tables[11] for N − 1 degrees of freedom at the selected probability range (usually 99% or $p = 0.01$). When the chi-square is within limits, the observed count rate does not differ significantly from what was expected. If the calculated chi-square falls outside the selected limits, the observed count rate differs significantly from that expected of a normal distribution, and the process should be repeated. The second time the criteria are not met, the instrument service representative should be notified.

A standard isotopic source (about 100,000 cpm) of the isotope of interest or one of similar γ ray energy should be counted often at the exact instrument settings used for routine clinical work.[5] Records should be kept and limits of count rate variability should be established by calculating the standard deviation (SD) as the square root of the mean counts. Because radioactive decay is a random event per time unit, the probability distribution of this random occurrence follows a Poisson distribution;[2] the SD of a Poisson distribution is the square root of the mean.[1] If the high voltage supply were to drift, the count rate of the standard source would fall outside the established day-to-day limits (*e.g.*, mean ± 6 SD of the initial standardization corrected for isotope decay). In multiwell γ counters, the standard source of the isotope of interest should be counted in each crystal; alternatively, a set of matched sources may be counted simultaneously. Any detector that differs more than 10% from the mean count rate of the others should be disabled and the service representative notified. After recording individual counts in each crystal, all crystals should be normalized within 1% to the crystal of lowest efficiency. Software for multiwell counters includes the normalization process.

A record of background counts in each crystal for each isotope used should be maintained. Background counts at the beginning and end of each batch of samples ensure that the crystal has not been contaminated. This is not as practical in multiwell instruments as it is in single-well instruments.

When both pulse-height analyzers are being used, the higher-energy isotopic standard should be counted and the spilldown into the lower-energy window should be noted and documented. If the high voltage supply has drifted and the two isotopes are no longer centered in the window, the spilldown into the lower window will have changed significantly and the voltage should be readjusted. When the spilldown is as expected, instruments with microprocessors correct samples and standards for the spilldown from the higher-energy isotope.

BETA COUNTERS

Records of counts obtained from standard isotopes of interest should be maintained. The value of the external standard for quench correction should be obtained at the same time and recorded; background counts in all channels should be used as well. The quench curve, if using quench correction, could be monitored at less frequent intervals.

References

1. Colton T: Statistics in Medicine, pp 77–78. Boston, Little, Brown, & Co, 1974
2. Harbert J, DaRocha AFG: Textbook of Nuclear Medicine, Vol 1: Basic Science, p 71. Philadelphia, Lea & Febiger, 1984
3. Howard PL, Trainer TD: Radionuclides in Clinical Chemistry, p 27. Boston, Little, Brown, & Co, 1980
4. Howard PL, Trainer TD: Radionuclides in Clinical Chemistry, p 38. Boston, Little, Brown, & Co, 1980
5. Johnson RF: Well-type scintillation counting systems and their care: A procedural approach. The Ligand Review 2:65–69, 1980
6. Kobayashi Y, Maudsley DV: Biological Applications of Ligand Scintillation Counting, pp 28–29. New York, Academic Press, 1974
7. Kolstoe RH: Introduction to Statistics for the Behavioral Sciences, Rev ed, pp 234–235. Homewood, IL, Dorsey Press, 1973
8. Price WJ: Nuclear Radiation Detection, pp 159–209. New York, McGraw-Hill, 1964

9. Quimby EH, Feitelberg S, Gross W: Radioactive Nuclides in Medicine and Biology, 3rd ed, p 65. Philadelphia, Lea & Febiger, 1970
10. Tietz NW: Textbook of Clinical Chemistry, p 192. Philadelphia, WB Saunders, 1986
11. Tietz NW: Textbook of Clinical Chemistry, p 1807. Philadelphia, WB Saunders, 1986

Suggested Reading

Bernier DM, Langan JK, Wells LD: Nuclear Medicine Technology and Techniques. St Louis, CV Mosby, 1981
Shapiro J: Radiation Protection: A Guide for Scientists and Physicians, 2nd ed. Cambridge, MA, Harvard University Press, 1981

16

AUTOMATED HEMATOLOGY SYSTEMS
Joan F. Mares

Definitions

Aperture: An orifice through which cells pass to be counted.

Beam Splitter: A device used in the H6000* optics that, by means of reflection, deflects light upward to the absorption-detection system and allows light to pass through to the scatter-detection system.

Burn Circuit: Electrical pulses generated to electrically burn off protein from the apertures.

CBC: Complete blood count.

Channel: The area between two threshold settings.

Coefficient of Variation: The degree of spread around the mean.

Coherent Light Beam: All photon waves are in phase.

Coincidence Counts: Cells that pass through the aperture together but are counted as one cell.

Dichroic Mirrors: Filters coated with a material allowing them to reflect and absorb selectively.

Electronic Editing: The method of excluding pulses produced by cells that pass through the aperture at the edge or at an angle, rather than through the center.

Femtoliter (fl): A unit of volume equal to one-quadrillionth of a liter (10^{-15}l). It is the recommended unit for expressing mean cell volume (MCV) and is equal to the formerly used measure, the cubic micron.

Firmware: Electronic components of a computer containing fixed instructions to perform certain functions.

Floppy Disk: A portable, flat, circular recording surface used in computer systems to store instructions or information.

Hct: Hematocrit.

Hgb: Hemoglobin.

Histogram: A bar chart with equal width to each bar, often depicting the number of cells in a particular size range.

Hydrodynamic Focusing: Centering something (cells) with the use of sheath fluids around the sample.

Laser: The acronym for *l*ight *a*mplification by *s*timulated *e*mission of *r*adiation.

LED: Light-emitting diode.

MCH: Mean cell hemoglobin.

MCHC: Mean cell hemoglobin concentration.

MCV: Mean cell volume.

Mean: Arithmetic average.

Median: The data item found in the middle of a distribution.

Mode: The data item that occurs with the greatest frequency.

MPV: Mean platelet volume.

Noise: Any unwanted disturbance or spurious signal within an electronic component. Noise is an unintended addition to the needed signal independent of that signal's presence.

PDW: Platelet distribution width. It is an indication of size variation.

Photodiode: A detector that converts photon energy to electrical energy (emf).

P-LCR: Platelet large cell ratio. Used to detect platelet aggregation or overlap of platelets with red blood cell (RBC) fragments.

PLT: Platelet.

RBC: Red blood cell.

RDW: Red cell distribution width.

RCMI: Red cell morphology index.

Software: The programs or instructions that cause data to be processed in a computer, and their associated documentation.

Sweep Flow: A steady stream of diluent that flows behind the RBC apertures during the sensing period and carries cells immediately away from the sensing zone.

Threshold: An electronically set size limit above which the pulse is analyzed and below which it is ignored.

WBC: White blood cell.

W-LCR: WBC large cell ratio.

W-MCR: WBC middle cell ratio.

W-SCR: WBC small cell ratio.

$\overline{XB}$:   Weighted moving average concept.

Z-Score: A value obtained by normalizing a datum point (x) by subtracting the mean of the parent population and dividing by the standard deviation.

Introduction

Instrumentation in hematology* has advanced rapidly in the past 20 years. The technologist of today is no longer constrained by tedious and imprecise manual methods for doing red blood cell (RBC) and white blood cell (WBC) counts. Today, most laboratories have automated platelet counters, and some laboratories even have automated differentials counters.

Cell Counters

The real breakthrough for hematology blood counters came when Joseph and Wallace Coulter introduced their conductivity method of cell counting.[5] This

---

*Instruments initially followed by asterisks (*) appear with company names in the Appendix at the end of this chapter.

principle, with some improvements, is still the basis of many of today's single-parameter and multiparameter instruments. Recent advances in technology have added new characteristics to the classic Wintrobe indices by adding new parameters such as an index of anisocytosis, cellular histograms, and partial differentials. State-of-the-art instrumentation today gives a variety of information on leukocytes, erythrocytes, and platelets with internal quality control checks built directly into the system.

PRINCIPLES OF OPERATION

Cell counters basically use one of two physical properties as their principle of operation—electrical impedance or optical scattering.

The principle of electrical impedance is called the *Coulter principle,* because it was introduced by Joseph and Wallace Coulter. This principle is the basis of the majority of instrumentation on the market today. Operation is based on the electrical conductivity difference between particles and diluent. Particles act as insulators whereas the diluent acts as a conductor. The particles suspended in an electrolyte are made to pass through a small aperture through which an electrical current path has been established. As a dilute suspension of cells is drawn through the aperture, the passage of each individual cell momentarily increases the resistance of the electrical path between two submerged electrodes. One electrode is located inside the aperture and one outside. The number of pulses generated indicates particle count, and the amplitude of the electrical pulse depicts the cell's volume. On the more advanced models, different cell types are distinguished electronically by sorting the pulses they generate.

The other major method of cell counting is based on light scatter. These instruments are basically flow-through systems in which a beam of light is scattered by the passage of a particle (cell) through its path. This scattered light hits photodetectors, which causes an electrical signal. The size of the signal is directly proportional to the amount of scattered light, which, in turn, directly reflects the size of the cell. From the signals, the instrument senses the number of cells and the size. Some advanced instrumentation can also detect information about the granularity of cells by the type of scatter produced.

SEMI-AUTOMATED CELL COUNTERS

For purposes of this chapter, *semi-automated* refers to all instrumentation that requires an outside dilution of the blood to be made before it can be introduced into the instrument for counting. All the instrumentation in this category that is presently marketed is based upon the principle of electrical impedance.

The first cell counter, the Model A*, was introduced in the early 1960s. It was hand-wired and used vacuum tubes. In spite of problems with reagents, dilution, and glassware, these instruments were highly reliable. The most important change in this instrumentation was in electronics. Vacuum tubes were replaced with transistors, and printed-circuit boards were used throughout the units. The early units, including the model Fn*, had a tendency to pick up transient broadcast signals from electric motors and fluorescent lights, causing a high background count. This was resolved with better grounding in later models.

In the simpler systems on the market today, such as the models Fn and ZBI*, timing of the counting mechanism is accomplished by connecting a U-shaped glass tube partially filled with mercury to an aperture. Two mercury contacts are spaced a precise distance apart on the glass tube. The system is closed with a valve. The counting mechanism is started when the mercury in the tube contacts the first electronic contact and stops when it meets the second contact. During this time, the cells are counted in a volume of suspension exactly equal to the volume of the glass tubing between the two electronic contacts (Fig. 16-1).

If two or more cells enter the aperture simultaneously, they will be counted as one pulse. This produces a coincidence error for which a correction must be made. Newer instrumentation uses various techniques to decrease coincidence. These techniques include decreasing the size of the aperture, decreasing the concentration of cells, electronic editing, and the use of a sheath fluid.

Because the height of each pulse spike is proportional to the size of the particle that produces it, the size of particles to be counted can be chosen by setting the size to be analyzed. To do this, thresholds are set. A threshold is an electronically set size limit above which the pulse is analyzed and below which it is ignored.

Figure 16-1. Simplified drawing of manometer measuring section and control section with electrodes—(A) aperture; (B) aperture tube; (C) internal electrode; (D) external electrode; (E) diluted sample; (F) vacuum line stopcock; (G) rinse-line stopcock; (L, M) start and stop electrodes; (K) mercury contact electrode; (O) rinse line; (P) vacuum line; (R) mercury column and reservoir. (After Mattern CFT, Brackett FS, Olson BJ: Determination of number and size of particles by electrical gating: Blood cells. J Appl Physiol 10:56, 1957)

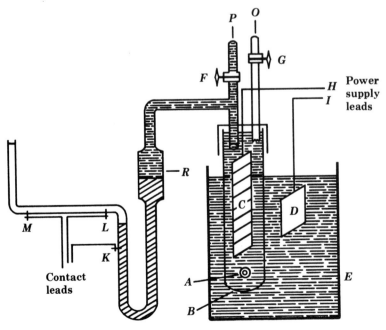

There are many semi-automated cell counters on the market today. These include the ZBI, the M430*, the Celltrak* systems, the HA-3D*, the 390A*, and the System 7000*, all of which have aperture clog indicators and automatic co-incidence correction. Some have automatic malfunction indicators, such as the Celltrak systems. The System 7000 includes automatic resampling if duplicate cell counts differ by more than 3%.

Some models of semi-automated equipment give as many parameters as the fully automated instruments, but are categorized here because of predilution of the blood sample. Some of these systems are quite sophisticated. For example, the System 8000* features eight parameters (WBC,RBC,hemoglobin [Hgb], hematocrit [Hct], mean cell volume [MCV], mean cell hemoglobin [MCH], mean cell hemoglobin concentration [MCHC], and platelet [PLT]), automatic reverse air-purge/fluidic-flush, platelet histogram, and a self-diagnostic program to alert the operator to such things as linearity range limits, abnormal population distributions, reagent status, flow errors, electronic reference values, and lysis errors. The Profile 750* also has self-diagnostic aids with 15 error messages.

AUTOMATED, MULTIPARAMETER CELL COUNTERS

The earliest, automated, multiparameter instrumentation measured seven hematology parameters: WBC, RBC, Hgb, Hct, MCV, MCH, and MCHC. This was followed by the addition of platelets. Today, almost all of these instruments feature at least the above eight parameters, and most give more. To better understand these instruments, we will look at some of them individually and describe their operation. There are many good cell counters that are not mentioned, but that are still excellent instruments.

S PLUS IV

The S Plus IV (S Plus Series)* is based upon the counting principle of electrical impedance. It consists of six main parts.

The power supply contains the vacuum and pressure pumps to move liquid through the diluter. It also supplies the voltages and currents needed by the electrical components as well as the current required for sensing the cells as they pass through the apertures. There are three sensing apertures in each bath. As diluent conducts current from the internal electrodes through the apertures to an external electrode, the cells are pulled through the apertures for 4-second intervals by a regulated vacuum of 152.4 mm Hg. Count and size information for each dilution is generated in triplicate, and this is sent to the analyzer in the form of electrical impulses.

The second part, or diluter, contains the ''hardware'' needed to aspirate, pipette, dilute, mix, lyse, and sense the sample (Fig. 16-2). Only 0.1 ml of blood is aspirated (earlier models used 1.0 ml whole blood or 44.7 μl prediluted). The blood sample is then divided into two aliquots, each of which is mixed with diluent to form the two primary dilutions. One dilution goes to the RBC aperture bath, where the RBC and platelet information will be generated. The other is delivered to the WBC aperture bath, where the WBC information will be sensed. A lysing

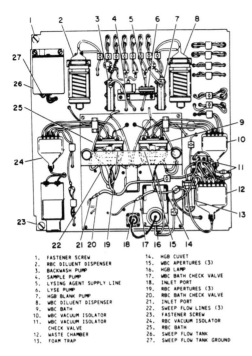

1. FASTENER SCREW	14. HGB CUVET
2. RBC DILUENT DISPENSER	15. WBC APERTURES (3)
3. BACKWASH PUMP	16. HGB LAMP
4. SAMPLE PUMP	17. WBC BATH CHECK VALVE
5. LYSING AGENT SUPPLY LINE	18. INLET PORT
6. LYSE PUMP	19. RBC APERTURES (3)
7. HGB BLANK PUMP	20. RBC BATH CHECK VALVE
8. WBC DILUENT DISPENSER	21. INLET PORT
9. WBC BATH	22. SWEEP FLOW LINES (3)
10. WBC VACUUM ISOLATOR	23. FASTENER SCREW
11. WBC VACUUM ISOLATOR	24. RBC VACUUM ISOLATOR
CHECK VALVE	25. RBC BATH
12. WASTE CHAMBER	26. SWEEP FLOW TANK
13. FOAM TRAP	27. SWEEP FLOW TANK GROUND

Figure 16-2. Schematic diagram of the S Plus IV diluter front center panel. (Courtesy of Coulter Electronics, Inc, Hialeah, FL)

agent is added to the WBC bath to lyse the red cells and release the hemoglobin. After counting the WBCs in the bath, the dilution is transferred to the built-in hemoglobinometer for hemoglobin determination. The RBC bath and Hgb cuvet then drain to the waste chamber. The burn circuit is activated to clear the apertures. The baths and Hgb cuvet are then rinsed. High vacuum is used to prime the sweep-flow lines and draw off any remaining cells into the vacuum regulator. The aspirator is backwashed to minimize carryover.

The analyzer is the third component. It contains the electronic and computing circuits needed to control the sequence of operations in the diluter and to process the data it generates. It is in the analyzer that size distributions are generated by the pulse size and individual pulses are categorized into size channels. Each channel on the X axis represents one femtoliter (fl). Each division on the Y axis represents one cell in that channel (Fig. 16-3). This size distribution forms a histogram that is used to determine the MCV and the red cell distribution width (RDW). The RDW is an index of the variation in red cell size or anisocytosis. On the Coulter S Plus II* and later models, it is computed directly from the histogram and represents the coefficient of variation of red cell volume distribution:

$$RDW = \frac{SD}{mean} \times 100$$

Oscilloscope

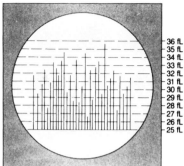

Histogram

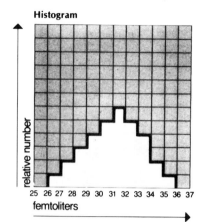

Figure 16-3. Individual pulses shown on oscilloscope are categorized into specific size channels forming the histogram. Each channel on the X axis represents size in femtoliters. Each division on the Y axis represents one cell in that channel. Histograms are used to determine the average size of the cells within a population, to determine the width of the distribution about the mean, and to analyze subpopulations within a main population. (Courtesy of Coulter Electronics, Inc, Hialeah, FL)

In the original S Plus, the RDW was obtained by the formula

$$RDW = \frac{A - B}{A + B} \times K$$

where A and B are the red cell volumes at which 20% and 80%, respectively, of the sampled RBCs are larger than that volume and K is a constant.

The analyzer also corrects the counts for coincidence and, using electronic editing, excludes pulses from cells that did not pass through the center of the aperture. It then compares the three corrected RBC counts; the same type of correction is made for WBC and platelet counts. If they are in close agreement, it reports an average. If only two are in agreement, the computer disregards the third count and reports an average of the two counts. If no values are within tolerance, it rejects the count.

The RBC dilution contains red cells, platelets, and white cells. To separate platelets from the other cells, the instrument takes advantage of the size difference between these particles. Particles between 2 μm^3 and 20 μm^3 are analyzed as platelets. Particles 36 μm^3 or larger are analyzed as red cells. Because the number of white cells (thousands) is normally insignificant as compared to red cells (millions), the analyzer does not attempt to remove them from the count. Therefore, the technologist must remember to subtract out the number of white cells when the number becomes significant (usually considered as >50,000/cmm), and to recalculate all indices because of sizing and Hgb turbidity errors.

In order to count platelets and compute the MPV, several improvements had to be made. These include smaller apertures (50 μm $\times$ 60 μm as opposed to

100 μm $\times$ 75 μm) to sense red cells and platelets, and improved statistical reliability by making more platelets available for counting. This was accomplished by decreasing the RBC dilution from 1:50,000 to 1:6,250 and extending the counting interval when the count was low. In addition, the swirling effect of diluent behind the aperture as particles are pulled through was eliminated by the installation of sweep-flow lines carrying diluent behind the apertures to sweep cells away from the sensing zone once they had been counted. This prevents larger cells from swirling behind the aperture, nicking the outside of the sensing zone and being counted again as a platelet. The addition of a built-in 64-channel pulse-height analyzer counting the number of particles in 64 equal-sized channels between 2 and 20 μm^3 allows the creation of a 64-channel histogram from the raw data. A computer then smoothes this histogram by using the moving average technique to identify two important points or valleys (minimums) immediately to the left and right of the mode. These valleys will become the thresholds between which data on this patient's platelet count will be based. The computer then generates a log-normal distribution curve based on the "raw data" between the two valley thresholds. This curve, referred to as the *fitted curve,* extends from 0 to 70 μm^3. If the valleys, mode, and histogram do not meet certain preset criteria, no platelet count will be printed.

Hemoglobin concentration is based upon photoelectric measurements of transmittance of light at a wavelength of 525 nm through a cuvet containing the lysed WBC dilution. While the WBC dilution is entering the WBC bath, the Hgb-blank pump transfers 5 ml of diluent into the Hgb cuvet. The Hgb blank is read by the photometer at the same time that the WBCs are being counted. The blank is then drained into the waste chamber and the remaining WBC dilution is transferred to the Hgb cuvet where it will be read. This voltage is compared to the reference voltage of the blank in the analyzer to calculate the Hgb concentration. This photometric measurement correlates well with the hemiglobin cyanide method.

The printer transfers the parameter values to printout cards, and an optional component, the data terminal, then displays the data captured and processed by the analyzer; displays the WBC, RBC, and platelet histograms; derives the lymph percent; computes the absolute lymphocyte count; and provides a quality control package. This extends the original eight parameters to 12. Those directly measured are the WBC, RBC, and Hgb. The computed parameters are the Hct, MCH, MCHC, and the lymphocyte number. The MCV and RDW are derived from the RBC histogram; the MPV, PDW, and PLT counts are derived from the PLT histogram; and the lymphocyte percent is derived from the WBC histogram. A three-part differential is an option that features four additional parameters: percent mononuclear cells, percent granulocytes, and absolute numbers for both. The final component, the matrix printer/plotter, provides a hard copy of the data displayed on the data terminal. This component is also optional.

Additional features found on the S Plus series above the Plus I* include $\overline{X}$B analysis, size reference histogram plots, user control of flagging limits, and nine quality control data files. The S Plus V* also includes a cap piercer, which permits aspiration directly from sealed collection tubes.

SYSMEX E-5000

The Sysmex E-5000* is an automated analysis system that is also based on electrical resistance. However, there is an added feature. The RBC and PLT counting systems employ hydrodynamic focusing to help eliminate coincidence. Hydrodynamic focusing is achieved by centering the sample stream into a sheath-flow configuration. The sheath fluid surrounds the sample stream and narrows it so that cells flow in single file through the aperture. This process accomplishes three things: first, it reduces coincidence counting and sizing because virtually all cells pass through single file; second, it reduces friction-caused interference on pulse height by focusing cells in the center of the stream; and finally, it eliminates recirculating cell paths because cells are carried away from the aperture before they can create a smaller pulse by swirling and nicking the sensing zone.

This system consists of a processor unit, a computer unit, a pneumatics supply, a ticket printer, and a graphics printer. It requires 200 μl of blood to yield 15 parameters (WBC, RBC, Hgb, Hct, MCV, MCH, MCHC, PLT, RDW, platelet distribution width [PDW], WBC small cell ratio [W-SCR], WBC middle cell ratio [W-MCR], mean platelet volume [MPV] and platelet large cell ratio [P-LCR]) along with histograms. The hemoglobin is determined by the cyanmethemoglobin method.

Additional features include a 300-sample memory, bar code reader, histogram recall from memory, nine quality control files, and $\overline{X}$m moving average. According to the manufacturer, the unit can process blood samples for 50 minutes without an operator because of the autosampler system. It can process up to 119 samples per hour.

ELT-8/WS

There are several models in the ELT line; the model discussed here is the ELT-8/WS*, but most of the principles apply to the other ELT models as well. The principle of cell counting in this instrument is based on light scatter. These instruments are basically flow-through cell-counting systems or cytometers, in which the light is scattered by the passage of blood cells, causing a signal detectable by the instrument. The light source used is a helium-neon laser (*laser* is an acronym for light amplification by stimulated emission of radiation). The lasers provide a very coherent emitted light and this characteristic allows the light beam, with the aid of lenses, to be focused so small that its intense light can illuminate a single red blood cell. In addition to the seven basic parameters plus platelets, the instrument provides histograms and a three-part differential screen.

At the heart of the ELT-8/WS system is the flowcell assembly, functionally consisting of three parts—a sample nozzle, a sheath funnel, and a quartz flowcell. The movement of blood and reagents through the counter is accomplished by a system of pumps and valves. The unit contains 12 pumps mounted on two drive units or cam blocks. There are two main parts—a sample handler and a data handler.

After aspiration of 100 μl of blood, the sample is split into two approximately equal aliquots. One portion is diluted and split to permit WBC enumeration. The second aliquot is diluted and split again. One portion of the second split is diluted to permit the hemoglobin determination via a modified cyanmethemoglobin method in a colorimeter. The other portion of this second split is diluted again and the cells are optically sized and counted to make RBC, Hct, and platelet determinations (Fig. 16-4).

We will trace the RBC/PLT aliquot to better understand the counting procedure. The sample stream is injected into the center of a flowing buffered saline sheath stream (hydrodynamic focusing). The sheath fluid narrows to a 250-μm stream with the sample stream narrowed to 20 μm. This hydrodynamic focusing of the sample stream is combined with the development of laminar flow causing the sample fluid to be surrounded by sheath fluid and centered within the quartz flowcell. In laminar flow, the fluid passing closest to a solid barrier is slowed by friction. Thus, the fluid becomes effectively "layered" in velocity with the center of the stream moving much faster than the periphery. The blood sample is, therefore, injected into and carried with the fastest moving part of the stream, the center portion. The high speed of the sample flow places cells in virtually single-file configuration allowing very little interference between cells. The cells are counted while incorporated in this laminar flow, which maintains the cells in an effective fluid aperture at the center of the laser beam. The RBCs, platelets, and WBCs are all counted in the flowcell; however, the WBC count is made later in time than the RBC/platelet determination.

The optical subsystem consists of a red helium–neon gas laser focused to the quartz flowcell. Two photoelectric sensors, one to detect forward scatter and the other to detect right-angle scatter, detect laser light scattered as the cell passes through the sensing zone. A narrow metal strip serves as a "blocker bar" to prevent the direct beam of laser light from reaching the forward scatter sensor (Fig. 16-5).

When no cells are in the sensing zone, the laser beam passes through the flowcell and falls onto a "blocker bar." Therefore, if no cells are in the chamber, there is no light scatter and no output from the photosensors. As a cell passes through the laser beam, a part of the light is scattered forward and at right angles by its interaction with the cell. The scattered light hits the photodetectors where it is changed to a voltage pulse representative of the cell. Each pulse is compared to threshold requirements and is classified. Red blood cells and platelets are counted at the same time and separated by pulse size. Only forward scatter is considered when determining these two cell types. (In models that do not have the three-part differential, forward scatter is all that is measured for WBCs also.) The Hct values are based upon pulse size measurements of the amount of laser light scattered during RBC counting. Indices are calculated in the data handler.

During the WBC count phase, electronic pulses are generated as a result of both forward and right-angle light scatter characteristics of the cells analyzed. Light scattered from a biologic cell or any object is not confined to forward scatter. This light scatter can also be useful in cellular determination. Low-angle light scatter intensity tends to be dominated by light bent by the outside surface of the cell (diffraction effects). Intensity at larger angles is due primarily to refraction

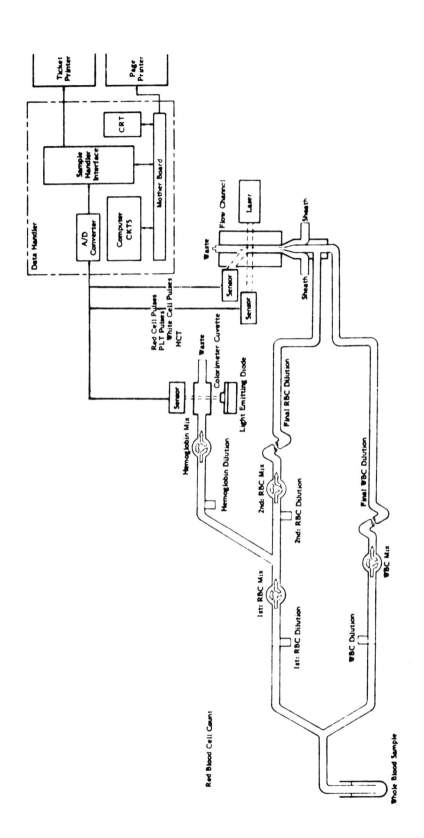

Figure 16-4. Schematic diagram of overall system of operation in the ELT-8/WS. (Courtesy of Ortho Diagnostic Systems, Westwood, MA)

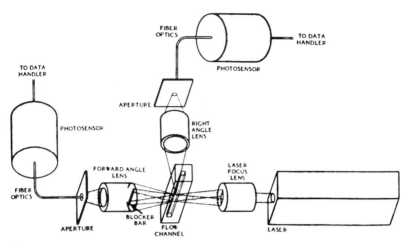

Figure 16-5.   ELT-8/WS optical subsystem. (Courtesy of Ortho Diagnostic Systems, Westwood, MA)

and reflection from reasonably large structures, primarily granules inside the cell. Therefore, granulocytes and monocytes tend to scatter more intensely at large angles than do lymphocytes. These pulses are transformed into a combined scatter histogram that displays debris, lymphocytes, monocytes, and granulocytes. A software algorithm locates the separation points between these categories. The total WBC count is the sum of the cells counted in the lymphocyte, monocyte, and granulocyte regions. The ratio of each cell type to the total WBC count determines the percentage of these cell classes.

The hemoglobin measurement is the result of a modified cyanmethemoglobin method in which light from a light-emitting diode is transmitted through a transparent cuvet to a light sensor. The output of the sensor when measuring the sample is compared to that when measuring the hemoglobin blank. The difference represents the hemoglobin value of the sample.

There is an elaborate quality control system for storage of control values, calculation of means, standard deviations, and coefficients of variation. Levy-Jennings graphs are charted, histograms are observed, and operator set flagging of abnormal specimens is done automatically. The patient population is also monitored to give mechanical information on the system by using Bull's formula (the $\overline{X}B$), called the moving average.[2] Instrument setup time is about 15 to 20 minutes. The instrument is then operational for runs and/or stat work.

The ELT-15 and ELT-1500 (the 1500 is faster than the 15) give 15 parameters: the standard seven parameters, relative and absolute values for the three-part screen, and an additional parameter, the red cell morphology index (RCMI). This parameter is a Z-score analysis of RBC dispersion. Like the RDW, it is an estimate of anisocytosis.

H6000 Counter

The other major cell-counting system based upon light scatter is the H6000. The electro-optical detection system is made up of four optical assemblies, which are axially positioned around a common tungsten-halogen light source. An overview of the system can be found in Figure 16-6.

The system gives the following parameters: WBC, RBC, Hgb, Hct, MCV, MCH, MCHC, PLT, and relative and absolute numbers for neutrophils, lymphocytes, monocytes, eosinophils, large unstained cells, cells with high peroxidase activity, and basophils. A RBC and platelet histogram are also produced. If the system is equipped with an Autoslide*, a labelled slide will be made on each patient that can be visually reviewed, when necessary.

A minimum of 2 ml whole blood is necessary for automatic stirring and sampling of the bloods to occur. Forty blood samples are identified by an optical reader that reads a printer label affixed to a holder into which the blood sample tube is placed. Each tube is mixed automatically by a paddle just prior to sampling. A sampling tube is lowered into the blood tube and aspirates 560 μl of blood if the system is equipped with the optional Autoslide system. If it is not, it aspirates 220 μl of whole blood.

The aspirated sample is diluted and divided into three streams, one for each of the three analytical manifolds: RBC/PLT/Hgb manifold, alkaline peroxidase manifold, and basophil manifold.

The RBC/PLT/Hgb manifold contains two channels—Hgb and RBC/PLT. Upon entering this manifold, the sample is diluted and resampled to each of the two channels. In the Hgb channel, the sample is added to a Hgb diluent reagent that lyses the RBCs and converts the hemoglobin to cyanmethemoglobin. This resulting solution flows to the Hgb colorimeter, which is also divided into two channels, a sample and a reference channel. The sample channel measures the absorbance at 550 nm of the sample stream as it passes through the flowcell. The reference channel is optically identical to the sample channel and is used to compensate for any variation in the output of the lamp. The electrical outputs from the sample and reference phototubes are sent to the log ratio module assembly for processing.

In the RBC/PLT channel, the sample is diluted and routed to the RBC/PLT optic's system. The flow rate of the sample stream is controlled by an individual peristaltic-type sample-stream pump, which provides a constant sample volume in the flowcell. Each sheath reagent is also controlled by a peristaltic pump. The sample stream enters the flowcell at point A, and the optically transparent sheath fluid enters at point B (Fig. 16-7). The velocities of the sample and sheath fluids are controlled so that laminar flow conditions exist. It is the hydraulic pressure of the sheath stream that constricts the sample stream to a diameter of 45 to 50 μm.

The RBC/PLT optics assembly has two detection channels—the photodiode scatter-detection channel to count RBCs and a photomultiplier tube (PMT) scatter-detection channel to detect platelets. In the photodiode scatter-detection channel, light passes through a beam splitter to a dark-field disk. The beam splitter deflects light upward by reflection toward the PMT while also allowing light to pass through to a dark-field disk directly behind and ultimately, if cells are present, to the photodiode. Direct light will be blocked from reaching the photodiode by the dark-field disk (Fig. 16-8). If a cell (RBC or WBC) is present in the flowcell, light is scattered through the annular opening in the dark-field disk and focused onto the

(*Text continues on p. 228.*)

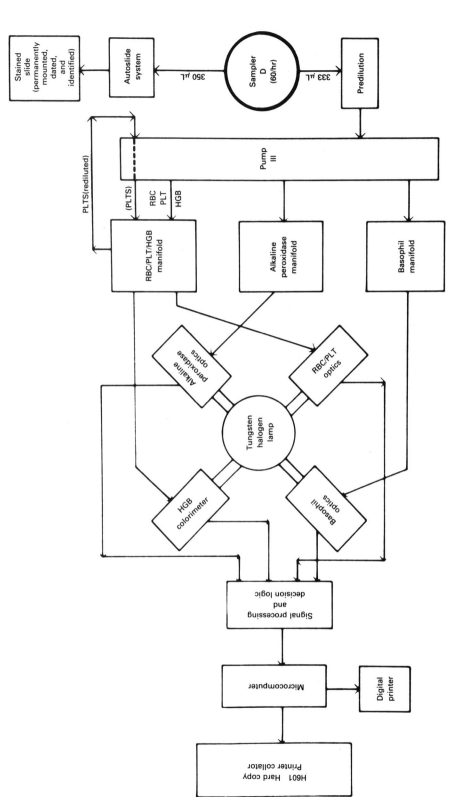

Figure 16-6. Schematic flow diagram of the H6000. (Reprinted from Hosty TA, Harris LG, Stonacek SM, Frazier B: Evaluation of an automated continuous-flow hematology instrument: The Technicon H6000. J Clin Lab Automation 2:408, 1982; courtesy of Appleton-Century-Crofts)

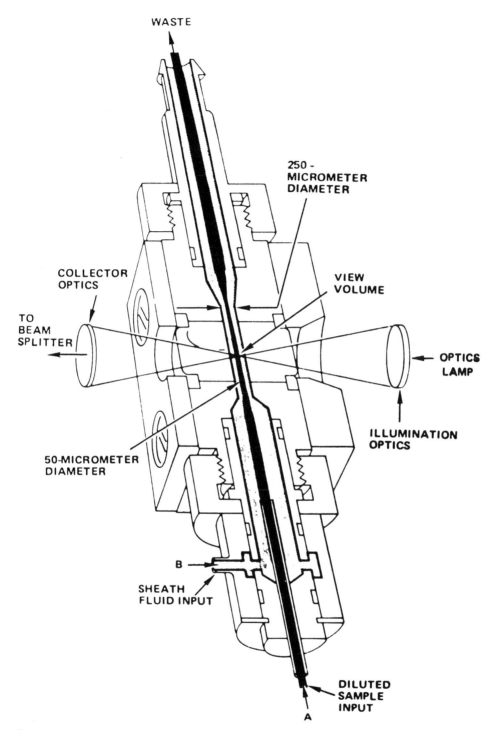

WASTE

250 - MICROMETER DIAMETER

VIEW VOLUME

COLLECTOR OPTICS

TO BEAM SPLITTER

OPTICS LAMP

ILLUMINATION OPTICS

50-MICROMETER DIAMETER

B

SHEATH FLUID INPUT

DILUTED SAMPLE INPUT

A

Figure 16-7. Sheath-stream flowcell in H6000. The sample stream enters the flowcell at point A and the optically transparent sheath fluid enters at point B. (Courtesy of Technicon Instruments Corporation, Tarrytown, NY)

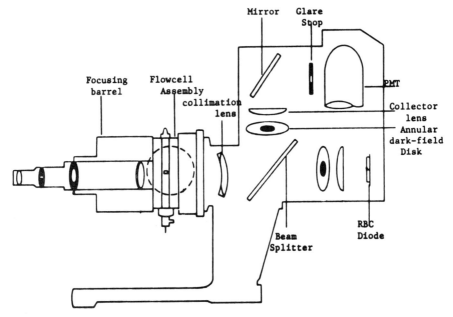

Figure 16-8. Flowcell and optical detection system for detection of RBCs and platelets in the H6000. (Courtesy of Technicon Instruments Corporation, Tarrytown, NY)

photodiode. The amount of scattered light and the pulse it generates are proportional to cell size. Platelet scatter is too weak to be picked up by the RBC photodiode.

The PMT channel is used to detect platelets. Light is reflected up by the beam splitter to a dark-field disk. Scattered light that passes this disk is reflected by a mirror toward the PMT. A glare stop prevents extraneous light (noise) from hitting the PMT. The PMT provides the sensitivity and amplification required to isolate platelet scatter signals from that of noise or from RBC scatter. The outputs from the photodiode and the PMT are sent to the RBC/PLT signal-processing circuits.

The WBCs are enumerated in the alkaline peroxidase optics assembly in much the same way as the RBCs are counted in the RBC/PLT optics. Red blood cells are lysed and the WBC count is derived from the scatter diode detection channel of the alkaline peroxidase optics assembly. When no cells are present in the sheath-stream flowcell, the dark-field disk in front of the lens collector prevents all light from reaching the photodiode. The scatter diode detects light only when a cell passes through the flowcell and scatters light through the annular opening around the dark-field disk. The photodiode produces an electrical signal proportional to the size (area) of the cell in the flowcell. The two WBC manifolds will be discussed further with automation of differentials.

Weighted Moving Average Concept on Multiparameter Counters
The concept of "weighted moving averages" is used as an immediate reacting, internally kept quality control mechanism for RBC parameters on several mul-

tichannel instruments. In the S Plus series with a data terminal, this concept is called $\overline{X}B$ (read X bar B); on the ELT-8/ds* and ELT-8/WS, it is termed *moving average library;* and on the System E-5000, the concept is termed $\overline{X}M$. Some differences will exist as to batch size, editing functions, and computer capabilities and print-outs, but the basic concept is the same.

The concept of using RBC indices (MCV, MCH, MCHC) as a means of quality control originated with Brian S. Bull.[2] Further studies indicate that red cell indices of the population of medium to large hospitals are stable over time.[4] This characteristic of stability is used in Bull's $\overline{X}B$ analysis algorithm as the basis of a quality control system that can be used on multichannel instruments. Its function is to enable reliable estimates of a population to be made from relatively small samples of that population. The formula trims the data by giving less weight to outliers, and smoothes it by incorporating information from the previous patient batch. The square root does the trimming function because it gives proportionally less weight to results that are farther from the expected mean.

Initially, population means are established by analyzing as large a sample population as possible, ideally 1000 blood samples. Once the population means have been established, the $\overline{X}B$ analysis can be applied using reasonably small patient samplings. The original means become the target values and are stored in the data terminal. The limits and percent differences are also stored. The indices determined are stable within 1% of the patient population mean. Some systems have broadened the limits to ±3% of the mean. As each sample is processed, the means of each of the red cell indices are subtracted from the corresponding mean established from the previous set of samples. The square root of the differences between these means is stored. After 20 patient samples (using 20 samples as the batch size) have been processed, the sum of these square roots is divided by 20. The result is squared to obtain the average (mean) deviation. The individual deviations carry a positive or negative sign, so they can be added to or subtracted from the corresponding previous means. The resulting new mean is then used for the succeeding batch of 20 samples. If the batch of patient samples falls outside the limits (3% of the mean), the batch is reviewed. If the $\overline{X}B$ is out owing to abnormal patient indices, these results can be edited out and the $\overline{X}B$ can be reaveraged by the machine. If all the results are somewhat abnormal, especially if more than one $\overline{X}B$ batch does not read, the instrument should be checked and controls should be run. The parameter that is out can also help pinpoint what direction to examine when trouble-shooting the instrument.

Calibration of Multiparameter Instruments

Automated hematology equipment presents a unique problem because, other than for hemoglobins, calibrator products do not meet the guidelines of being standards. As a general rule, it is best to follow the recommended procedure suggested by the instrument manufacturers.

Some guidelines have been established by independent groups. Usually, the recommended procedure by hematologists has been whole blood calibration, but studies have failed to show a significant difference between instruments that have been whole blood calibrated and those that have been calibrated with commercial calibrators.[3]

The current concept held by the Hematology Resource Committee is that fresh whole blood calibration is the standard against which other methods of calibration should be compared. However, they no longer hold that this is the method that must be required. Instead, they say that if commercial control material is used for calibration, the accuracy of the calibration must be verified. Recommended procedures to verify the accuracy of the control include (1) analyzing the manufacturer's stated values by analyzing the material with reference material, (2) demonstrating that the newly calibrated instrument gives results on commercial material produced by a second manufacturer that are in agreement with that manufacturer's stated values, or (3) by demonstrating that at least three whole blood specimens run on the newly calibrated instrument and on reference methods are within agreement.[3]

The ELT-8/WS and the H6000 require daily calibration checks. Adjustment is made when necessary. The manufacturers will suggest certain calibration materials that should be used. The S Plus series can be calibrated with S Cal* or with other products assayed on the reagent system in use on your instrument. Generally, the S Plus series is only calibrated if a shift in values exists, or if the blood sampling valve or apertures have been changed. If platelets are also done on back-up equipment, it may be advisable to do whole blood calibration on your platelet parameter, to retain consistency between methods.

PLATELET COUNTERS

Prior to 1910, platelets were presumed to be cellular debris originating from leukocyte destruction. In 1910, J.H. Wright reported that platelets were cytoplasmic fragments of megakaryocytes found in the bone marrow. Enumeration of these elements, which in 1912 were found to be involved in coagulation, was first reported by Dameshek in 1932.[6] The first methods involved examining stained blood smears.

Phase microscopy and the hemocytometer facilitated platelet counting. The use of anticoagulants allowed platelet-rich plasma (PRP) to be prepared by low-speed rapid centrifugation or sedimentation techniques from whole blood. Then, the Coulter counter was developed, which counted RBCs and WBCs. Reduction in the size of the aperture, use of PRP, and modifications in diluents facilitated platelet counting on the automatic cell counters. The first instrument for counting platelets used the cell-counting principle of electrical impedance. Modifications to this technique have made it possible for some counters to use whole blood instead of PRP. Hydrodynamic focusing has reduced coincidence and aperture plugging in several of these units.

Mean Platelet Volume

Pulse-height discrimination (thresholding) is essential for distinguishing debris from various cell types. Cell-size-distribution histograms can be constructed from pulse-height data. This information has gained importance during the past decade as people have looked into the possibility that mean platelet volume (MPV) may indicate age (bigger being younger), functional ability, and possibly a disorder.

Increased MPVs have been seen in the Bernard-Soulier syndrome, myelofibrosis, idiopathic thrombocytopenia purpura, splenectomy, chronic myelogenous leukemia, and sickle cell anemia.[4,8] Decreased MPVs have been noted in hypersplenism, postchemotherapy, the Wiskott-Aldrich syndrome, aplastic anemia, and megaloblastic anemia.[4,8] The exact value is somewhat difficult to determine because size distributions and survival data have to be correlated with the MPV. Most multiparameter automated systems that give platelet counts can also give the MPV. The value is calculated from the platelet histogram in the same fashion as the MCV is derived from the RBC histogram.

The normal range in platelet size varies with the platelet count. There is an inverse relationship between platelet count and size in normal patients (*i.e.,* the size increases as the count decreases). This relationship is shown by nomogram (Fig. 16-9).[1,4]

The nomogram shows that an MPV between 9.0 and 9.8 fl is normal, but that other values may or may not be, depending upon the platelet count. Exact values of the MPV verses count will vary with the brand of instrument, but the shape of the nomogram will remain the same.

One should also be aware that platelets undergo a swelling and shape change in EDTA anticoagulant.[7] This causes the platelets and, therefore, the MPV to increase in size about 20% during the first hour or so, after which the MPV will remain stable for about 12 hours. Evaluation of MPV should be done within 1 to 4 hours after the blood is drawn.[4]

Platelets as Counted on Multiparameter Instruments

Platelet counting on the multiparameter instruments is discussed under specific cell counters. To summarize briefly, the S Plus series uses the principle of electrical impedance to count platelets. A histogram is formed from which the platelet count, MPV, and PDW are derived (Fig. 16-10). The Sysmex E-5000 also uses this principle, with the addition of hydrodynamic focusing. The ELT-8 series

MPV Nomogram

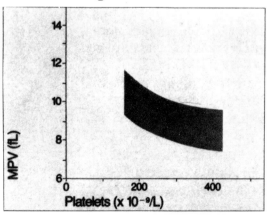

Figure 16-9. MPV nomogram. In normal patients there is an inverse relationship between platelet count and size, as depicted by this nomogram. (Courtesy of Coulter Electronics, Inc, Hialeah, FL)

Normal Platelet Histogram

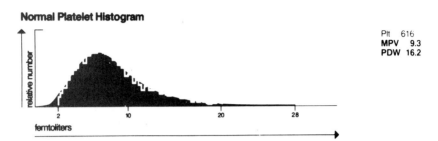

Plt   616
MPV 9.3
PDW 16.2

Figure 16-10. Normal platelet histogram as seen on the S Plus series. The computer counts particles between 2 and 20 femtoliters. The raw data, shown as a solid line, is tested against a set of mathematical criteria and fitted to a log normal curve from 0 to 70 femtoliters represented by the shaded area. The platelet count, MPV, and PDW are derived from this histogram. (Courtesy of Coulter Electronics, Inc, Hialeah, FL)

determines platelets based on the principles of laminar flow hydrodynamic centering of cells prior to counting using a laser optics system. The operator is informed if giant platelets (or microcytic RBCs) represent greater than 4% of the patient population. The H6000 uses light scatter to determine platelet count.

Dedicated Platelet Counters

The dedicated counters all use the electrical impedance principle of counting platelets. Several systems such as the Celltrak-Plt counter, the MK4/HC*, and the Thrombocounter-C* use PRP for the specimen. The whole blood value is derived by using the patient's hematocrit and a special thumbwheel correction chart. The Celltrak-Plt counter also has error alert indicators and power orifice clog removal. The Series 810* is a microprocessor-controlled electrical impedance counter that uses hydrodynamic focusing and flush and air purging cycles between assays. It has a "micro RBC" alert that tells the operator of a significant number of particles greater than 30 fl. A "macro Plt" and noise alarm are also included to aid the operator. A "micro Plt" count mode is used if giant platelets are present. It can use either whole blood or PRP samples, as can the Cell-Dyn 100*.

The Ultra-Flo 100* is an electrical impedance counter that also uses hydrodynamic focusing. The operator uses a thumbwheel setting on the instrument to enter the patient's RBC count. The system has two electronic windows. One is used to count platelets and the other is used to count RBCs. A 1:910 dilution of patient blood and diluent is made in a special counting unopette. The instrument's counting chamber has a pressurized hydrodynamic focusing aperture with front and back fluid sheaths. A pressurized container of sheath fluid provides the hydrodynamic focusing action. During counting, the cells suspended in diluent are focused by sheath-fluid action through the central axis of a 60-μm diameter aperture. The back sheath fluid removes the counted sample from the back of the aperture to prevent the generation of a second pulse from one particle. Amplitude discrimination allows platelets and blood cells (RBCs mainly) to be sorted and accumulated in separate channels. Particles between the thresholds of 3.25 to 40 fl are normally counted. If excessive noise exists between 1.75 to 3.25, a "lower valley" alarm lights on the front panel. If excessive numbers of particles exist between 40 and 43 fl, an "upper valley" alarm alerts the operator to the presence of microcytic RBCs or giant platelets. A second counting mode, the "micro" mode, can then be used to shift the upper threshold of platelets from 40 to 30 fl. After a number of RBCs equal to 1% of the RBC count has been reached, the counting process stops. The raw count from the platelet window is divided, processed, and reported on the light-emitting diode as platelets $\times$ 10^9/liter. The system is equipped with several alert levels, an audible cadence counter, and flow gauge to alert the operator to system and specimen irregularities. Counts with persistent alarms should be verified by phase microscopy.

Not all patient specimens can be counted on electrical or automated counters. Some counters reject the majority of problematic specimens; others do not. Nevertheless, aside from running known controls on your instrument, all reported platelet counts should be correlated against an estimate of platelet number on the peripheral smear to detect any individual patient platelet problems. The bottom line is that, although platelet instrumentation has greatly improved speed and precision in the majority of the patient population, no instrument is infallible. Cytoplasmic fragments, schistocytes, electronic noise, platelet clumps or satellitism, rouleaux, drugs, and so forth can affect an occasional count.

Differential Counters

Automated differentials were first attempted in the mid-1960s. However, the technology at the time prevented the development of a practical instrument. The first instrument was manufactured by Perkin-Elmer and was essentially an automated microscope attached to a computer. Although a 100-cell differential took many hours to perform, it could recognize lymphocytes, monocytes, and neutrophils with 90% accuracy. In the 1970s, technology of sophisticated cameras, integrated circuits, computer speed, and advanced measuring techniques allowed for a more practical approach to this form of instrumentation. In October 1972, the Hematrak* Differential Counter and the Larc* (Leukocyte Automatic Recognition Computer) were introduced. They were based on the principle of pattern recognition. Later, the Diff 3*, the ADC-500*, and the Diff 350* and Diff 4* were introduced. The Diff 350 and Diff 4 were updates on the Diff 3, which Coulter aquired from Perkin-Elmer. In 1975, another differential counter was introduced, the Hemalog D*. This instrument was based on a different principle of operation, which was flow cytochemical analysis.

Today, only the Hematrak and the H6000 instruments and updated models are marketed, although some of the others may still be in operation.

In addition to the complete differential systems, an abbreviated differential or screening system was developed in 1983. This screen divides cells into three cell populations. The S Plus IV and V, ELT-8/WS, and Sysmex E-5000 can all give a three-part differential screen in addition to at least eight other cell-counting parameters.

Automation of differentials was attempted for many reasons, such as for speed, improved precision and accuracy, and to reduce differential fatigue. The largest sources of error with manual eye-count differentials deal basically with three factors: slide-distribution errors, cell-recognition errors, and statistical sampling errors. Automated differential counters had to deal with the same problems. The slide-distribution problem was dealt with by "automating" the slide-making process, or, in the case of the Hemalog D, by eliminating the slide. Statistical sampling was aided by counting larger numbers of cells in short periods of time, and cell recognition was standardized to deal with subjectivity of cell call.

There are two basic approaches to automation of differentials: pattern recognition (image processing) and flow-through cytochemical instrumentation. *Pattern recognition* can be briefly defined as a process of capturing a cell image electronically and extracting features to classify cell type by computer-assisted image analysis. Most instruments utilize the principle of pattern recognition. The other approach seen in the Hemalog D and H6000 is *flow-through cytochemical determination*. In brief, this can be defined as a process in which determination of cell type is done by selectively staining cells based on enzyme or heparin components, and analyzing these stained cells electro-optically in a flow-through system.

PATTERN-RECOGNITION DIFFERENTIAL AUTOMATION

The concept of pattern recognition is not new. Man-made symbols such as numbers have been read by computers for some time. Reading zip codes or checking account numbers is pattern recognition in its simplest form. The shape of each number is stored by using a series of masks. Numbers are identified by passing the mask over the image to see if there is a match. Machine classification of objects based on their characteristics uses a television-type camera to receive and transmit an electronic image to a computer, which processes the image and extracts the required data.

Despite this technology, applying the principle of pattern recognition to biologic cells is not as simple. Numbers or letters used in pattern-recognition systems are evenly spaced, always oriented in the same direction, and identical in shape, size, and color. Biologic cells, on the other hand, are never predictably spaced or oriented, are three-dimensional, and vary in size, shape, color, and texture. Consequently, it would take an infinite number of masks to handle every subtle difference. Another approach had to be used. Automated differential counters use a computer program to identify cell type, instead of masking techniques, in conjunction with high-speed cameras and feature extraction. Because the only instrumentation utilizing pattern recognition that is on the market today is the Hematrak, the following discussion will apply directly to the mechanics used in the models now marketed: the Hematrak 450*, 450QP*, and 590*.

HEMATRAK SYSTEMS

To accomplish its objective of determining a differential, the Hematrak is essentially doing three processes simultaneously: optical imaging, cellular recognition, and data output. These processes are accomplished by two computers and four (or five) microprocessors (five, if the model has a bar code reader). The microprocessors control functions such as printing, slide movement, focusing, high-speed scanning, operator interaction with the system, and the bar code reader. One computer is termed the *morphological analyzer,* which extracts features by electronic probing. The other is the *recognition computer,* which takes numbers from the morphological computer and, from this, analyzes and determines cell type.

The instrument can use either a wedge smear, if made by an automated slide-maker, or a spun smear. The slide is positioned below the objective by the system, it is oiled automatically, and the appropriate working area is found. This working area is determined by the unit if a wedge smear is used, or a particular Y-coordinate is located if the smear used is spun.

Location of cells is accomplished utilizing a flying spot. The light source for the flying spot is a cathode ray tube, which generates a beam of white light that moves back and forth across the microscope field (Fig. 16-11). In search mode, the light beam sweeps across the field at 1-micron spacings until it locates a nucleus of a cell (change in optical density). It then builds a 24 × 32 micron electronic window around the cell and the scan line spacing is decreased to 0.25 micron.

Light is focused down through the condenser where special filters called *dichroic mirrors* separate out three colors: green, blue, and red. Three separate photomultiplier tubes measure and convert this light energy into electrical energy. These three colors are each further divided into six levels (quantization). This provides 18 signals at every 0.25 × 0.25 block based on color and density alone.

Figure 16-11.   Cell location and scanning on the Hematrak system. When a dark object is located (nucleus), the scan sweep is reduced from 1 μm to every 0.25 μm and a 24 × 32 μm electronic window is built around the object. (Courtesy of Geometric Data, Wayne, PA)

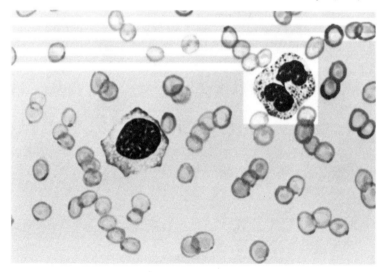

The lowest density level corresponds to cytoplasmic detail, the middle depicts the nucleus as a whole, and the highest density level depicts the darkest density portions of the chromatin pattern within the nucleus. Electronic images are transformed into digital signals and stored in image memory circuits.

A procedure called *line dropping* is also occurring. The microprocessors make measurements by placing lines or patterns across these images at many angles (Fig. 16-12). As the lines are electronically moved across the image, a statistical tally is made of the number of times both ends of the line either fit or do not fit inside the image. These lines vary in length from 0.25 micron to 10 microns. The smallest lines reveal information about the texture of the cell, middle size lines reveal information about the nuclear shape, and the longer lines tend to indicate the outer shape and the amount of cytoplasm.

In a matter of 17 milliseconds, 3,000,000 bits of data are generated for each cell examined. This raw data is processed to provide distinguishing features for each WBC. Many of these numbers correspond to cell size, chromatin pattern,

Figure 16-12.   Line dropping on the Hematrak system. As the lines are electronically moved across the image, a statistical tally is made of the number of times both ends of the line either fit or do not fit inside the image. The line represented by A to B would be a "hit" or "count," whereas the line C to D would not. The data is processed to generate the features of a cell. (Courtesy of Geometric Data, Wayne, PA)

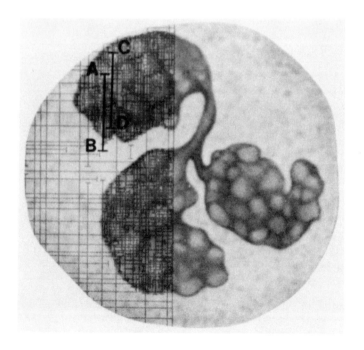

nuclear shape, nuclear/cytoplasmic (N/C) ratio, granularity and vacuolization—
things technologists judge also by sight. Other numbers generated have no visual
perception under the microscope. Red blood cells and platelets are processed
essentially the same way as WBCs. The morphological computer analyzes RBCs
for size, shape, and hemoglobin density. Platelets are judged on nuclear density
and size information. Platelets are counted as particles from 0.4 to 4 microns in
diameter in the first 30 fields.

The recognition computer is a programmable minicomputer that develops
mathematical parameters for each cell and compares this to data in step-by-step
logic-tree fashion with data stored in memory. Cells that do not fit within stringent
classification criteria will be relocated during cell review and presented to the
operator for classification. Up to 50 unclassified cells can be stored per differential.
If more than 50 are found, manual review is necessary. This program is also stored
on a floppy disk so that it can be reloaded and normal function can be resumed
in case of power failure.

After the analyzer has processed the slides, the operator must review all
suspect cells and slides that have exceeded the user's flagging limits. The results
appearing on the monitor always represent 100%. Extra normal cells to equal the
number of abnormals classified are identified during the automatic scanning cycle.
At the time of operator review, these abnormal white cells are added to the
unclassified cell category. As the technologist identifies the unclassified cells, they
are sequentially added to the differential and the extra normal cells are removed.

The system's operating program is part of the software (floppy disk), which
makes many updates possible simply by changing to an updated disk. However,
some updates do require firmware changes.

The system has user-selectable thresholds for differentiating neutrophils into
segmented and band forms. It utilizes user-selectable flagging criteria, generates
Levy-Jennings quality control charts, and has a cell recall system that stores in
memory the location of a cell you wish to review at a later time. Additional
programs can be purchased for the system. These include a teaching pack, retic-
ulocyte counting, and T and B labelling utilizing the Immunogold technique.

The unit is calibrated in the factory and then tested in the field against factory
and local reference slides. These local reference slides are analyzed manually by
technologists in the user hospital. The results of each parameter are plotted on
scattergrams to determine if values fall within 95% confidence limits. The unit
should then be checked routinely by quality control slides. The parameters printed
are polys, bands, lymphs, monocytes, eosinophils, basophils, platelet estimates,
poikilocytosis, anisocytosis, microcytosis, macrocytosis, polychromasia, and hy-
pochromia. The following parameters will be printed on the auxillary printer, but
must be verified (identified) by the operator: atypical lymphocytes, immature
granulocytes, blasts, nucleated RBCs, unclassified cells, spherocytes, and target
cells. There are limitations to cell identification that the operator has to recognize;
toxic granulation and vacuolization of neutrophils, for example, can cause erro-
neous call. As a general rule, the WBC recognition program appears to be more
highly developed than that of abnormal RBC morphology.

FLOW-THROUGH CYTOCHEMICAL DIFFERENTIAL COUNTER

The flow-through cytochemical differential counter on the market today is the H6000. The system has evolved from a purely differential system to one that performs a complete blood count: WBC, RBC, Hgb, MCV, MCH, MCHC, RDW, PLT and absolute and relative percentages of neutrophils, lymphocytes, monocytes, eosinophils, basophils, and large unclassified cells. The counting portion has been discussed previously. This discussion will deal with the differential portion—the alkaline peroxidase manifold and the basophil manifold.

By definition, a *flow-through cytochemical differential counter* selectively stains cells on the basis of enzyme reactions and analyzes them by electro-optical means in a flow system. A minimum of 2 ml of blood collected in EDTA is required when using automatic sampling. Blood samples are placed in a sample tray and are identified by an optical reader that reads a printer label affixed to a holder into which the blood sample tube is placed. Each tube is mixed automatically just prior to sampling. A sampling tube is lowered into the tube and aspirates 220 μl of blood or 560 μl if equipped with the Autoslide system. The sample is divided into three streams and pumped to the three manifolds.

The common steps in the two leukocyte manifolds are (1) fixation to preserve cellular enzymes and to maintain cellular shape, (2) erythrocyte lysis to minimize optical interference, (3) cell staining, (4) cell counting, and (5) cell classification.

The staining in the alkaline peroxidase channel is from the reaction of 4-chloro-napthol with peroxidase. This cellular enzyme is present in neutrophils, monocytes, and eosinophils. When the reaction is carried out at a pH of 9.7, the staining is intense in eosinophils, moderate in neutrophils, light in monocytes, and nonexistent in lymphocytes. The sample stream from this manifold is routed to the alkaline peroxidase optics (Fig. 16-6). This optical assembly contains an absorption channel and a scatter channel (Fig. 16-13). Light from the exciter lamp passes through two lenses and apertures to be focused into an optical view cell. Light passing through the optical view cell is collimated and focused onto a beam splitter that sends light to each of the two detection channels. The scatter-detection channel measures the light-scattering characteristics of the cells, which are used to determine cell size and total number. In this channel, when there are no cells present, light passes through the illumination barrel onto the flowcell, through the collimation lens to the beam splitter. The dark-field disk will block out all direct light, and no light will strike the scatter diode. However, when cells are present in the optic path, they act as secondary sources of light. Light bouncing off the cell will scatter around the dark-field disk, be condensed, and strike the scatter detector. The greater the amount of light striking the scatter detector, the larger the cell. Therefore, the signal is directly proportional to the size of the cell. In the absorption channel, when no cells are present, all the light from the light path hits the beam splitter and passes upward to the absorption diode, resulting in 100% of the light striking the absorption detector. However, if the particular cell in the light path has staining quality, light will be absorbed into the cell and there will be less light striking the absorption detector. This will cause a decrease in the absorption photodiode output, which is proportional to the amount of light

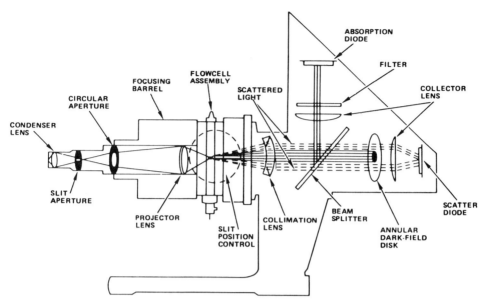

Figure 16-13. Alkaline peroxidase flowcell and optics detection system. (Courtesy of Technicon Instruments Corporation)

absorbed by the cell and, therefore, to the degree of cell staining. The outputs from the diodes are routed to the alkaline peroxidase signal processing circuits and decision logic circuits.

Absorption and scatter generated by each cell passing through the flowcell are plotted on the X-Y display. *Scattered* light (which depends on cell size) is measured along the Y axis. *Absorption* (representing enzyme activity) is measured along the X axis. In this peroxidase channel, there are two thresholds for scatter, low and high (S_L and S_H), and two for absorption, low and high (A_L and A_H). There are also two moving thresholds that automatically adjust to the slight differences in peroxidase staining qualities of each individual patient's neutrophils (Fig. 16-14). Signals falling below S_L are due to noise, platelets, or red-cell stroma. Signals between S_L and S_H are small cells; those above S_H are large cells. Cells to the left of A_L are unstained; those between A_L and A_H are moderately stained; and those to the right of A_H are intensely stained.

Staining in the basophil channel is the result of the reaction of alcian blue dye with heparin bound in the granules of basophils. The sample stream from this manifold is routed to the basophil optic assembly. The basophil optic assembly contains two scatter channels; one channel measures the light-scattering characteristics of the sample stream of red light and the other channel measures the light-scattering characteristics of green light. The outputs from each diode are sent to the basophil signal processing and decision logic circuits.

The X-Y display from the peroxidase channel shows seven regions corresponding to (1) neutrophils, (2) high peroxidase activity (HPX), frequently as-

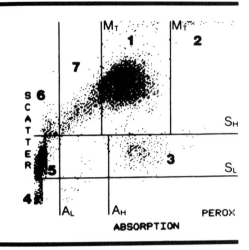

Figure 16-14. An X–Y display from the peroxidase channel of the H6000. Scattered light is measured along the Y axis and absorption is measured along the X axis. The threshold locations and cell types are depicted as follows: (*1*) neutrophils; (*2*) high peroxidase (HPX); (*3*) eosinophils; (*4*) platelets, erythrocyte stroma, noise; (*5*) lymphocytes; (*6*) large unstained cells; (*7*) monocytes and basophils; S_L = scatter low; S_H = scatter high; A_L = absorption low; A_H = absorption high; M_T = moving threshold. (Courtesy of Technicon Instruments Corporation, Tarrytown, NY)

sociated with immature cells, (3) eosinophils, (4) platelets, RBC stroma, and noise, (5) lymphocytes, (6) large unstained cells, and (7) monocytes and basophils. The monocyte value is obtained by subtracting the basophil count from the basophil channel out of the monocyte-basophil region derived from this histogram.

No assessment of RBC morphology is made; however, RBC indices, RDW, and RBC and platelet histograms are given.

The instrument must be recalibrated after each shutdown, and start-up takes about 30 minutes. If the instrument is left operational, it will continue to use reagents. Therefore, the instrument is best suited for batch work.

The unit can store up to 250 patient results and also stores quality control results with calculations of moving averages and graphic displays. All can be printed out.

PARTIAL DIFFERENTIALS ON MULTIPARAMETER COUNTERS

In 1983, three manufacturers announced the addition of a partial differential to their multiparameter cell counters. Cell counters with the three-part differential potential are S Plus IV/V/VI* and the ELT-8/WS. The Sysmex CC-800* with PDA-410* system provided a two-population screen, which has been updated to a three-population screen on the Sysmex E-5000. The full potential or exact extent of use has not been definitely established yet. The principle of operation for each of the three-population differential screens follows.

The S Plus IV, V, and VI three-part differential is based upon the Coulter principle of cell counting and sizing (electrical impedance). This, in brief, states that as a dilute suspension of cells is drawn through a small aperture, the passage of each individual cell (a nonconductor) will momentarily increase the resistance of the electrical path between two submerged electrodes located on each side of the aperture. Whereas the number of pulses indicates the particle count, the amplitude of the electrical pulse indicates cell volume or size. Each pulse is sorted by a series of thresholds according to its size. The individual pulses received from each of the three WBC apertures in the WBC bath are shown on the oscilloscope and categorized into specific size channels to form the WBC histogram (Fig. 16-3). Each channel on the X axis represents size in femtoliters. Each division on the Y axis represents one cell in that channel. The histogram, then, gives information to calculate the count, to average the size of the cells within the population, and to analyze subpopulations within the main population. To obtain the three-part differential on the S Plus systems, a special lysing reagent is used that acts on the cell membrane and cytoplasm, causing differential shrinkage of the cell types. This allows cells to be classified by their relative sizes. Although the WBC histogram displays all cells as small as 30 fl, only those greater than 35 fl are tallied. The lymphocytes are smaller than the mononuclear cells, which are smaller than the granulocytes (including eosinophils). Mononuclear cells are monocytes in normal patients; however, in abnormal patients, the mononuclear cell region includes blasts, promyelocytes, myelocytes, metamyelocytes, and other abnormal forms as well as monocytes. The WBC histogram is divided into four regions (Fig. 16-15). The total number of cells in these regions equals the total WBC count. Cells between 36 and 99 fl are classified as lymphocytes, cells between 100 and 200 fl are classified as mononuclear cells, and cells greater than 200 fl are classified as granulocytes. Abnormal subpopulations present in significant numbers may cause characteristic patterns in the histogram, which will cause the failure of certain mathematical criteria. This failure will cause a flag as indicated by an R to the right of the parameter. The number next to R (1, 2, 3, or 4) will indicate the region of failure. If more than one region shows interference, the multiple regions (RM) flag will print. In Figure 16-15, the R_1 flag indicates that the problem is in region 1, which might indicate nucleated RBCs. Any flagged results would warrant a manual differential.

The ELT-8/WS system uses an optical system for counting and differentiating cell types. Cells in laminar flow are hydrodynamically focused in a flowcell and

Figure 16-15. A WBC histogram from the S Plus IV equipped with an optional three-part differential screen. When the histogram fails certain mathematical criteria, the subpopulation percentages and numbers are flagged R_1, R_2, R_3, or R_4, indicating the region of interference. (Courtesy of Coulter Electronics, Inc, Hialeah, FL)

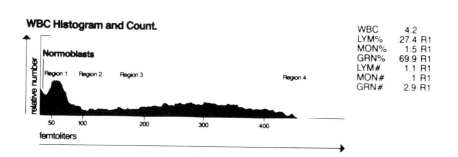

are illuminated by a helium-neon laser. The size of the cell is measured by the amount of light scattered by the cell at low-forward angle scatter as the cell passes through the laser beam. Intensity of low-angle scatter from cell-sized objects at visible wavelengths tends to be dominated by diffraction effects (light bent by the outside surface of the cell). Intensity at larger angles is due mainly to refraction and reflection from reasonably large structures inside the cell. Hence, monocytes tend to have more visible intracellular structure (complex nuclear shape and granules) than lymphocytes and granulocytes.

The first step in data analysis is to transform a two-parameter cytogram to a one-parameter histogram (Fig. 16-16). Because the light-scatter measurement of cells is made on intact, whole cells, the only purpose of the lysing reagent is to lyse RBCs. The reported screen consists of relative and absolute number values for lymphocytes, mononuclears, and granulocytes.

The Sysmex-E5000 is a newly introduced 15-parameter cell counter that also gives a three-part differential screen. The WBC detection system is based on electronic resistance utilizing hydrodynamic focusing. A special WBC lysing agent shrinks the cell membranes and cytoplasm, causing them to collapse and shrink down around the nucleus of the cell. This accentuates the size difference between

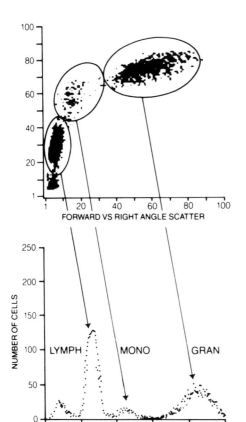

Figure 16-16. A cytogram-to-histogram transformation on the ELT-8/WS. (Courtesy of Ortho Diagnostics Systems, Westwood, MA)

lymphocytes and mature neutrophils. A third population falls into the center, which includes monocytes, immature granulocytes, blasts, eosinophils, and basophils. These populations appear on the histogram as small cells (W-SCR, meaning WBC small cell ratio), middle cells (W-MCR, meaning WBC middle cell ratio), and large cells (W-LCR, or WBC large cell ratio). The Y axis of the histogram represents relative cell number and the X axis shows cell volume. The trough between the cell populations is detected by the computer and not by the assignment of a specific point or cell-size threshold.

Summary

The production of cell-counting instruments based on the theory of electrical conductivity was revolutionary for the hematology laboratory. Cell counters today are based on one of two principles: electrical impedance and light scatter. Representative instruments were presented to demonstrate how these principles are utilized in operation. Special features of this instrumentation such as new parameters (RDW, MPV), sophisticated internal quality control programs ($\overline{X}B$), hydrodynamic focusing, and partial differentials were also presented and explained.

The second major advancement of hematology instrumentation was the automated differential system. The systems available today utilize either pattern recognition (image processing) or flow-through cytochemistry as their principles of operation. Both concepts were discussed in theory and operation.

The field of hematology seems to be exploding with new features and parameters. It is yet too early to know how some of these parameters, such as the MPV and partial differentials, will be utilized by the clinician.

Appendix

Trade Name	Company
1. ADC-500	Abbott Laboratories, Abbott Park, IL
2. Celltrak system	Angel Engineering Corp, Trumbull, CT
3. System 7000	Baker Instruments Corp, Allentown, PA
4. System 8000	Baker Instruments Corp
5. MK 4/HC	Baker Instruments Corp
6. Series 810	Baker Instruments Corp
7. Model HA-3D	Clay Adams, Parsippany, NJ
8. Ultra-Flo 100	Clay Adams
9. LARC system	Corning Medical & Scientific, Park Ridge, IL
10. Model A	Coulter Electronics, Inc, Hialeah, FL
11. Model Fn	Coulter Electronics, Inc
12. Model ZBI	Coulter Electronics, Inc
13. Model M430	Coulter Electronics, Inc
14. S Plus series (Models I through VI)	Coulter Electronics, Inc
15. S Cal (calibrator)	Coulter Electronics, Inc
16. Thrombocounter-C	Coulter Electronics, Inc
17. Diff 350	Coulter Electronics, Inc
18. Diff 4	Coulter Electronics, Inc
19. Hematrak systems, Models 450, 450QP, and 590	Geometric Data, Inc, Wayne, PA

20. Miniprep slidemaker	Geometric Data, Inc
21. Profile 750	Mallinchrodt, Inc, Marietta, OH
22. Profile 390 A	Mallinchrodt, Inc
23. ELT Series, Models ELT-7, ELT-8, ELT-800, ELT-8/ds, ELT-8/WS, ELT-15, ELT-1500	Ortho Diagnostic Systems, Westwood, MA
24. Diff 3	Perkin-Elmer, Oak Brook, IL
25. Cell-Dyn 100	Sequioa-Turner Corp, Mountain View, CA
26. Hemalog D	Technicon Instruments Corp, Inc, Tarrytown, NY
27. H-6000	Technicon Instruments, Corp, Inc
28. Autoslide slidemaker	Technicon Instruments, Corp, Inc
29. Sysmex series, models CC-800 and E-5000	TOA Medical Electronics, Inc, Carson, CA
30. PDA-410	TOA Medical Electronics, Inc

References

1. Bessman J, Williams LJ, Gilmer PR: Mean platelet volume: The inverse relation of platelet size and count in normal subjects and an artifact of other particles. Am J Clin Pathol 76(3):289, 1981
2. Bull BS, Elashoff RM, Heilbron DC, Couperus J: A study of various estimators for the derivation of quality control procedures from patient erythrocyte indices. Am J Clin Pathol 68:185, 1977
3. College of American Pathologists: Summing Up, Spring, 1985
4. Coulter Electronics Inc: Significant advances in hematology, pp 1–30. Hematology Education Series, May, 1984
5. Coulter WH: High speed automatic blood cell counter and size analyzer. Proc Natl Electron Conf 12:1034, 1956
6. Dameshek W: Method for simultaneous enumeration of blood platelets and reticulocytes. Arch Intern Med 50:579, 1932
7. Lippi V, Cappelletti P, Schinella M, Signori D: Mean platelet volumes: Facts or artifacts? Am J Clin Pathol 84:111, 1985
8. Roper PR, Johnston D, Austin J et al: Profiles of platelet volume distributions in normal individuals and in patients with acute leukemia. Am J Clin Pathol 68:449, 1977

Suggested Reading

Koepke JA: Laboratory Hematology. New York, Churchill Livingstone, 1984
Lee LW, Schmidt LM: Elementary Principles of Laboratory Instruments, 5th ed. St Louis, CV Mosby, 1983

17

AUTOMATED COAGULATION SYSTEMS
John D. Olson

Definitions

Conductivity: The ability of a substance to conduct an electric current.

Elasticity: The property that enables a substance to change its shape in response to a force and then to recover its original shape when the force is removed.

Impedance: The ratio of the force on a system undergoing harmonic motion to the velocity of the fluid in the system.

Light Scattering: The process in which light is diffused or deflected by particles in the medium that it traverses.

Polymerization: The combination of similar molecules to form a more complex, higher molecular weight product.

Synthetic Substrate: A compound formed in the laboratory that can act as a substrate for one or more enzymes. As used in this chapter, the synthetic substrate contains a chromogenic or fluorogenic component that is released by enzymatic cleavage.

Viscosity: The property of a fluid that resists the forces tending to cause it to flow.

Introduction

Plasma coagulation is a complex process that changes blood from a liquid to a solid when the soluble molecule, fibrinogen, is converted by the enzyme, thrombin, to an insoluble polymer, fibrin. *Thrombin generation* is the product of a highly complex and delicately regulated sequential activation of serine proteases and their cofactors. The details of the coagulation mechanism are of great interest but extend beyond the scope of this chapter.

There are some features of the coagulation mechanism, however, that are of interest in understanding the operation of the instruments to be described. It is important to realize that the conversion of fibrinogen to fibrin is a two-step reaction. First, fibrinopeptides are cleaved from the fibrinogen molecule by thrombin to form the fibrin monomer. The second step is the polymerization of fibrin monomers into a highly organized structure. This polymer of fibrin monomers (clot) is strong enough to withstand low levels of mechanical stress and can be measured. The formation of a stable covalently linked fibrin clot is dependent upon a second enzymatic reaction catalyzed by a plasma transaminase, fibrin-stabilizing factor (factor XIII). Once factor XIII has carried out its function and cross-linked the fibrin molecule, the fibrin clot becomes very rigid and resistant even to very high mechanical stress.

Instruments that measure the coagulation mechanism are all, in general, dependent upon the formation of the enzyme thrombin and most instruments subsequently measure the polymerization of the endogenous fibrin monomer (*i.e.,* the fibrin monomer derived from fibrinogen in the patient plasma). The formation of cross-linked fibrin (which is dependent upon the activated form of factor XIII) is usually not measured well by these instruments.

The mechanisms for the measurement of the coagulation endpoint can be categorized as follows: (1) conductivity, (2) elastic modulus or mechanical resistance, (3) turbidity, and (4) absorbance and fluorescence spectroscopy. These categories will each be discussed.

Measurement of the Coagulation Endpoint

UTILIZING CONDUCTIVITY

In the course of the last 20 years or more, several instruments have been developed that take advantage of the conductivity of plasma and the formation of the fibrin for measuring the coagulation endpoint (Fig. 17-1). In these more recent procedures, the patient's specimen is placed in the reaction cup. The reaction is then started by the addition of an appropriate activator and, simultaneously, the electrodes are submerged in the plasma and the timer begins. During the course of the reaction, one of the two electrodes is mechanically lifted above the surface of the plasma, breaking the electrical circuit. This action occurs at approximately 1-second intervals. As long as the circuit is broken at each cycle of the electrode, the instrument continues to function. When the fibrin forms and has sufficient tensile strength to be lifted from the plasma, the electrical conductivity is maintained throughout the entire cycle of the up-and-down stroke of the moving electrode. Then the instrument stops and the timer records the amount of time required for the reaction to occur. The principle components of this type of instrument are represented in Figure 17-1. The cup in which the reaction occurs is disposable and rests in a heat block that maintains the temperature of the reaction at 37°C. The electrodes need to be easily accessible or easily removable from the instrument in order to allow for their effective cleaning between measurements. There is an electric motor to develop the up-and-down stroke cycle of the moving electrode. Finally, the switching device provides a mechanism to stop the instrument when the electrical current between the two electrodes is maintained throughout a cycle and a timer to measure seconds elapsed to the endpoint.

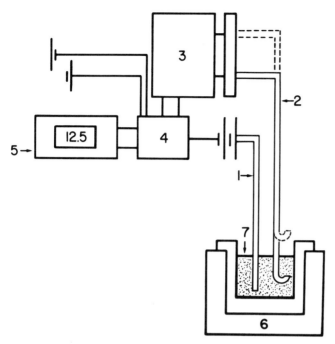

Figure 17-1. Components of instruments used for measuring coagulation endpoints by conductivity: (*1*) stationary electrode, (*2*) electrode with a cycling up and down motion, (*3*) motor for cycling the mobile electrode, (*4*) switching device, (*5*) timer, (*6*) temperature-controlled block for specimen container, and (*7*) specimen. The reaction in this instrument is started by simultaneously activating the start switch and adding activation material to the specimen. During the reaction, the motor cycles the mobile electrode in and out of the specimen, continually breaking the current between electrodes 1 and 2 at about 1-second intervals. When fibrin monomer polymerization occurs, the fibrin monomer attaches to the mobile electrode and maintains the electrical conductivity between electrodes 1 and 2 throughout the entire cycle of the mobile electrode; this action then activates the switch, shutting off the motor and stopping the timer.

UTILIZING INCREASING VISCOSITY AND ELASTICITY

As fibrin monomer is generated by thrombin and polymerization of the fibrin monomer proceeds, there is a continuing increase in the viscosity of the specimen and in the tensile strength of the resulting polymer. The development of this tensile strength can be measured in devices that are designed for the measurement of viscosity or elasticity. These instruments use the piston and cylinder or a vibrating probe technique. In the piston and cylinder technique, the piston and cylinder are approximated, with the specimen providing the only contact between them. The device can then function by automatically oscillating the cylinder through a pre-

scribed rotational angle at a predetermined rate. The amount of resistance provided by the specimen in the cup is then measured by determining the force that
is applied to the piston. An example of one of these devices and its output is
depicted in Figure 17-2. One can see, for example, that if there is no specimen
in the cup and the only contact between the piston and the cylinder is air, then
there is virtually no influence of the motion of the driven component (the cylinder)
upon the measuring component (the piston). If fluids of varying viscosity are
added to the instrument, one can reflect that viscosity by the ease with which the
oscillating cylinder can exert a force through the fluid upon the measuring piston.
This principle is then extended to the reaction of coagulation by the continually

Figure 17-2. Essential components of piston-cylinder instruments for measuring coagulation endpoints (rotational
arc-type): (*1*) cylinder drive, (*2*) cylinder, (*3*) piston, (*4*) mirror, (*5*) light source, (*6*) photodetector, (*7*) recorder, (*8*) a
sample record, and (*9*) specimen. The specimen and its appropriate activators are added to the cylinder, and the piston
is lowered into the specimen inside the cylinder. The drive
is started and the cylinder is rotated through a predefined
arc of approximately 4° to 5° at a constant rate. As the fibrin
monomer polymerization proceeds, the viscosity and elasticity of the specimen increase with increasing rotation of
the piston. Rotation of the piston causes deviation of the
light striking the mirror and the light is reflected in increasing
arcs in the photo detector. The signal is transmitted to a
recorder that generates the resulting record.

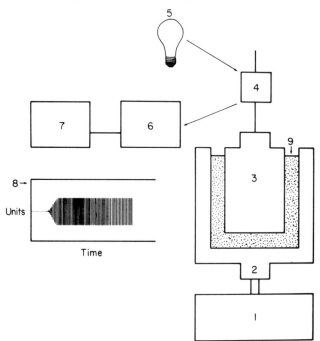

increasing resistance of the specimen that is between the piston and the cylinder as fibrin monomer polymerization proceeds and the specimen changes from a liquid to a solid. These devices allow a mechanism to graphically represent the tensile strength of the forming fibrin clot as well as the rate of its formation.

A second method for measuring the coagulation endpoint is the impedance method (Fig. 17-3). It uses a specimen cup in which a disposable vibrating probe is suspended. The movement of the probe is continually measured and, as fibrin monomer polymerization proceeds and viscosity increases, there is increased resistance to the movement of the probe. This impedance to the movement of the probe is recorded graphically.

The principal components of the piston–cylinder instruments include a specimen cup that becomes the cylinder in the instrument, a mechanism to drive that cup at a constant rate of oscillation, a piston that is engineered to fit with precise clearances inside the cylinder, and, finally, a mechanism to detect the movement of the piston that is suspended in the specimen in the cylinder. The piston motion can be detected by shining light upon a mirror that reflects upon a photo detector or photosensitive paper in a recorder. This light beam, of course, will then move

Figure 17-3. Components of a mechanical impedance instrument for measuring coagulation endpoints: (*1*) cylinder cup, (*2*) vibrating probe, (*3*) probe vibration and device to measure increasing impedance, (*4*) recorder, (*5*) specimen, and (*6*) sample record. The specimen and activator are added to the cup, and the probe is lowered into the specimen. The drive is activated, and the probe is vibrated at a constant rate. As fibrin monomer polymerization proceeds, the viscosity and elasticity of this specimen increase, providing a gradually increasing resistance to the vibration of the probe, which is measured and reflected in the recording.

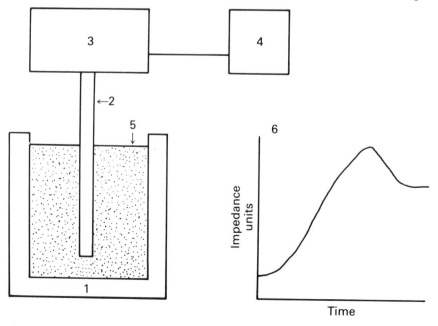

through the rotational angle of the movement of the piston as that movement is generated. The piston motion can also use a position transducer to send a signal to the recorder.

The principal components of the impedance instruments include a temperature-controlled specimen cup. The probe is lowered into the specimen and is vibrated by a mechanical drive. The vibration is measured and resistance to its motion imparted by the specimen is recorded graphically.

When compared to the system described utilizing conductivity, one can see the similarity between these instruments in that they depend upon increasing viscoelastic properties in order to make the measurement. The devices using the piston–cylinder or the vibrating probe add a second dimension to this process by supplying a method for graphically visualizing the polymerization process.

UTILIZING TURBIDITY

When thrombin generates fibrin monomer from fibrinogen and fibrin monomer begins to polymerize, the growing polymer will take on light-scattering characteristics and, ultimately, the resulting fibrin clot will be opaque. This characteristic of the fibrin monomer polymerization can be exploited in instruments that measure the changing turbidity of the plasma sample and use that change in turbidity to reflect the growing fibrin polymer.

The techniques of turbidometric measurement are discussed in Chapter 5 and will therefore not be addressed here. The instruments that exploit turbidometry for measuring coagulation endpoints are available in a wide variety of configurations. These range from instruments that make single specimen determinations with manual addition of activating reagents to complex instruments that allow the loading of many (more than 20) specimens simultaneously onto a specimen tray, automatically adding the activating agent and measuring and recording the coagulation time. Many of these instruments can also be interfaced directly to laboratory computers. These larger and more complex instruments also provide a mechanism for continually chilling the specimens waiting for measurement as well as appropriately warming them to 37°C prior to the addition of the activating agent. They also allow for appropriate activation times as indicated.

UTILIZING ABSORBANCE AND FLUORESCENCE

As mentioned above, the generation of fibrin from fibrinogen is the result of the complex and orderly activation of a series of enzymes present in the plasma. These enzymes are mostly serine proteases with restricted substrate specificities. Efforts in organic chemistry in the past 10 years have led to the development of a number of synthetic substrates that mimic the physiologic substrate of these enzymes. The chromogenic or fluorogenic compound is linked to a synthetic peptide, ester, or amide. When the enzyme cleaves this substrate and releases the compound, the chromogen can be measured spectrophotometrically or the fluorogen can be measured fluorometrically. Although the utilization of these

Table 17-1
Examples of Synthetic Substrates in Use

Synthetic Substrate	Enzyme Measured	Clinical Assays
Chromozyme-TH H-D-Phe-Pro-Arg-AIE	Thrombin	Antithrombin III Prothrombin Heparin Prothrombin time
Chromozyme-PL H-D-Val-Leu-Lys-AIE	Plasmin	Plasmin Plasminogen α_2-antiplasmin

synthetic substrates is still limited to only a few enzymes, this technology is likely to develop further in the coming years.

Depending upon the configuration of the synthetic substrate, the techniques of either absorbance or fluorescence spectroscopy can be used to measure the endpoint of these reactions. Absorbance and fluorescence are adequately discussed in Chapters 5 and 8 and the principles and techniques discussed in these chapters apply to the utilization of absorbance and fluorescence for measuring coagulation enzymes. Table 17-1 provides a very brief list of some synthetic substrates that are currently utilized. In general, these synthetic substrates are used to measure the enzymatic activity of thrombin or plasmin. Exploiting the ability of thrombin or plasmin to be detected by this technique, it is also possible to measure plasma inhibitors of these enzymes utilizing modifications of the same assay techniques. Therefore, assays for antithrombin III activity, heparin quantification, and α-2 antiplasmin activity in plasma are also available.

Advantages of the Varying Techniques

Those instruments that measure the endpoint either by conductivity or by reflecting the elasticity have advantages in relation to the versatility of specimen and activator that can be utilized. These instruments can make measurements on purified components in buffered solutions, in plasma, or in whole blood. In addition, they are capable of utilizing many activators regardless of the turbidity that they may impart to the specimen.

The instruments that reflect the changing elasticity of the clot provide a graphic demonstration of fibrin polymerization. This has been claimed to make possible the measurement of more than simply the clotting endpoint. It may also afford information related to platelet function, clot stability, clot lysis, and the cross-linking of the fibrin clot, reflecting factor XIII activity.

The impedance instrument that utilizes the vibrating probe technique to reflect the elasticity of fibrin monomer polymerization can also be modified to make measurements of the viscosity of serum, plasma, or whole blood.

The distinct advantage of instruments that utilize turbidity as the endpoint measurement is their ability to prepare multiple specimens for automatic determination. In laboratories in which a large volume of testing is necessary, this becomes a distinct cost-saving advantage.

The use of synthetic substrates for the measurement of absorbance and fluorescence in coagulation provides advantages related to the assay of specific enzymes and their inhibitors. These techniques have been expanded to reflect the entire plasma-coagulation mechanism similar to the activated partial thromboplastin time and prothrombin time; however, these techniques are still not widely utilized.

Disadvantages of the Varying Techniques

Instruments that use conductivity and depend upon the mechanical formation of the fibrin clot, and that do so utilizing the patient's endogenous fibrinogen, will tend to have an increased sensitivity to decreased concentrations of fibrinogen or to abnormal fibrinogens. It is debated whether this increased sensitivity represents an advantage or a disadvantage when screening for coagulation defects. Since specific assays for fibrinogen are available in the laboratory, some may argue that the screening tests (prothrombin time and activated partial thromboplastin times) would be better if they reflected earlier phases of the coagulation cascade. Whether increased sensitivity to fibrinogen reflects an advantage or a disadvantage in these instruments depends upon the interpretation of the data that is generated. Nevertheless, the instruments that measure the clotting endpoint by the turbidity technique tend to be less sensitive to decreased concentrations of fibrinogen.

The instruments that measure the clotting endpoint utilizing elasticity or conductivity techniques do not lend themselves well to batch-assaying techniques applicable to large numbers of specimens. They tend to be more labor-intensive and, on a per-test basis, more costly.

In contrast, the instruments that measure the endpoint by the turbidity technique have considerable limitations in that they cannot utilize whole blood; they are also limited in the activating reagents that can be used in individual tests. Those reagents that increase the turbidity of the specimen can present problems. In addition, specimens that have elevated levels of chylomicrons with opacity of the plasma cannot be measured by this technique.

Those reactions that utilize absorbance or fluorescence spectroscopy tend to be highly specific reactions, and their utilization for screening procedures has not yet been fully developed. Synthetic substrates have been developed to be specific targets for selected enzymes. There is, however, a small amount of cross-over to other enzymatic activities, which can, in rare cases, create some problems. There have been encouraging developments in the area of synthetic substrates and the movement of plasma coagulation testing into more specific enzymology. However, it is still early in the development of this field, and only the future will determine whether or not these technologies will be heavily utilized. Because of their limited use, the substrates are expensive reagents at this time.

Suggested Reading

Starrett D: Application of thromboelastograph. American Clinical Products Review 3:34–43, April, 1985

Svendsen LG et al: Newer synthetic substrates in coagulation testing: Some practical considerations for automated methods. Semin Thromb Hemost 9:250–262, 1983

Von Kalla KN et al: The impedance machine: A new bedside coagulation recording device. J Med 6:73–87, 1975

18

AUTOMATED CONTINUOUS FLOW CHEMISTRY ANALYSIS
Thomas L. Williams

Definitions

Accuracy: A measure of the ability of an analytical system to produce the "correct" answer as determined by such means as primary and secondary standards, calibrated reference materials, and comparison with an accepted reference method for the same analysis.

Analytical Cartridge: A component of SMA series and SMAC systems where a dialyzer, heating block, mixing and/or phasing coils, and other apparatus, all pertaining to a given analyte (or channel), are found.

Base-Line Steady State: The steady level of transmittance obtained with the system pumping, mixing, and presenting to a detector all reagents, water, and air segments except for standards, controls, or unknowns.

Calibration Curve: A concentration–transmittance or concentration–absorbance curve obtained by introducing standards of known value into the system.

Control: Material of a source similar to those specimens under analysis (plasma, serum, urine) with a relatively well-established value for the substance under analysis (blood urea nitrogen [BUN], sodium) that is introduced periodically as an unknown sample to determine precision at a certain analytical level as well as to evaluate the analytical system for potential systematic errors.

Cocurrent: Parallel flow in the same direction. This term is usually applied to the direction of the liquid stream traveling on either side of the dialyzing membrane.

Countercurrent: Parallel flow in the opposite direction.

Detector: A final readout system that may be a colorimeter, spectrophotometer, fluorometer, flame photometer, or atomic absorption spectrometer.

Dialysis: The separation of a crystalloid from a colloid (generally plasma proteins) in solution by the interposition of a membrane with small pore size between the crystalloid-colloid solution (*e.g.*, plasma or urine) and a solution that is relatively hypotonic to the crystalloid. In actual practice, the amount of material dialyzed varies from 5% to 30% of the total.

Drift: A continuous steady gentle increase or decrease in the %T reading while determining base-line or steady-state.

Noise Level: Irregularities in base-line or steady-state determinations. Noise may be caused by precipitation, irregular mixing, incomplete reactions, irregular pulsation, or electronic failure.

Precision: A measure of reproducibility of an analytical determination without regard to accuracy. Some authors describe repeatability as in-run precision and reproducibility as inter-run precision.

Sample Interaction: The effect that each preceding sample has on the succeeding sample; that is, whether a low sample causes the subsequent high sample to appear significantly lower than the actual value and vice versa (also referred to as *carryover*).

Sample Steady State: A steady level of transmittance obtained when the system is pumping, mixing, and presenting to a detector all reagents, water, and air segments as well as continuous aspiration of a standard or sample.

Standard: Material utilized in calibrating the instrument. These are usually aqueous or protein-base materials that contain known amounts of the substance under analysis. They are utilized to determine the concentration-versus-transmittance or concentration-versus-absorbance curve for comparative analyses of unknowns.

Wash Time: The length of time required to wash out remnants of each preceding sample. The wash time often determines the maximum rate of analysis in that a short wash time reflects little specimen interaction and suggests that more specimens per hour may be evaluated.

Introduction

The idea of "assembly-line" automated analysis, executed by passing a series of different samples via the same tubing through a modular analytical instrument, was originally developed by Leonard Skeggs, Ph.D. The subsequent marketing of the Technicon AutoAnalyzer in the late 1950s represented a historical and technical landmark in the evolution of laboratory instrumentation. With the AutoAnalyzer, increased total work production without a great increase in personnel or fatigue, decreased glassware utilization, and decreased cost per test for higher volume analyses were accomplished. Instrumental descendants of the original AutoAnalyzer remain widely used today and multichannel continuous flow analysis (CFA) has made possible the automated processing of up to 150 samples per hour for a variety of analytes. Continuous flow analysis is the concept fundamental to understanding the AutoAnalyzer, SMA series, and SMAC instruments.* In CFA, samples are separated, dialyzed, mixed with reagents, incubated, and identified, and analytes are measured while being continuously pulled through a tubular pathway.

The text to follow will explain how CFA performs various functions; it will describe the single-channel (single-analyte) AutoAnalyzer; and it will extend these concepts to multichannel analyzers (SMA series and SMAC). Some perspective regarding applications of CFA instrumentation will be offered.

*Trade names of Technicon Corporation, Tarrytown, NY.

Attributes and Functions of Continuous Flow Analysis

The attributes of CFA are as follows:

1. All samples (standards, controls, and patients) are inflexibly processed in an identical manner.
2. Different samples are continuously carried one after another through the same tubing throughout the instrument.
3. All functions necessary for analysis can be performed while the series of samples is continuously moving through the instrument.

Functions performed within the tubing in CFA include sample transport, sample separation, reagent introduction, and mixing. Other functions (incubation, heating, and dialysis) are performed as the sample passes through tubing or tube-like pathways in components of the instrument. In the original AutoAnalyzer, these components were separate pieces of equipment known as modules.

SAMPLE TRANSPORT

Samples are carried through plastic tubing that approximates 0.05 inch inside diameter. Because the flow rate (volume/time) through a tube segment is directly determined by its size, tubing having a wide range of calibrated inside diameters is available for use as needed in various analyses. Tubing having special chemical composition is available for corrosive reagents. Basically, two functional types of tubing exist; these are pump tubing and transport tubing. Pump tubing is precisely calibrated to yield predictable flow rates and transport tubing should not be used on pump manifolds.

SEPARATION

The integrity of different liquid samples serially propelled through a length of tubing can be maintained. These samples (also standards and controls) are introduced into the tubing, one after the other, in the sampler module.

Mutual contamination of each sample by its neighbor is minimized by the incorporation of air bubbles at regular intervals within and moving with the sample stream (Fig. 18-1). Each standard, control, and patient sample is interposed between two bubbles and is, in turn, separated from adjacent samples by a segment of "neutral" wash solution. Regularly spaced air bubbles are also added within individual sample segments (Fig. 18-2). These bubbles pass through all modules of the instrument to the detector module input point, where they are removed (except SMAC). The effect of air bubbles on the rapidity by which samples reach steady state (*i.e.,* time to wash out a previous sample or truly plateau a new one) is graphically demonstrated (Fig. 18-3). A series of properly separated samples

Figure 18-1.   Regularly spaced air bubbles minimize intersample contamination.

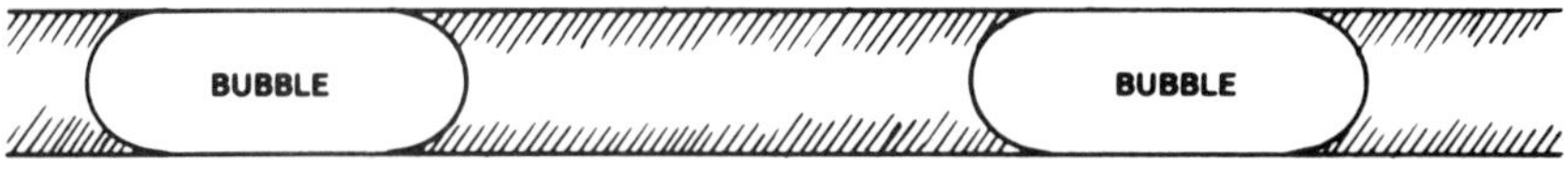

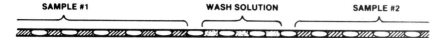

SAMPLE #1   WASH SOLUTION   SAMPLE #2

Figure 18-2. Intersample and intrasample air bubbles.

will have a characteristic signal profile at the detector (Fig. 18-4). The bubbles also provide an observable monitor of flow dynamics within the tube system. A minimum of pulsatile flow is an indicator of good sampler, pump, and dialyzer function.

The bubble patterns for the original AutoAnalyzer, SMA systems, and SMAC have been generated by different means. In the sampler module, regular sampler probe aspiration of air between sample and wash solution provides some bubbles in all systems. A unique feature of the SMAC sampler is that it introduces four intrasample air bubbles by pecking rather than continuously aspirating each sample. These are subsequently replaced by larger bubbles via the liquid-out-air-in (LOAI) pump before samples ascend the vertical riser. The volume of air in each bubble ensures that a portion of each is resampled by each analytic cartridge. Smaller bubbles are also produced in SMAC by a pressurized air-metering system. Proportioning Pump III, used in SMA series instruments, has an "air bar" system, which introduces bubbles in a precise manner to further minimize the mildly pulsatile flow dynamics of the pump system.

It should be mentioned that a bubble-free form of flow analysis, called *flow injection analysis,* has been studied.

SAMPLE SPLITTING AND REAGENT INTRODUCTION

Reagents can be added to samples by merely joining reagent and sample tubing. Samples within tubing can be equally or unequally diverted into a desired

Figure 18-3. Effect of air bubbles on system wash time. (Principles of Operation: Basic AutoAnalyzer System. Technicon Corporation, Tarrytown, NY)

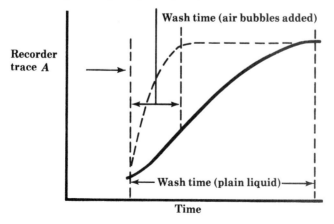

Recorder trace *A*

Wash time (air bubbles added)

Wash time (plain liquid)

Time

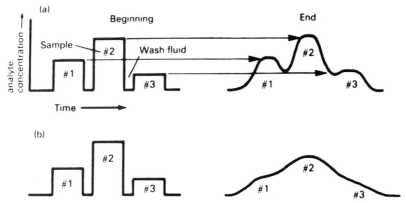

Figure 18-4.   Effect of dispersion during continuous-flow analysis on sample concentration curve shape—(*a*) acceptable dispersion: analyte and analyte–chromogen concentrations plotted on molar basis; (*b*) unacceptable dispersion. (Snyder L, Levin J, Stoy R, Conetta A: Automated chemical analysis update on continuous-flow approach. Anal Chem 48:944A, 1976)

number of other tubes. A selection of connectors having known flow characteristics and various configurations is available for these different requirements.

MIXING

During transit through a horizontal glass coil (Fig. 18-5), sample and reagent mixtures are continually inverted, end over end, enhancing mixing.

Modules

The original AutoAnalyzer incorporated six separate modules, each of which performed a specific function: sampler, proportioning pump, dialyzer, heating bath, detector (specifically, a colorimeter or flame photometer), and recorder. These functions have been retained in subsequent multichannel systems in more compact, technically advanced, and decentralized form. Though not an original

Figure 18-5.   Schematic diagram of mixing coil.

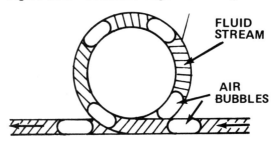

AutoAnalyzer module, the programmer/computer control console will also be introduced here.

SAMPLER

The original AutoAnalyzer sampler and succeeding models II, III, and IV are similar in design and function. Functional components of Sampler II and later models consist of a sample probe, sample cups, revolving sample wheel, wash receptacle, and optional sample mixer built into a motorized unit. The sampler probe alternately aspirates sample, air, wash solution, air, next sample, and so on from the revolving sample tray. The sampling frequency and ratio of sample to wash volume are determined by an internal sampler cam in the single-channel AutoAnalyzer and in multichannel systems by a separate mechanical or computerized programmer module.

The original AutoAnalyzer sampler held 40 sample cups with a volume of 0.5 to 3 ml each. Samples were aspirated by a hinged crook that dipped into successive cups without an interposed wash cycle. The volume of sample/air aspirated approximated 2:1 and varied with the sampling rate. The Sampler II held 40 sample cups (0.5 to 8.5 ml) and offered sampling of from 10 to 120 samples per hour with sample/wash ratios of between 1:1 and 6:1 as determined by the selection of a fixed cam, and even an adjustable cam, when used with an AutoAnalyzer system. Intersample aspiration of wash solution was routine, and vibrating mechanical sample mixer arms were optional. A metal sample probe was used and its action minimized the effect of sample fill volume on aspiration volume present with the original AutoAnalyzer sampler. Samplers III and IV retained these features. After Sampler II, a routinely refilling wash receptacle, an optional rotary mixer, a selection of sample probes, and an optional automated sample-identification system (routine with SMAC) were introduced. Sampler II and later model samplers have been used with AutoAnalyzer and SMA systems. Larger capacity samplers such as the T-40 were offered.

The SMAC sampling system is described in the section reviewing SMAC multichannel operations.

PROPORTIONING PUMP

A functionally similar pump mechanism has been used in all systems (AutoAnalyzer through SMAC). Lengths of tubing mounted on a manifold and carrying samples and reagents are compressed between a series of regularly spaced, moving rollers and a nearly flat stationary plate ("platen"). The manifold consists of a pair of grooved plastic end blocks that hold parallel sample and reagent tubes by small external sleeves placed equidistant on each tube to ensure uniform stretching when the end blocks are attached to the proportioning pump. The pump mechanism is schematically illustrated in Figure 18-6. This shows the platen-above-roller arrangement of pump models II and III, which followed the original AutoAnalyzer proportioning pump (roller above platen). The maximum number of pump tubes that can be used varies from one pump model to another. In a multichannel (SMA) system, more than one pump module is required owing to

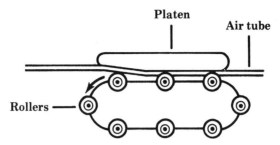

Figure 18-6. Schematic diagram of proportioning pump—Models II and III. (After Programmed Instruction Manual for SMA 12/60. Technicon Corporation, Tarrytown, NY)

the number of reagent and sample tubes. The SMAC utilizes two racks of six pumps each, mechanically linked to a single motor, built into the analytical console.

Because all tubes in a pump are compressed by rollers moving at the same rate, the rate of flow in a tube is determined by the pump tube diameter. A selection of pump tubing having different, precisely calibrated diameters is available for various analytic requirements. The pump produces minor peristalsis in flow patterns that can be visualized as slight, regular surges in bubble flow rate throughout the system. There is no backflow traversing the pump(s) during normal operation.

A series of proportioning pump models was introduced. Proportioning Pump II had a capacity of up to 28 tubes, 13 more than the original AutoAnalyzer pump, and introduced an optional leak detector. Proportioning Pump III is equipped with a leak detector and has a similar tube capacity and an air bar assembly for generating air bubbles within tubing traversing it. With all pumps, rollers and platens can be separated for access to the roller mechanism and to relieve point-to-point compression of pump tubing when the instrument is turned off. All pump models offered optional two-speed motors to decrease time required for system wash and manifold changeover. Special pumps were designed for industrial and hematologic applications.

DIALYZER

Dialysis is used to remove interfering substances and protein during analysis of low-molecular-weight organic and inorganic molecules. Properties affecting dialysis are time, temperature, membrane surface area, concentration, coefficient of dialysis, membrane pore size, particle size, ionic strength, and ionization constant. Rates of dialysis vary considerably among molecules and ions of clinical interest, and, generally, only a fraction of a desired analyte is actually recovered in the recipient stream. Obviously, all standards, controls, and samples must have similar dialysis properties. This requirement bears upon the use of aqueous or other standards or controls in light of effects of protein concentration, relative protein binding of the unknown, relative hydrophilia, and relative solubility in both sample and recipient stream that may be unique to such material.

Dialysis is performed by passing the sample (donor stream) along one-half of a tubular pathway, which is bisected throughout its length by a semipermeable membrane. Opposite the membrane, in the other half of the tubular pathway and moving at the same speed, is a bubbled recipient stream (Fig. 18-7). This cocurrent, parallel-flow dialysis cell is formed by a cellophane membrane pressed between two plastic plates that have mirror-image grooving. The grooving has a semicircular or "U" pattern to increase the length of dialysis exposure within a small dimensional area.

The original AutoAnalyzer dialysis module consisted of relatively large dialysis plates that were suspended in a thermostatically controlled, motorized-stirrer–equipped water bath. Membrane replacement was difficult. Two dialysis plate sets (*i.e.,* two analytes) could be submerged per bath. Newer SMA series dialysis plates are smaller (groove lengths of 3 to 12 inches versus the Auto-Analyzer's 87 inches), membranes are accessible for observation of bubble patterns in the dialyzer and for easy maintenance, and donor stream temperature is controlled by a heating block. In SMA series systems and SMAC, dialyzers are now integrated within individual analytical cartridges, as required. Two types of membranes are available—cellophane, and silicon rubber for gas dialysis (CO_2 content).

HEATING BATH

The original AutoAnalyzer heating bath module consisted of a double-walled, insulated, thermostatically controlled vessel equipped with a motorized stirrer and housing a coiled sample tube generally approximately 40 feet long. Various temperatures (*e.g.,* 37° or 95°C) were maintained for uniform hydrolysis, digestion, enzymatic reaction, or color development. The heating bath module was replaced in SMA series analyzers by small, short-path, thermostatically controlled heating blocks incorporated into individual analytical cartridges. Small, thermostatically controlled heating baths are used in appropriate SMAC analytic cartridges.

DETECTOR

Analytic methods incorporate colorimetry, fluorometry, flame photometry, nephelometry, and potentiometry. Continuous flow analysis colorimetry and flame photometry will be presented here.

Figure 18-7. Cocurrent dialysis.

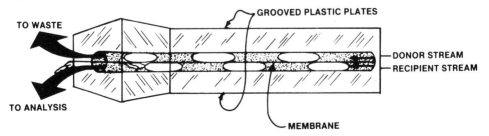

Colorimeter

The endpoint of most analyses in the clinical laboratory is a colored product having, at a specific wavelength, an intensity related to the concentration of the desired analyte. By interpolating the color intensities (absorbances) of unknown samples with those produced by standards and controls against a reference or blank channel, sample analyte concentrations can be determined and quality control can be achieved.

The colorimeter 5A, widely used with SMA series systems, has one reference and four sample channels arranged centripetally in a quarter circle around a single tungsten light source. In each sample or blank channel, light from a tungsten lamp passes through two lens assemblies, an interference filter assembly, a flowcell assembly, and an adjustable aperture to a phototube-housing assembly. The reference channel has no flowcell or lens assembly. More than one colorimeter module is required to accommodate all channels in a typical SMA system. Each sample channel produces an uninterrupted photodetector output that is continuously monitored to detect abnormalities in curve contours or phasing. Continuous flow analysis colorimetry requires a flow-through cuvette called a flowcell. Figure 18-8 shows a colorimeter 5A flowcell featuring simple one-piece design and self-debubbling.

In SMAC, a single visible light source is partially surrounded by 26 fiberoptic cable inputs representing 23 sample and three blank channels. A separate arc lamp provides an ultraviolet-rich light source in SMAC for up to 12 sample channels and one reference channel. SMAC colorimetry is also unique in that flowcells are not proximate to the light source but are separately located in the appropriate analytic cartridges. Incident and transmitted light are respectively passed to and from these flowcells by fiberoptic cables to a central photomultiplier tube that operates in a time-sharing fashion. In SMAC, bubbles pass through the flowcell and their signals are electronically removed.

Flame Photometer

The AutoAnalyzer and all SMA systems have determined sodium and potassium via flame-emission photometry. Four flame photometer models were introduced, incorporating certain technical advancements. Major improvements in-

Figure 18-8. Flow cuvette for an SMA system.

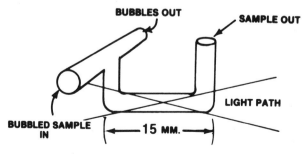

cluded the use of compressed air instead of oxygen and either propane or natural gas fuel, improved atomization and adjustable burner, a quieter flame, and a flameout detector alarm with automatic fuel shut-off. All models have measured sodium and potassium simultaneously against a lithium reference. The input line is debubbled immediately prior to flame injection. Flame IV has been widely used in SMA 6/60, SMA 12/60, and SMA II applications. Chapter 6 presents theoretical and technical aspects of emission flame photometry.

RECORDER

The original AutoAnalyzer recorder incorporated a slide-wire potentiometer into a pen-servomotor system, which balanced the input voltage from a sample channel against the reference channel. Because the recorded signal was a linear representation of the photodetector output (proportional to % transmittance), logarithmic conversion of the data (proportional to absorbance) was required for the determination of the concentration of unknown samples and controls. This was accomplished via a transparent logarithmically calibrated overlay called a comparator, or by semilog absorbance paper. Logarithmic amplifiers in SMA systems produce output signals that can be directly penned to linear graph paper labelled in concentration units; in SMA II systems, these signals can be fed through an analog-digital converter to a computer for data storage, quality control, and hardcopy.

Programmer/Computer Control Console

All multichannel systems share the common technical problems of collating signal outputs from multiple detector channels so that each sample "peak" can be identified, quantitated, and recorded; efficiently organizing more complex operating controls and indicators; and continuously presenting data monitoring the operational status of the instrument. The SMA programmer, or SMA II or SMAC computer control console unit, is an operator's "module" that provides these functions.

Essential components of an early SMA series programmer included a mechanical timing cam that controlled sampling and coordinated input of data from the detectors into the chart-recorder, the chart-recorder itself, and miscellaneous controls and indicators for calibrating, phasing, and monitoring individual channels. The SMA 12/60 introduced a cathode ray tube that continuously displayed detector output patterns for all channels simultaneously to allow convenient inspection for any anomalies of phasing or curve contour. During operation of an SMA 12/60, in addition to monitoring curve characteristics, the operator repetitively both reviews analog chart-recorder calibration data and manually recalibrates all analyte channels. This requires considerable dexterity. In the computerized SMA II and SMAC, sampling and data recording/storage are automated; calibration, phasing, and qualitative curve inspection for all channels are performed by the computer.

Single-Channel Analysis

Figure 18-9 shows the original AutoAnalyzer system, with the indicated modules in series. The sampler cam governed sample introduction frequency and the sample/wash ratio. The colorimeter or other detector output was continuously recorded. At the detector, each sample produced a progressive increase toward steady-state (maximum) absorption followed by a steady fall toward basal (reagent) levels near the end of its wash phase. The percentage to which peak absorbance approached steady state varied widely with the procedure. Judicious use of standards and controls minimized the effect of instrumental drift to achieve acceptable precision and accuracy.

AutoAnalyzers were combined in groups such as two or four. Various combinations of sampler, pump, detectors, and recorders allowed the simultaneous determination of such combinations as electrolytes, BUN, and glucose. After several prototype models combining eight, ten, and twelve channels, Technicon marketed the SMA 12/30 and 12/60.

The AutoAnalyzer II represents an updated AutoAnalyzer that applies analytic cartridge technology to provide single-channel or several-channel analysis with graphic or digital data accumulation.

Multiple-Channel Analysis

The development of multichannel systems required numerous technical improvements. The introduction of electromechanical and computerized programmers allowed centralized monitoring and control of a relatively large instrument by a single operator. Sensing systems for crude module malfunctions, such as proportioning pump tubing leaks and flame photometer flame-out, were expanded

Figure 18-9. Original AutoAnalyzer system. (Courtesy of Technicon Corporation, Tarrytown, NY)

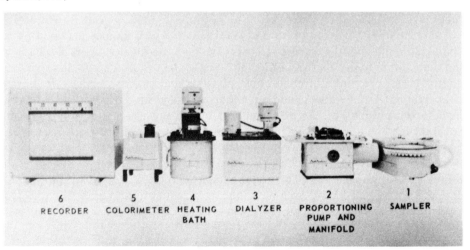

| 6 | 5 | 4 | 3 | 2 | 1 |
| RECORDER | COLORIMETER | HEATING BATH | DIALYZER | PROPORTIONING PUMP AND MANIFOLD | SAMPLER |

to include automated quantitative and qualitative monitoring of individual analytic channel functions. Increasingly compact and simple heating bath and dialyzer modules for each analyte were physically incorporated into individual sample "modules" known as analytic cartridges, which conserved tubing and space, and eased maintenance. Stable reagent systems using enzymes immobilized within reaction coils have simplified measurement of some analytes. Specially designed reagent containers fitted refrigerated and unrefrigerated storage consoles. Data management became computerized with the provision of results and quality control information.

Multichannel analyzers have applied the above continuous flow analysis (CFA) principles and modules to multiple, simultaneously operating analyte channels. Unlike single-channel analysis, sequential multiple-channel analysis requires the development of a steady state or plateau (*i.e.,* "flat top") in each sample peak. Thereafter, the fundamental challenge unique to CFA multichannel systems is that of identifying and compiling data from multiple samples as they continuously flow through all the detectors (a noncomputerized SMA 12/60 chart recorder can pen data from only one analytical channel at a time).

These problems were overcome in such a system through a synchronization of sample flow through all analytic channels with the programmer-recorder channel recording cycle known as *phasing*. Each channel receives standards, controls, and samples as a series of sample segments that arrive in a known sequence and have a certain sampler-to-detector transit time. By inserting one of a selection of phasing coils into the flow path of any channel, the arrival of its sample at its detector can be delayed by a desired amount. Because a noncomputerized SMA system has a recorder that is programmer-directed to metronomically record serially from all system channels in a predetermined cycle again and again, the channels are so phased (*i.e.,* variably delayed) that for each analyte channel, the optimal portion of the plateau of each sample peak passes its detector just as its detector is being recorded by the programmer (Figs. 18-10 and 18-11). In other words, a specimen from each patient, control, or standard is split into sample segments that enter each analytic channel, and all of a given specimen's sample segments arrive at the detectors of all channels at *nearly* the same time. Arrival times, by phasing, are staggered by precise amounts relative to one another to allow sequential recording of data from each sample/channel peak by a single recorder, as described above. The chart recorders of these instruments are then continuously recording data from *some* channel, but *each* channel is actually recorded only briefly (*e.g.,* 5 seconds for SMA 12/60). Computerized systems (SMA II and SMAC) do not require manual phasing.

THE SMA 12/60 AND SMA II

The SMA 12/60 typically incorporates a programmer (including cathode ray tube [CRT] and chart-recorder) with sampler IV, four Proportioning Pump IIIs, four Colorimeter 5As, 16 analytic cartridges, and a Flame Photometer IV. It processes 12 analytes at 60 samples per hour.

The SMA II (Fig. 18-12) basically replaces the SMA 12/60 programmer with

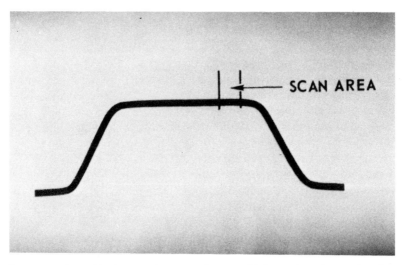

Figure 18-10. Single sample curve from multichannel analyzer showing the plateau and the optimal portion for recording data. (Courtesy of Technicon Corporation, Tarrytown, NY)

a computer and analyzes 18 tests at 90 samples per hour. During operation, the computer controls sampling, electronically phases and monitors the instrument, and provides hardcopy results and quality control data summaries via a printer. Calculations such as anion gap, serum osmolality, and so on can be routine. Automated monitoring for selected electronic, hydraulic, and sampler identification malfunctions is coupled with peak and function monitors to review each detector output. All channels are monitored continuously. Electronic phasing is carried out by means of a red dye that, being instilled in the first sample cup, allows calibration of a relative detector arrival time ("dwell time") for each sample in all channels in each run. A typical SMA II system incorporates a sampler IV, six Proportioning Pump IIIs, a Flame Photometer IV, six Colorimeter 5As, and 20 or more analytic cartridges plus computer console and printer. The computer also provides patient data storage and quality control functions.

SMAC

The SMAC sampler utilizes rectangular carrier blocks that hold eight samples each, carry machine-readable sample identification labels, and migrate in rectangular patterns about the Linear Sampler module. If a sample position is empty, wash solution will be aspirated during the 24-second sampling interval. Eight empty sample positions or an absent carrier block are interpreted by the instrument as the end of a run and sampling is terminated. The proportioning pump mechanism and bubble-generating systems have been described. Twenty analytes are analyzed at 150 samples per hour.

The analytic console (Fig. 18-13) contains a predilution cartridge and up to

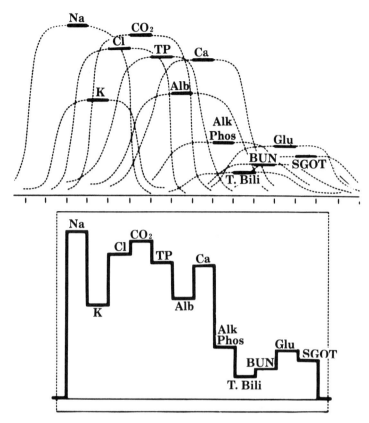

Figure 18-11. Continuous monitor of some channels of SMA-12. Sample aspiration fixed at 1'50" steady-state curves for some determinations given by "phasing"; the various curves are interrelated as shown in time sequence. By serially monitoring the various phototubes during the 9-second interval, shown on the upper chart, the line graph shown below may be obtained. (Whitehead EC: Sequential multiple analysis. Technicon Symp I:437, 1965)

23 analytic cartridges, each of which variably contains a dialyzer assembly, heating bath assembly, mixing coils, and one or more flowcells. Each flowcell has a squared "U" configuration, with the base of the "U" constituting a 7-, 10-, or 12-mm light path. The light path is within a frosted glass barrel. Light is passed to and from the flowcell by sapphire rods fused to each end of the barrel. Sodium and potassium are potentiometrically determined by ion-specific electrodes within separate analytic cartridges. Each patient channel is scanned (colorimeter system previously described) every 0.2 second, as controlled by a revolving chopper (a disk bearing a U-shaped notch). Separate photomultiplier tubes and filter systems register ultraviolet and visible wavelength flowcell transmissions. These outputs are fed to log preamplifiers and then through additional circuits to the computer.

Sections	Description
1.	ANALYTICAL CARTRIDGES
2.	6- and 12-CHANNEL PREDILUTION MANIFOLDS
3.	6- and 12-CHANNEL CHEMICAL CONSOLE HYDRAULICS
4.	6- and 12-CHANNEL CHEMICAL CONSOLE ELECTRICAL
5.	6- and 12-CHANNEL REAGENT/WASH VALVES
6.	6- and 12-CHANNEL DRIP TRAYS
7.	CHOLESTEROL VALVE
8.	REFRIGERATOR
9.	PUMP III
10.	COLORIMETER, 5A
11.	SAMPLER IV
12.	FLAME PHOTOMETER IV
13.	ELECTRONICS CONSOLE
14.	LINE PRINTER

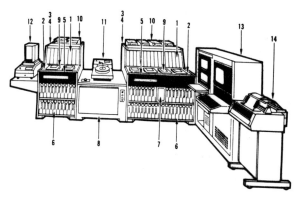

Figure 18-12.   The SMA II system and its components. (Courtesy of Technicon Corporation, Tarrytown, NY)

The system is operated via the primary control panel and alphanumeric keyboard/CRT. An error panel informs the operator of module or chemistry channel errors. Hardcopy of results and quality control data are generated by the computer module.

SMAC II has been combined with the RA-1000 discrete analyzer to achieve increased analytic flexibility.

Conclusion

The evolution of continuous flow analysis instrumentation has reflected changes in laboratory needs, clinical demands, available technology, and reimbursement that have occurred since the introduction of the AutoAnalyzer in 1957. The AutoAnalyzer introduced the concept of single-analyte (per instrument) automated analysis. It provided higher sample throughput, with lower cost and personnel time. As more than one AutoAnalyzer was combined, multiple-channel analysis and the possibility of multichannel profiling and screening were introduced. High-test-volume multichannel profiling has been efficiently provided via evolving SMA series instruments and SMAC. These and other instruments permitted clinical

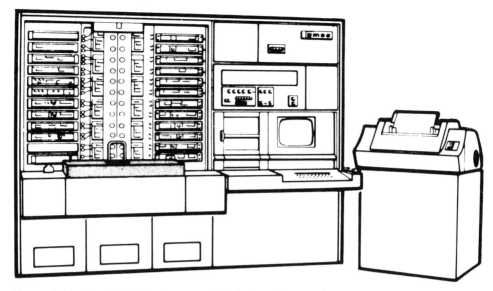

Figure 18-13. SMAC I. (Courtesy of Technicon Corporation, Tarrytown, NY)

laboratory test volume to more than double in the United States between 1970 and 1977. The overall diagnostic impact of multiple-channel screening has been somewhat controversial, however.

In recent years, the need for highly flexible profiling/discrete instruments has strengthened. These requirements are antithetical to standard continuous flow analysis methodology. Presently, the newly introduced Technicon Chem I has incorporated continuous flow analysis with discrete analysis using a scheme referred to as *capsule chemistry*. All nonelectrolyte samples with, but separate from, reagents required for various discrete analyses are introduced into the tubing system as a sample-reagent packet or "capsule." The capsule specifically consists of the sample plus first reagent, a small or "vanishing" air bubble, second reagent, air bubble, buffer, and air bubble. There is a single tubular flow path for all optical channels with nine detectors placed strategically along its length in the analytic chamber. As the sample capsule enters the analytic chamber, a slight increase in tubing diameter breaks the vanishing bubble barrier allowing mixing of sample/first reagent and the second reagent, initiating the desired chemical reaction. The entire system uses small-bore Teflon tubing. All tubing and probe surfaces are coated with liquid fluorocarbon, preventing actual contact between the tubing walls and the samples and reagents needed for each analyte. Intersample carryover is virtually eliminated. The electrolytes and CO_2 content are analyzed in a separate potentiometric pathway. The system is computerized to provide sample identification, resulting hardcopy and storage, and quality control information. This system is suitable for multichannel profiling or discrete analysis, and, with the usual test mix, can provide approximately 1000 tests per hour.

Suggested Reading

Benson E: Initiatives toward effective decision making and laboratory use. Hum Pathol 11:440, 1980

Cassaday M, Diebler H, Herron R et al: Capsule chemistry technology for high-speed clinical chemistry analyses. Clin Chem 31:1453, 1985

Finkelstein S: Technological change and clinical laboratory utilization. Med Care 18:1048, 1980

Levine J: Continuous flow analyzers. In Werner M (ed): CRC Handbook of Clinical Chemistry, p 483. Boca Raton, FL, CRC Press, 1982

Seitz WR, Grayeski ML: Flow injection analysis: A new approach to laboratory automation. J Clin Lab Autom 4:169, 1984

Skeggs LT Jr: An automated method of colorimetric analysis. Am J Clin Pathol 28:311, 1957

Skeggs LT Jr, Hochstrasser H: Multiple automatic sequential analysis. Clin Chem 10:918, 1964

Synder L, Levine J, Stoy R, Conetta A: Automated chemical analysis: Update on continuous-flow approach. Anal Chem 48:942A, 1976

Thiers RE, Cole RR, Kirsch WJ: Kinetic parameters of continuous flow analysis. Clin Chem 13:451, 1967

19

DISCRETE CHEMISTRY ANALYZERS, PART I
Batch Systems
Wesley K. Tanaka
David L. Witte

Definitions

Abbott Bichromatic Optics: A patented optical system that measures the absorbance difference between two wavelengths as a means to quantitate analyte concentrations.

A/D Conversion: The conversion of a continuously variable parameter (*e.g.*, voltage, current) to digital values.

Batch Analyzer: An instrument in which all samples are loaded at the same time and a single analysis is performed on each sample.

Centrifugal Analyzer: An instrument that uses centrifugal force to mix sample and reagent and a spinning rotor to pass reaction cuvettes through a light beam.

Dilution Ratio: The volume of a sample divided by the volume of sample plus reagent expressed as a ratio (*e.g.*, 1:101 dilution).

Discrete Analyzer: An instrument that compartmentalizes each sample reaction.

EMIT (Enzyme Multiplied Immunoassay Technique):   A homogeneous immunoassay using enzyme-labeled ligand to compete with unlabeled ligand.

Linear Fitting Routines: Computer software used for finding the straight line that best represents a collection of data (*e.g.*, least squares analysis).

Multichannel Discrete Analyzer: An instrument that is capable of performing multiple simultaneous analyses on a sample using segregated modules for each analysis.

Multitest System: An instrument that is capable of performing multiple analyses on a sample.

Nonlinear Fitting Routines: Computer software for finding the curved line that best represents a collection of data.

Random Access Analyzer: An instrument that is capable of selecting a sample for analysis and of sequentially performing selected analyses on that sample.

Rotor: A specially molded holder containing light-transmitting windows for measuring spectral changes in a sample and used to compartmentalize sample and reagent.

Sample Carryover: The contamination of one sample by the preceding one.

Selectivity: The capability of performing multiple tests on a sample using only sample and reagent for those tests requested.

Signal Averaging: Repeated measurements of a signal to enhance it over noise.

Signal-to-Noise Ratio: The ratio of the magnitude of the signal to the magnitude of the noise. An indication of the sensitivity of measurement.

Introduction

The clinical laboratory has had to respond to changing demands over the years. The need to improve productivity and precision led, in part, to the development of continuous flow analysis used in the Technicon AutoAnalyzer. Changes in reimbursement and concerns over rising health-care costs have increased pressures to reduce reagent costs, decrease staffing, and increase flexibility in test ordering. These demands have had to be met while maintaining high quality and providing timely support of patient care. All of these factors plus the introduction of microprocessor-controlled instrumentation have led to the development and widespread acceptance of automated discrete analyzers. In contrast to continuous flow, discrete analyzers place each sample in a separate reaction cuvette. Because of this characteristic, most discrete analyzers are selective, using only the reagent and sample necessary to perform the requested tests.

Discrete analyzers can be classified somewhat arbitrarily into two basic groupings—multitest systems and batch analyzers. The distinction is made on the basis of sample flow during analysis. There are two classes of multitest systems. Multichannel discrete analyzers permit simultaneous analysis of multiple analytes by taking multiple aliquots of each sample and independently performing each test selected in a dedicated channel (Fig. 19-1*A*). Random-access test systems permit analysis of different analytes by taking single aliquots and performing the test selected (Fig. 19-1*B*). While the first analysis is being incubated, a second analysis with another test and/or sample can be started. In a discrete batch analyzer, all samples are loaded at the same time and the same analysis is carried out for all samples (Fig. 19-1*C*). A sample requiring a variety of tests requires repeated batches.

This chapter will discuss two of the most common discrete batch analyzers available, the bichromatic analyzers, manufactured by Abbott Diagnostics, and centrifugal analyzers, using the Multistat III F/LS (Instrumentation Laboratory, Inc) as an example. The capabilities of these analyzers are representative of the capabilities of modern microprocessor-controlled discrete analyzers. They exemplify the application of this technology to instruments that demonstrate high precision, reliability, low reagent consumption, ease of operation, and rapid data reduction.

The Abbott bichromatic analyzers are the commercial application of the design concepts of Dr. Max Liston, Liston Scientific, Newport Beach, California. Liston Scientific was awarded patent rights for this concept in 1968. Abbott Diagnostics acquired those patent rights, refined the original design, and has produced four analyzers, the ABA-50, ABA-100, ABBOTT-VP, and ABA-200. The ABA-50

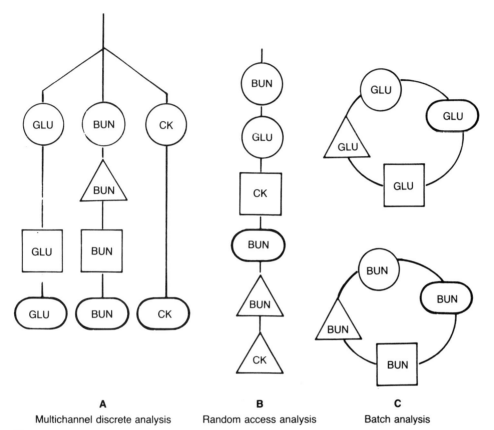

A
Multichannel discrete analysis

B
Random access analysis

C
Batch analysis

Figure 19-1. Figures schematically represent the sequence of test analyses (glucose [GLU], blood urea nitrogen [BUN], creatine phosphokinase [CK]). Different shapes represent different patient samples. In *A* and *B*, the order of test and patient analyses is shown from top (first) to bottom. In *C*, connected shapes represent analyses done together.

is a smaller, less automated version of the ABA-100. The ABBOTT-VP, a second-generation instrument, shares many design and operational characteristics with the ABA-100 but includes an integral syringe for a second reagent, a diluter capable of detecting liquid levels, logic to calculate results using multiple standards, additional error-detection capabilities, fluorescence-measuring capability, and choices of reaction times. The last instrument introduced, the ABA-200, has added flexibility in dilution ratios, times of reagent addition, and computational capabilities. Collectively, this group will be referred to as the Abbott analyzers except where reference to a particular model is made.

Centrifugal analyzers are the result of the developmental work started by Dr. Norman G. Anderson of the Oak Ridge National Laboratory in 1967. Commercialization of centrifugal analyzers resulted in the first prototypes displayed by Electro-Nucleonics (GeMSAEC) and Union Carbide (CentrifiChem) in 1969. Table 19-1 lists the five companies currently marketing centrifugal analyzers in the

Table 19-1
Table of Various Centrifugal Analyzers

Manufacturer	Model	Rotor
Baker Instruments Corp	CentrifiChem	30 cuvette Reusable
	Encore System II	30 cuvette Reusable
Electro Nucleonics Inc	Gemeni	20 cuvette Disposable
	Flexigem	20 cuvette Disposable
	Gem Profiler	20 cuvette Disposable
Instrumentation Laboratory, Inc	Multistat III MCA	20 cuvette Disposable
	Multistat III F/LS	20 cuvette Disposable
	Monarch	39 cuvette Disposable
Roche Analytical Instruments	Cobas Bio	30 cuvette Disposable
	Cobas FARA	30 cuvette Disposable
Travenol Laboratories, Inc, Instrument Division	Rotochem CFA 2000	36 cuvette Reusable

United States. Like the Abbott bichromatic analyzers, centrifugal analyzers have evolved from the early models. The first-generation instruments featured a reusable rotor to hold sample and reagent, dynamic photometric monitoring of multiple cuvettes, and simultaneous adding and mixing of sample and reagent by rapid acceleration and deceleration of the rotor. Second-generation instruments featured component miniaturization, disposable rotors, automated delivery systems for sample and reagent, multiple optical configurations for fluorescence and light-scattering measurements, and an increase in the number of applications. Recently, third-generation instruments have incorporated centrifugal analysis technology into complete systems, which include additions such as ion-selective electrodes. These systems can identify samples and results by patient, can perform simultaneous multiple analyses, and can print summary reports.

Operating Principles

Automated analyzers use unique approaches to the automation of steps done during manual test analysis. The batch analyzers can be compared and contrasted with respect to the mechanization of measuring sample and reagent, mixing, incubating, measuring spectral changes, calculating results, and identifying interfering substances.

Centrifugal analyzers and Abbott analyzers both have several functionally separate parts: (1) a 32-position multicuvette (Abbott) or 20-cuvette rotor (Multistat), (2) a sample and reagent measurement and delivery system, (3) a spectrophotometric measurement system, and (4) a programmer module that the operator uses to control the instrument.

SAMPLING SYSTEM

Both types of instruments use instrument-controlled syringes to aspirate the correct volume of reagents and sample. Both have less than 0.2% carryover between samples. The Multistat III F/LS uses separate syringes and probes to deliver sample and reagent to the appropriate compartments of a specially designed disposable rotor where they are kept separate until sample analysis is initiated (Fig. 19-2). Sample carryover is minimized by cycling the sample and reagent probes through a wash station where they are immersed and rinsed out with saline. On the Abbott analyzers, sample and reagent are aspirated by separate syringes but solution is delivered through a single probe. When the reagent syringe is ready to expel reagent, a valve is rotated so that the reagent is pumped through the sample syringe and the probe (Fig. 19-3). Sample carryover is minimized by the high reagent to sample ratio (*i.e.*, a large volume of reagent is used to rinse the sample from the sample probe). Both analyzers can accurately deliver sample volumes as small as 1.25 μl and can accommodate reagent volumes of 250 μl. Both have the capacity for a second reagent. The small reagent volumes used on both analyzers reduce reagent costs and minimize sample size requirements.

MIXING AND INCUBATION

The 32-position multicuvette is one of the unique features of the Abbott analyzers. Ejection of reagent and sample through the narrow diameter probe causes turbulence and mixing. Reactions are initiated as soon as they are ejected into a cuvette. Each cuvette holds a separate reaction mixture. On the ABBOTT-VP and ABA-200, a second reagent is added by a separate probe. Times for addition of the second reagent can be varied owing to the open cuvette design of the reaction cuvette. The temperature of the cuvette and reaction mixture is maintained by a constant-temperature water bath. On the Multistat III F/LS, the

Figure 19-2. Cross section of Multistat III rotor. This figure shows one section of the various compartments making up a 20-sample rotor.

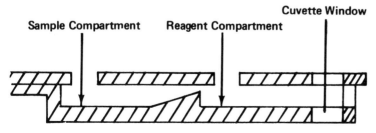

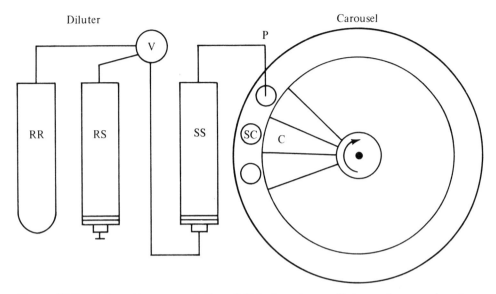

Figure 19-3. Schematic representation of Abbott analyzer, diluter, and carousel system: RR = reagent reservoir; RS = reagent syringe; SS = sample syringe; V = valve; SC = sample cup; C = cuvette segment; P = sample probe.

rotor, into which reagent and sample are placed, has three major functions. Like the Abbott multicuvette, the Multistat rotor is a cuvette to hold the reaction mixture while photometric readings are being made. The rotor is also designed to hold the sample and reagent in separate compartments while temperature is equilibrated at a preselected value. The addition of sample to reagent to initiate reaction occurs when the rotor is spun. Rotor design is unique to each centrifugal analyzer. Rotors can be permanent or disposable (Table 19-1). Permanent rotors are designed to be washed and rinsed between runs. Rotors also vary in the number of cuvette positions. All rotors have two compartments as typified by the Multistat III disposable rotor shown in cross-section in Figure 19-2. The sample is delivered to the sample compartment. If two reagents are required, the loader will also put the secondary reagent in the sample compartment. The other reagent solution is delivered to the reagent compartment. The disposable rotor is placed in the rotor chamber of the analytic unit. Prior to sample analysis, rotor, samples, and reagents are rotated slowly until temperature is equilibrated by forced air from a compressor-type refrigerator or a radiant (infrared) heat lamp. If a second reagent is included in the sample compartment, preincubation will occur. When the desired temperature is reached, the rotor is accelerated to 4000 revolutions per minute (rpm) and then brought to a sudden stop. The sequence of sudden acceleration and stop occurs in approximately 2 seconds. The acceleration results in the simultaneous addition of sample to reagent in all cuvettes. The turbulence created in stopping the rotor results in mixing. Simultaneous initiation of all reactions at a precisely determined point in time is a unique feature of centrifugal analyzers.

Once mixing is accomplished, the rotor is spun at 1000 rpm. At this speed, the reaction mixture is pushed by centrifugal force to the outer edges of the rotor where it lies between the cuvette windows (Fig. 19-2). It is during this time that data collection takes place. The Multistat collects data on all reactions simultaneously as the rotor spins at 1000 rpm. The Abbott analyzers collect data on each reaction in sequence, advancing the cuvette one position every few seconds. Both types of instruments are flexible in the number and interval of measurements possible.

SPECTROPHOTOMETRIC MEASUREMENT

The single most distinguishing feature of the Abbott bichromatic analyzers is the optics system that measures the difference in absorbance between two wavelengths (A_d). This system is represented schematically in Figure 19-4. Light of two different wavelengths is alternately sent through the cuvette. This design results in the enhancement of spectrophotometric precision, the minimization of errors due to filter or cuvette defects, and the minimization of other light-scattering contaminants. The bichromatic optics on these instruments is not designed to eliminate spectral interferences and is not an alternative to a serum blank. The measurement of each wavelength separately is most optimal for serum blanking. Blank reactions that occur in the standard methods will also affect the Abbott analyzers.

The measurement of A_d by these instruments is electronically complex. It will be discussed here only in general terms. For additional detail, references are listed. As shown in Figure 19-4A, the Abbott photometer has two pairs of filters arranged in a wheel, with the identical filters opposite each other. As the wheel spins, the detector sequentially sees light of the primary wavelength, darkness due to the opaque wheel between the filters, and then light of the secondary wavelength. This cycle repeats itself as the wheel spins at 1800 rpm on the ABA-100 and 3600 rpm on the VP and ABA-200. Figures 19-4B and 19-4C show the response of the two detectors, one sensing light transmitted through the cuvette and the other sensing filter-wheel position. On the VP and ABA-200, measurements at a particular wavelength are taken every 8.3 msec (2 measurements at each wavelength per revolution). A total of 330 data points are averaged and the mean is sent as a dc voltage to an A/D converter.

The Abbott analyzers have excellent photometric precision. The heart of this system is the unique A/D conversion, which divides the absorbance range into 10,000 divisions and allows more precise measurements to be made of absorbance. This capability can be appreciated using a ruler analogy. A more precise measurement can be made with a ruler having 10,000 divisions than one with only 100 divisions. Precision for the photometer shows a coefficient of variation of 0.10% with a linearity to 2.5 A_d. Cuvette pathlength is 1.0 cm.

As shown in Figure 19-4, the light beam passes through two filters of the same wavelength. This design allows the use of less expensive filters (because the unwanted wavelengths are more effectively absorbed), it corrects for minute holes present on those filters, it decreases the effective bandpass by $1/\sqrt{2}$, and, perhaps most interestingly, it allows these systems to perform spectrophotometric mea-

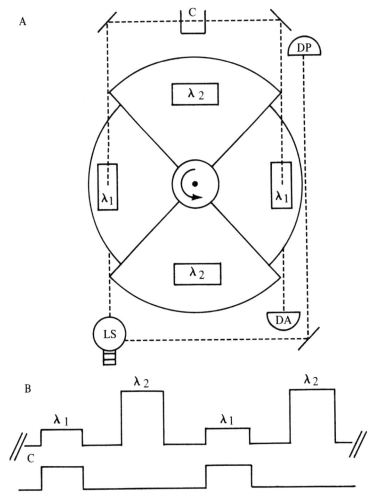

Figure 19-4. Optical diagram of the ABA bichromatic photometer with the filter wheel rotating in a plane perpendicular to the light beam— (*A*) the filter wheel, which rotates at 1800 rpm ([λ_2] the filter that transmits secondary wavelength, [λ_1] the filter that transmits primary wavelength, [LS] light source, [DA] detector for analytic measurements, [C] cuvette, [DP] detector for filter wheel position); (*B*) light arriving at the analytic detector; (*C*) light arriving at the detector for filter-wheel position; because the filter wheel has a larger diameter in the sectors containing the λ_2 filters, the light is blocked when the λ_2 filters are in position.

surements in cuvettes open to room light as opposed to the usual light-shielded sample compartments.

The Abbott analyzers are marketed with four wavelength pairs—340/380 nm (for NADH), 450/415 nm (for paranitrophenol), 500/600 nm, and 550/650 nm. The wavelengths in the first two pairs are relatively close together. As a result, light scattering at the two wavelengths will be nearly equal and will cancel when an absorbance difference (A_d) is measured. This will not be true when the wavelengths are further apart.

Because the Abbott photometer is designed to measure absorbance difference (A_d) and not absorbance, it is useful to consider how this relates to our understanding of the Beer–Lambert law. Consider the following reaction as measured in a bichromatic photometer. Species, X, is a colored reactant that is converted to a colored product, Z, by a constituent, Y, in serum. The amount of Z formed is proportional to the amount of Y.

$$X \xrightarrow{Y} Z$$

Where

a_{X1} = absorptivity of species X at wavelength 1
a_{X2} = absorptivity of species X at wavelength 2
a_{Z1} = absorptivity of species Z at wavelength 1
a_{Z2} = absorptivity of species Z at wavelength 2
$a_{Xd} = a_{X1} - a_{X2}$
$a_{Zd} = a_{Z1} - a_{Z2}$
C_X = concentration of species X, and so on
SB_1 = absorbance contribution due to serum blank at wavelength 1
SB_2 = absorbance contribution due to serum blank at wavelength 2
A_1 = absorbance at wavelength 1
A_2 = absorbance at wavelength 2
$A_d = A_1 - A_2$
$A_1 = a_{X1}C_X + a_{Z1}C_Z + SB_1$
$A_2 = a_{X2}C_X + a_{Z2}C_Z + SB_2$
$A_d = a_{Xd}C_X + a_{Zd}C_Z + (SB_1 - SB_2)$

To appreciate the concept, let us consider the following quantitative example. Let

$C_X + C_Z = C_{total} = 100$
$a_{Z1} = 10 \qquad a_{X1} = 2$
$a_{Z2} = 2 \qquad a_{X2} = 1$
$a_{Zd} = 8 \qquad a_{Xd} = 1$
$SB_1 = SB_2 = 0$

Using these values and the equations above, the data in Table 19-2 is generated. When $SB_1 = SB_2 = 0$, A_d will be directly proportional to the amount of Z and therefore to the amount of Y in the serum sample. The above example can be simplified if X is uncolored; then, A_d is directly related to C_y or C_z. If the absorptivities of Z are known at wavelengths 1 and 2, the analysis can be calibrated from these physical constants in combination with the volume of the sample and reagent and the pathlength of the cuvette.

Measuring spectral changes on the Multistat III F/LS contrasts sharply with the approach used on the Abbott analyzers. As described earlier, the Abbott

Table 19-2
Example A$_d$

% Conversion $X \longrightarrow Z$	A$_d$ Predicted	Relative Concentration of Y
0	100	0
5	135	5
25	275	25
50	450	50
80	660	80
100	800	100

analyzers monitor each reaction cuvette in sequence. In the Multistat, the reaction cuvettes are rotated through the light beam, allowing for monitoring of all reactions simultaneously. Light is passed from one side of the rotor to the photodetector located below the rotor (Fig. 19-5A). Light strikes the photodetector only when a cuvette window comes between the light source and the detector. The photodetector then produces a current proportional to the amount of light transmitted through the rotor and sample. Where the light beam is blocked, the photodetector produces dark current. A water or other appropriate blanking solution is placed in cuvette number 1 and is used to set 100%T. The Multistat III F/LS collects data from a maximum of 64 successive revolutions to generate a single point. Like the Abbott analyzers, successive measurements of the same sample are taken over a short period (0.06 second) of time, permitting signal averaging to enhance the signal-to-noise ratio. The single-beam optics system of the centrifugal analyzer can be contrasted to that of a more sophisticated dual-beam spectrophotometer. In the centrifugal analyzer, the light beam is essentially "split" as it passes through

Figure 19-5. (*A*) Optical configuration used on the Multistat III for measuring absorbance or transmittance; (*B*) optical configuration used on the Multistat III for measuring fluorescence or light scattering.

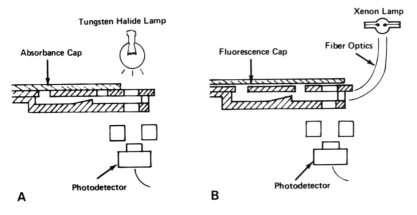

each cuvette. Once every 60 milliseconds, the beam is referenced and a dark current measurement is made. This allows for corrections in light source variations and photodetector noise in much the same way as a dual-beam spectrophotometer. Precision for the photometer shows a coefficient of variation of approximately 0.1% with linearity to 2.0 A. Cuvette pathlength is 0.5 cm. For absorbance spectroscopy, the Multistat is equipped with eight interference filters—340, 380, 405, 500, 520, 550, 620, and 690 nm with band passes ranging from 7 to 12 nm.

Both the Multistat III and the newer Abbott bichromatic analyzers have fluorescence-measuring capability. The VP and ABA-200 have a "straight-through" fluorescence optics system. The filter wheel used for fluorescence includes filters that transmit the excitation wavelength and emission wavelength for the fluorophor. When the filter wheel lines up in the light path with excitation filter first and emission filter second, fluorescence is measured. Other orientations of the filter wheel allow measurement of reference and stray light signals. The Multistat III F/LS uses a more traditional approach to fluorescence measurements. Light is passed from a high-intensity xenon lamp through a fiberoptic bundle to the optical surface at the edge radially out from the rotor. Fluorescence is measured at 90° to the excitation light using the same photodetector used for absorbance measurements (Fig. 19-5*B*).

CALCULATION OF RESULTS

Both the Multistat III and the Abbott analyzers have sophisticated data-calculation capabilities. Both have linear and nonlinear fitting routines for dealing with multiple standards and all of the necessary computational abilities necessary for doing equilibrium, kinetic, EMIT, and fluorescence immunoassay analyses. The Multistat III Plus F/LS has 32K of memory and, when equipped with a terminal, is user programmable. The VP and ABA-200 can both be interfaced to IBM-PCs.

INTERFERENCES

The most commonly encountered spectral interferences in the clinical laboratory are hemolysis, icterus, and lipemia. The effects of these interferences are somewhat predictable. Lipemia causes a monotonic increase in absorbance with a decrease in wavelength. Hemoglobin has a sharp absorbance peak at approximately 415 nm (Soret band). Bilirubin has a broad absorbance peak at 460 nm. Single wavelength determinations in an equilibrium measurement will be affected near the absorbance maximum as shown in Table 19-3, column 2. Bichromatic measurements will also be affected as shown in Table 19-3, columns 3 to 6. Reaction rate (kinetic) measurements are not affected unless the reaction conditions alter the spectra of the interferents. For example, reagent systems have been shown to cause the clearing of lipemic turbidity. Bilirubin is oxidized by the hydrogen peroxide generated in the cholesterol-oxidase based cholesterol determination. Interference occurs in these cases because the spectral properties of the interferents are changed in the reaction. In addition to spectral interferences, analysis on centrifugal analyzers must also be concerned with centrifugation ef-

Table 19-3
Effect of Interferents on Spectral Measurements

Interferent	A_{max}	340–380	415–450	500–600	550–650
Lipemia	Short wavelengths	+ + + +	+ + +	+ +	+
Hemolysis	415	0	+ + + +	0	0
Icterus	460	+	+ +	+	0

fects, such as a decrease in turbidity due to particle sedimentation or flotation. These examples should caution the laboratorian to investigate interferences in all laboratory methods rather than assume that the interferences are predictable.

Applications

Both the Multistat III F/LS and Abbott analyzers have reagents designed especially for them. Because of their flexibility and widespread acceptance, many reagent manufacturers have adapted their reagents for these instruments. The main advantages of these instruments are the small reagent and sample volume required, easy programmability for development of new procedures, and the ease of adapting user-selected reagents.

For manual analyses not yet adapted for either of these instruments, careful attention to the details of the analysis and to the operating principles of each instrument must be given. For example, do existing filters or filter pairs allow determination of reaction chromophores with sufficient sensitivity? Are the reaction times available on the instrument sufficient? What type of reagent addition is necessary and when can reagents be added to the reaction mixture? What type of interferences are expected? What type of blank is necessary to correct for interferences?

Quality Control

The discrete analyzers provide a unique opportunity for the design of quality control schemes. In the continuous flow analyzer, the inference is made that if the control samples are analyzed correctly, the patient samples are also correct because the cuvette is monitored continuously. The inference from the quality control sample to the patient sample is less robust in discrete analyzers. The discrete nature of each analysis creates the possibility that an error in one sample, like inadequate sampling, can go undetected. This is not to detract from the other advantages of a discrete analyzer, but the reader should be aware of the difference.

Summary

Discrete batch analyzers fulfill a useful role in the hospital laboratory. For less frequently requested tests, batch analyzers make efficient use of the technologist's time. For large-volume single-test requests, batch analyzers are as efficient as random-access analyzers. Because of their flexibility, batch analyzers are useful as back-up instruments to perform tests while a large primary laboratory instrument is being repaired. Some newer automated analyzers capable of random-access testing can be operated in a batch mode to better meet the workflow needs of the laboratory.

Suggested Reading

Bradley, CA: Centrifugal analysis in the clinical laboratory. In Stefanini M, Gorstein F, Fink L (eds): Progress in Clinical Pathology, Vol IX, pp 225–246. New York, Grune & Stratton, 1984

Khalil OS, Routh WS, Lingenfelter K et al: Automated in-line ratio-correcting filter fluorometer. Clin Chem 27:1586–1591, 1981

Pesce MA: Evaluation of the Multistat III fluorescence/light scatter centrifugal analyzer. J Clin Lab Autom 3:327–339, 1983

Price C, Spencer K (eds): Centrifugal analyzers in clinical chemistry. In Methods in Laboratory Medicine, Vol I. New York, Praeger, 1980

Savory J, Cross RE (eds): Methods for the Centrifugal Analyzer. Washington, DC, American Association for Clinical Chemistry, 1978

Witte DL, Neri BP: Bichromatic analysis: The design and function of the ABA-100. In Hercules DM, Hieftje GM, Snyder LR, Evenson MA (eds): Contemporary Topics in Analytical and Clinical Chemistry, Vol 4, pp 37–54. New York, Plenum Press, 1982

Witte DL, VanDreal PA: Bichromatic automated chemical analyzers. In Race GJ (ed): Laboratory Medicine, Vol I, Chap 35. Philadelphia, Harper & Row, 1984

Young DS, Tracy RP: Instrumental developments in clinical chemistry. In Stefanini M, Gorstein F, Fink L (eds): Progress in Clinical Pathology, Vol VIII, pp 136–138. New York, Grune & Stratton, 1983

20

DISCRETE CHEMISTRY ANALYZERS, PART II
Sequential Analysis of Multiple Analytes

Catherine Leiendecker–Foster
John H. Eckfeldt

Definitions

Data Stream: The string of data bits sent sequentially from instruments in a manner defined by a standard computer communications protocol (*e.g.*, RS 232).

Direct Costs: Costs that can be attributed to the analysis of specific tests (*e.g.*, reagents, labor, equipment depreciation).

Discrete Analyzer: An analyzer that performs only the tests actually requested on a clinical specimen, rather than a fixed profile of tests.

Indirect Costs: Costs that are generally not assignable to the analysis of specific tests (*e.g.*, building overhead, laboratory supervisory costs).

Random Access: The ability to utilize any given reagent and/or any given sample at any time in any desired order.

Sequential Analysis: On a given clinical specimen, more than one test analyzed one after another.

Simultaneous Analysis: On a given clinical specimen, more than one test analyzed concurrently.

Throughput: The total number of tests or specimens that can be analyzed in a given time (usually per hour).

Turnaround: The time between the receipt of a specimen and the reporting of analytic test results on that specimen.

Introduction

Continuous flow technology hearlded the onset of clinical chemistry automation, which was followed shortly thereafter by single-analyte automated batch analyzers. More recently, "discrete" analyzers with random access to specimens

Table 20-1
Effect of Number of Tests Per Specimen on "Sequential"
and "Simultaneous" Discrete Analyzer Throughput

Discrete Analyzer Type	Average Number of Tests Per Specimen	Total Specimens Per Hour	Total Tests Per Hour
"Sequential" (1000 Tests Per Hour)	2	500	
	5	200	
	10	100	
	20	50	
"Simultaneous" (100 Specimens Per Hour)	2		200
	5		500
	10		1000
	20		2000

and to reagents were introduced. With the advent of legislative and economic changes, along with the age of computer technology, laboratories are witnessing the emergence of highly sophisticated discrete analyzers as the major type of chemistry instrumentation. These analyzers are designed to allow a high throughput of specimens and to analyze only those tests that are actually requested on each specimen. This chapter will discuss those discrete analyzers that perform the bulk of their tests sequentially (*i.e.*, each test is performed one after another). Chapter 21 will discuss those discrete analyzers that perform all tests on a given specimen simultaneously. This separation is a bit arbitrary, as many of the "sequential" discrete analyzers that we will discuss perform some of their tests simultaneously (*e.g.*, electrolytes with ion-selective electrodes). However, the distinction is useful when one considers instrument speed, as shown in Table 20-1. The "sequential" analyzers are generally test-per-hour limited, whereas the "simultaneous" analyzers are specimen-per-hour limited. The following discussion of "sequential" discrete analyzers will include basic components common to all analyzers, followed by a description of representative instruments that are currently available.

General Principles

The dictionary defines the word *random* as "without careful plan, not uniform"; *discrete* as "separate and distinct, not attached to others"; and *access* as "a way or means of approaching, getting, using." These definitions aid the reader in understanding the basic principle common to all sequential random-access discrete analyzers (*i.e.*, testing is performed in a nonuniform, nonbatch manner, with one test after another being performed on each specimen until those tests requested on that specimen are completed). A few instruments are exceptions to this general principle in that only the requesting of tests is random (*e.g.*, Electronucleonics ALTAIRE), but actual performance of the tests is grouped into batches. Such instruments have random access to specimens, but not to reagents.

Nonetheless, because the operator may request tests on individual samples in a "nonuniform" manner, these instruments still fit into a loose definition of *random-access discrete analyzers*.

Basic Instrument Components

SPECTROPHOTOMETRIC MEASUREMENT SYSTEMS

All instruments' optics consist of the following basic components: (1) a light source, (2) a spectral isolation unit, (3) a reaction cuvette, and (4) a photodetector. The manner in which these components are combined may vary from one system to the next, but in all cases the operation of this system is microprocessor-controlled to allow automatic analysis of a variety of tests at differing wavelengths. For most systems, the light source is a tungsten-halogen lamp, and narrow band-pass interference filters are used to select appropriate wavelengths. However, a few systems use diffraction gratings for spectral isolation.

Another variable between systems is the type of reaction cuvette. Some instruments use glass or quartz cuvettes that are cleaned and reused. Such cuvettes are intended to be replaced only very rarely. Other instruments use cuvettes referred to as semidisposable. They are generally plastic and, as the name implies, are cleaned and reused, but unlike glass or quartz cuvettes, they require replacement on a regular basis (weekly to monthly) and become a consideration in direct operating costs. Finally, other instruments use disposable cuvettes that are used only once and are discarded. With these instruments, cuvette costs are a major factor in determining direct operating costs. Regardless of the type of cuvette used by a given instrument, cuvette blanking is always performed. For the non-disposable quartz and semidisposable cuvettes, a blank measurement is required to determine cleanliness from one filling to the next. For all types of cuvettes, a blank measurement is required to correct for any differences in spectrophotometric matching that may exist between cuvettes.

Depending upon the system design, there can be one or more photodetectors used to accumulate data from one or more cuvette positions at multiple wavelengths. Each system has various options for measurement, dependent upon the instrument design. Kinetic and endpoint measurements are available in all cases. Bichromatic, and occasionally trichromatic, measurements are available on most systems. One system (Abbott SPECTRUM) provides for "polychromatic spectral mapping," which allows the system to simultaneously monitor a reaction over a broad spectral range. These measurement options are usually selected via a parameter table for each test that is to be performed on the instrument.

ION-SELECTIVE ELECTRODE SYSTEMS

Ion-selective electrodes (ISE) for the measurement of electrolytes have been included, at least as an additional purchase option, with all the sequential random-access discrete analyzers presently on the market. All instruments use ISEs for sodium and potassium. Some instruments use ISEs for chloride, whereas others use them for total carbon dioxide. In most cases, these ISE systems operate simultaneously with the spectrophotometer analysis, allowing for some increase in maximum test-per-hour throughput. A few instruments use "direct" ISE potentiometry in which undiluted serum is in direct contact with the electrodes. However, most manufacturers have chosen "indirect" ISE potentiometry in which the serum is prediluted with buffer prior to the potentiometric measurements.

REAGENT SYSTEMS

With very few exceptions, all of these instruments are designed to run with reagents from the instrument manufacturer or other specified company. However, adaptation of reagents from nonspecified manufacturers is possible in most cases. The major limitation is the form the reagent takes as it is placed on the analyzer. For certain instruments that use dry chemicals or special packaging (*e.g.,* DuPont *aca* and Dade PARAMAX), it is not practical for the user to develop alternate reagents. Other systems use reagent concentrates (*e.g.,* Olympus DEMAND) that make applications of reagents from other vendors difficult, but not impossible. Still other manufacturers have encouraged users to develop reagents by designing the system to accommodate a wide variety of sample volumes, reagent volumes, and reaction times.

Analysis temperature varies between instruments. Many systems allow operation at more than one temperature, generally either 30° or 37°C. In different instruments, temperature may be set by the operator, a service engineer, or the factory. It is generally impractical to operate these analyzers at more than one temperature, because the principle of their operation is based on rapid, sequential analysis of different analytes on a given sample. However, it may be useful to be able to select the analysis temperature.

SAMPLE-REAGENT DISTRIBUTION SYSTEM

Most analyzers deliver reagents and samples with precision-bore syringes driven by microprocessor-controlled stepping motors, an arrangement that has proven very reliable in terms of accuracy and precision of delivery volumes. Less commonly used are displacement pumps (Technicon RA-1000) or pneumatically controlled digital diaphragm pumps (Baker SPIRIT). Because the reagent and sample probes are usually reused, carryover between specimens or reagents must be minimized. Most systems provide a wash of the outside and inside of the probes. Use of additional diluent following dispensing of reagent and specimen provides further insurance against reagent or specimen carryover. An alternate approach is the introduction of a "slug" of air or diluent into the probe immediately prior to reagent and specimen aspiration. The Technicon RA-1000 uses a unique approach to maintain specimen and reagent integrity. By coating the internal and external surfaces of the probe with an inert immiscible fluid, Technicon Random Access Fluid, the sampled liquid is protected from contact with the walls of the probe and therefore does not carryover to the next sampling.

SPECIMEN IDENTIFICATION–TEST REQUESTING

Because these analyzers are designed for high throughput, positive identification of the sample becomes an important concern. Each system has its own method of specimen identification. The most recent approach is bar-coding. Although this type of identification is used in only a few of the sequential random-access analyzers on the market to date, it is quickly becoming the favored technique. Bar-code labels on serum-separator tubes collected directly from the patient can be decoded by a bar-code reader on the instrument at the time of actual sampling. Not only does this afford nearly infallible specimen identification, but, in most cases, it allows the operator to load samples onto the instrument in a random order. Other forms of sampling, such as from numbered carousels, trays, or break-apart chains, do not provide the same degree of confidence in specimen identity as does the bar-code system.

A keyboard is provided on all systems for test requesting. Generally, this requires an operator to type in a specimen identification number and those tests requested on the specimen. With some instruments, a "touch-sensitive" screen or a light-sensitive pen may be used to test request. Of course, the ultimate in test requesting is via two-way communications from the laboratory's mainframe computer, in which the computer requests those tests desired on each specimen without operator intervention.

DATA OUTPUT SYSTEM

Test results can be produced either by a printer incorporated into the instrument itself or by an accessory printer in a form suitable for placement directly into the patient's medical record. Some systems offer both options for printing. In addition, essentially all of these systems have the capability of an RS 232 serial interface to a mainframe computer, which will allow test result information to be transferred directly to patients' computer files. However, in such situations, mainframe computer or interface software able to interpret the discrete analyzer's "data stream" must generally be purchased or developed.

Sequential Random-Access Discrete Analyzers

The market is rapidly becoming inundated with random-access discrete analyzers, as industry responds to the laboratory need for rapid turnaround, low-cost, low-maintenance, user-friendly instrumentation. As a result, it is becoming more and more difficult to select a system that will meet all the needs of an individual laboratory. Table 20-2 presents data regarding several systems that are currently available. Although it is not possible to discuss all instruments in detail, the following sections will discuss representative instruments and will attempt to review some of their unique aspects.

OLYMPUS DEMAND

The Olympus DEMAND is imported into the United States from Japan by Cooper Biomedical. The instrument is composed of two floor-standing consoles:

Table 20-2
Discrete Analyzers Performing Sequential Analysis

Instrument	Price $	Maximum Test/hr*	ISE Option	Reaction Vial or Cuvette	Cuvette Minimum Volume (μl)	Maximum Number of Different Reagents	Reagent Storage Temperature	Specimen Container
737 (Hitachi [BMD])	182,000	1200	Na, K, Cl	Reusable	350	23	4°C	Blood collection tubes
PERSPECTIVE (Am Monitor)	135,000	1000	Na, K	Disposable 2¢/cuvette	200	68	RT and 4°C	Special cup 3¢/cup
PARAMAX (Dade)	160,000	720	Na, K, Cl	Disposable 4¢/cuvette	300	32	4°C	Blood collection tube
SPECTRUM (Abbott)	115,000	600	Na, K, Cl	Disposable (can wash)	250	23	4°C	Special cup 3¢/cup
DACOS (Coulter)	142,000	450	Na, K	Reusable	300	28	15°C	Special tray 1¢/well
DEMAND (Cooper)	110,000	400	Na, K, Cl	Disposable 3¢/cuvette	250	32	4°C	Special cup 3.5¢/cup
ALTAIRE (ENI)	93,000	360	Na, K, Cl	Reusable	300	37	4°C	Blood collection tube
PROGRESS (Kone [ASP])	90,000	350	Na, K, Cl	Disposable 6¢/well	250	24	10°C below RT	Standard cup < 1¢/cup
SPIRIT (J. T. Baker)	55,000	320	Na, K	Disposable 3¢/well	400	12	RT	Standard cup < 1¢/cup
RA-1000 (Technicon)	83,000	240	Na, K, CO_2	Disposable 5.3¢/well	300	12	RT	Special cup 1¢/cup
GENESIS (IL [Fisher])	80,000	200	Na, K, Cl	Reusable	200	24	4°C	Standard cup < 1¢/cup
705 (Hitachi [BMD])	99,000	180	Na, K, Cl	Reusable	300	16	RT and 4°C	Special cup 3.3¢/cup

*The analyzer speeds (test/hr) listed are for spectrophotometric tests using a single cuvette without the ion-selective electrode (ISE) attachment operating. Tests using more than one cuvette slow the throughput and use of ISE may increase it as much as twofold.

the analyzer console and the system control console. Reagents are stored in the analyzer console as a fivefold concentrate in a refrigerated compartment, allowing for reagent stability of 5 days. However, the use of refrigerated, concentrated reagents limits adaptability of reagents from other manufacturers, due to solubility problems. Concentrated reagents and serum are both diluted with four volumes of wash water upon addition to the reaction cuvette. All reagents must be added at the beginning of the reaction. The disposable 1-cm pathlength plastic cuvettes, which also serve as reaction vessels, rotate on a 37°C cuvette wheel past 15 photometer stations. All spectrophotometric measurements are made bichromatically. The 72-position cuvette wheel moves one position once every 9 seconds, and therefore requires almost 10 minutes for the first test result, followed by one result every 9 seconds. Different tests may be processed in adjacent cuvettes of the cuvette wheel, allowing for true random-access testing. There is a special sampler for stat specimens that can interrupt routine operation. The system can perform up to 20 different tests (23 tests if ISE option is added) at one time. By using a second reagent carousel and program disk, additional tests can easily be performed. The system control console allows the operator to request tests individually or by user-defined panels, to edit patient or quality control data, to adjust test parameters, to set limits for reference ranges, and so forth. Results can be printed either on the compact instrument printer or in chartable form on an accessory printer. A computer interface is available that allows for two-way communication, so that not only can patient results be sent to a mainframe computer, but the mainframe computer can also identify those tests requested on each specimen, eliminating the need for operator test requesting.

ELECTRONUCLEONICS ALTAIRE

Like the DEMAND, the ALTAIRE is composed of two units: an analyzer console and a communication console. Reusable reaction vessels are automatically emptied, cleaned, and dried prior to use. Sample and reagents are added to the reaction cups as they pass the appropriate dispenser. A second reagent station offers delayed addition of a second reagent if desired. There are four 0.25-cm spectrophotometric flowcells and photodetectors that take 60 absorbance readings over 30 seconds regardless of the test being performed. Tests are performed in batch manner even though test requesting and sampling is performed randomly. The time required for the first result is about 12 to 14 minutes, with an additional result every 10 seconds thereafter. The reaction cups are incubated at an operator-selectable temperature of 25°, 30°, or 37°C. The instrument is capable of performing 16 different assays, but there is no provision for handling stat specimens. Test requesting is performed by the operator using either the keyboard, the communication console, or a light pen that can read bar-coded patient identification and test request information. This communication console handles the input of test parameters, review of results, editing data, printout of patient, and quality control results. As with all of these instruments, a two-way RS 232 interface to a mainframe computer is an available option.

ABBOTT SPECTRUM

The SPECTRUM is one of the newer discrete analyzers on the market. This instrument is composed of a single unit that may be placed on a bench top or support module. The reagent vessels are bar-coded for identification within the reagent carousel. Although reagents from manufacturers other than Abbott can be adapted to the SPECTRUM, empty reagent containers must be purchased in order to have the proper bar-code. One of the unique features of this system is a linear photodiode array, which, in conjunction with a holographic grating, can simultaneously monitor 16 different wavelengths. This feature, called *polychromatic spectral mapping*, results theoretically in the ability to assay more than one analyte within a single reaction vessel. Another feature unique to the SPECTRUM is *tandem access scheduling*, in which the instrument's computer schedules the test sequence based on the length of reaction for each assay in order to yield the most rapid production of test results. With tandem access scheduling, the lag time for the first test result depends upon the combination of tests that are requested. The system can perform 20 different tests (23 tests with ISE) without changing reagents. The operator communicates with the analyzer through a touch-sensitive screen that permits test requesting, access to test results, production of a variety of workload and quality control reports, and so forth.

AMERICAN DADE PARAMAX

This instrument is a newcomer to the category of dry reagent analyzers. The system is contained in a single stand-alone unit. The photometric unit utilizes fiberoptic bundles connected to a single light source to transmit pulses of seven different wavelengths of light to eight separate photodetectors. Reagents in the form of dry tablets are dispensed from the rotating reagent carousel. One tablet is dispensed into each reaction cuvette, diluent is added, and the reagent tablet is dissolved, aided by an ultrasonic probe. Additional dispensers are provided so that user-determined liquid reagents may be used. Disposable cuvettes, which are also used as the reaction vessels, form a continuous belt, and are incubated in a water bath set at either 30° or 37°C. The cuvettes move one position every 5 seconds. During the 5-second pause at the photodetector station, 100 readings are taken at each wavelength, are integrated, and are used to produce bichromatic absorbance measurements as specified by the test parameters. The first result is available in approximately 14 minutes after sampling and every 5 seconds thereafter. The PARAMAX can perform 32 different assays in a random access mode and stat specimens are easily requested on the system. The operator can select tests using a light-sensitive pen touched to a cathode ray tube display of the available tests. Specimens can be placed on the analyzer in any order, because they are identified by a bar-code reader at the time of sampling. Bar-code labels may be printed by the operator in a predetermined sequence. Results can be printed in a chartable form, as well as sent to a mainframe computer via a serial RS 232 interface.

DUPONT *aca*

This name has been known for several years to the majority of clinical laboratorians, who are most familiar with the *aca* I, II, and III. The latest additions to this family are the *aca* IV and V. The latter two systems are more compact than their predecessors: the *aca* IV is a bench top unit and the *aca* V is a floor model. The reagents for each individual test are packaged in separate bar-coded plastic packs. The sample is added to this reagent pack, which moves on a chain in a 37°C temperature-controlled air chamber. The sealed reagent compartments are broken and mixed with the specimen and diluent at one or both of two breaker-mixer stations. The plastic pack forms its own cuvette, and spectrophotometric readings are taken at either one or two wavelengths as specified by the individual test. The first test result is available about 6 minutes after sampling, with an additional result every 37 seconds. Results are printed on a separate report slip for each specimen. Because the reagent packs and specimens are placed on the analyzer manually by the operator, the order of sampling and reagent access is random, and the number of different tests is limited only by the analyzer's computer capabilities (particularly with the *aca* I and II) and the test packs that are available. Compared with the other discrete analyzers discussed above, the DuPont *aca* throughput is very low, approximately 97 test results per hour, and the cost per test is quite high. However, there are over 50 different tests available for the DuPont *aca*, of which many are unavailable on any other automated chemistry analyzer. All stat specimens can be manually introduced into the sampler at any time and there is need for only limited communication with the system, because the bar-coded reagent packs are placed behind each specimen cup to identify the tests desired for each specimen. The major difference between the *aca* IV and V, other than size, is that the *aca* V has ISE capability for sodium and potassium analysis.

Suggested Reading

Davis JE: Automation. In Kaplan LA, Pesce AJ (eds): Clinical Chemistry: Theory, Analysis, and Correlation, pp 261–272. St. Louis, CV Mosby, 1984

21

DISCRETE CHEMISTRY ANALYZERS, PART III
Simultaneous Analysis of Multiple Analytes

Ronald D. Feld
Jim Noffsinger

Definitions

Bar Coding: A system in which information is encoded in a series of lines or bars. The spacing and thickness of these lines are sensed by a reader system and this information is then relayed to a computer. This system allows quick input of information into a computer without the need for a keyboard.

Discrete Analysis: Analysis in which each test is compartmentalized and separated from preceding and subsequent tests.

Ion-Selective Electrode: An electrode with a unique phase that allows it to respond selectively to the concentration of a single ion in the presence of others.

Random-Access Analyzer: An analyzer capable of performing single or multiple tests on each sample, but performing only those tests requested on each sample. Samples and reagents in the analyzer menu that are not requested are not utilized for tests.

Throughput: The maximum number of tests that can be processed in a unit of time, usually 1 hour.

Introduction

The previous three chapters have all discussed types of automated chemistry analysis. Chapter 18 described the first automated colorimetric analysis of Skeggs in 1957 and modifications of this continuous flow technique. In Chapter 19, Tanaka and Witte classified the various types of discrete analyzers as multitest systems and batch systems and limited their focus to batch systems. Chapter 20 followed by further dividing the multitest systems into those instruments that perform all tests requested on a given specimen simultaneously and those that perform the tests sequentially while describing the latter. In this final chapter on automated chemistry analyzers, the emphasis will be on automated multichannel discrete analyzers that permit simultaneous analysis of multiple analytes by taking multiple aliquots of each sample and independently performing each test selected in a dedicated channel (see Fig. 19-1A).

There are several of these multichannel discrete analyzers on the market, but this chapter will discuss only three of them—the American Monitor Parallel, the Beckman Astra, and the Eastman Kodak Ektachem. The three were selected because of their uniqueness and/or acceptance in the clinical laboratory. Because the instruments are quite dissimilar, they will be discussed separately.

Parallel

When one compares the myriad of discrete, random-access chemistry analyzers available on the market today, the American Monitor Parallel* certainly seems to be in a class by itself. Its ability to process 240 samples per hour with up to 7200 test results per hour and its size (288 square feet of floor space and nearly 5000 pounds of shipping weight) immediately convince you that this instrument is not meant for the 100-bed hospital.

INSTALLATION REQUIREMENTS

The analyzer itself consists of several units. The chemistry unit contains the serum sampler mechanism, reagent storage and dispensing mechanism, reaction vessels, spectrophotometers, and flame photometer. The electronic unit consists of two cabinets, one of which contains a DEC PDP 11/23 with 256K kilobyte random access memory (RAM) and two 10 megabyte DEC hard disk drives. The other cabinet contains a Computer Automation minicomputer that controls the chemistry analyzer under instruction from the DEC computer. There are also three cathode ray tube (CRT) terminals associated with the system; one has an associated optical card reader and one has an optional bar-code reader wand. A high-speed printer and an air compressor are also part of the analyzer.

Installation of the system requires 288 square feet of floor space with adequate service clearances. Because of the weight of the components, the floor must be sturdy and uncarpeted, and precautions must be taken to eliminate static electricity. Operating temperatures are between 68° and 77°F with relative humidities between 34% and 80%. The unit itself, with the flame photometer in operation, generates 35,000 BTUs/hr and special precautions may be necessary to dissipate this heat load. Two 240-volt outlets are required and a 110-volt dedicated grounded circuit is required for the database cabinet. Type II College of American Pathologists (CAP) grade water must be supplied to the instrument at pressures between 35 and 60 psi and at a rate of 1.2 liters/minute with an extra 25% contingency for peak demand periods. A floor drain is required. Compressed air and vacuum for controlling functions such as reagent and sample dispensing, spectrophotometer transfer, and reaction vessel washing are supplied by the air compressor/vacuum

*American Monitor Corporation, Indianapolis, IN

pump. The flame photometer requires an oxygen and propane source. Oxygen consumption is 10 to 12 cubic feet per hour whereas that of propane is 3 cubic feet per hour.

CHEMISTRY ANALYZER OPERATION

An overview of the operating principles of the chemistry unit will be presented, and each of the various subsections of the chemistry unit will then be discussed in more detail. The key to understanding the chemistry unit is the 15-second cycle of the analyzer. During this 15-second cycle, various functions are occurring simultaneously in different areas of the instrument. An aliquot from as many as 30 specimens is introduced into 30 reaction vials. Reagents are dispensed into reaction vials that have received specimens during a previous cycle. Reaction vial contents are mixed, incubated for a variable number of 15-second cycles, and aspirated into spectrophotometers for absorbance determinations. Reaction vials whose contents have been aspirated are then washed three times with deionized water and evacuated during a series of cycles before reuse.

Specimen Sampling

Specimens, either in specimen cups or spun blood collection tubes, are introduced into the system by a continuous loop of 150 carriers located at the front of the instrument. Input as to specimen identification and tests ordered on that particular specimen is carried out by a bar-code reader. Alternatively, specimens may be scheduled via one of the terminals and the computer generates a printed pour list. Specimens are placed in the transport chain according to this pour list.

Specimen aliquots are transferred to the reaction vials via a sample bar that contains 30 sample probes. The sample bar moves out and over the sample transport chain, and the sample bar with probes is lowered into 1 to 30 sample cups, depending upon chain position, every 15 seconds. Sample probes are connected to precision microsyringes that are filled with deionized water down through the sample probe. During specimen transfer, the syringe aspirates a specific amount of sample that has been preset for that particular chemistry. The sample bar then moves over the reaction vials and dispenses the sample aliquot and a deionized water flush that washes out the probe. During each 15-second cycle, the sample probes are dipped in a sample wash reservoir of deionized water that rinses the outside of the sample probes. If one of the chemistries is not ordered on a particular specimen, deionized water is placed in the reaction vial to prevent air from being transferred to the spectrophotometer flowcells. The specimen aliquot does not come into contact with the sample syringe itself, which contains only water. This minimizes wear on the syringe by not having it in contact with serum proteins.

Specimen volume range is 1 to 100 μl, with a precision of $\pm 0.5\%$ at 10μl. Just as in several other parameters, specimen sample volume is under user control so that additional chemistries may be adapted by the user.

Analysis

Reaction vials are contained in 68 reaction vial bars, each containing a linear array of 30 2.0-ml reaction vials. The reaction vials are not disposable and, barring breakage, should not have to be replaced. The reaction vial bars are distributed in two rows of 34 bars and are in a bath that maintains the vial temperature at 37°C ± 0.2°C. During each 15-second cycle, a reaction vial bar with freshly washed and dried vials moves into proximity of the sample bar so that specimen aliquots can be dispensed. The specimen vial bar that had been filled with specimen in the previous cycle moves back one position in the right row of 34 reaction vials. After each cycle, the reaction vial bar moves back one place in the row. After the 34th position in the right-hand row, the bar is moved to the back of the left row and then the bar moves forward one position in the left row. Because one reaction vial bar moves into position every 15 seconds, it takes 16 minutes for each bar to complete the counterclockwise rotation. The bars on the right move from front to back while those on the left move back to front. Each row of reaction vials is exposed only to the reagents of a single chemistry, which minimizes contamination. Therefore, in each reaction vial bar, up to 30 chemistries are proceeding in parallel fashion (Fig. 21-1).

Mounted above the reaction vial bars is a fiberglass platen that contains a circular hole corresponding to each reaction vial. Placed on the platen are the reagent dispensing lines, spectrophotometers, and mixers as well as tubes for aspirating and washing reagent vials. During each 15-second cycle, the platen is raised and lowered above the reaction vials. Depending upon where a vial is in the cycle it could be stirred, mixed, read for absorbance, incubated, or aspirated and washed.

Reagents are dispensed by a fluidic system in which the amount of reagent is controlled by varying the length of time a valve is held open under constant

Figure 21-1.   Schematic diagram of the Parallel showing the sample transport, aspirate/dispenser probes, reaction vial bars, and platen. (Courtesy of Macor Publishing Co, New York)

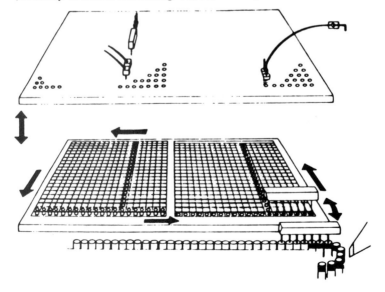

pressure. The solenoid valves are under computer control and reagent volumes can vary from 50 to 1300 μl with a precision of $\pm 0.2\%$. Again, reagent volumes are user-programmable for adapting test methodologies to the instrument. Up to six reagents may be dispensed in a channel. Reagents are stored in two cabinets located in the rear of the chemistry analyzer. The cabinet at ambient temperature has room for 32 reagent bottles and the refrigerated cabinet has room for 24.

Mixing is accomplished by a motor with a mixer blade located in the platen at appropriate locations for a particular chemistry. The motors are under computer control so that the duration of stirring during each 15-second cycle is preprogrammed.

Specimens are transferred from reaction vials to spectrophotometers by means of a test transfer assembly, which is controlled by air pressure. The spectrophotometers are mounted on the platens at appropriate positions depending upon the individual chemistry, and these positions are flexible so that the user can adapt other test methodologies. Each spectrophotometer unit serves two channels and, therefore, contains two one-centimeter quartz flow-through cuvettes having a volume of 0.076 ml. A tungsten-halogen lamp serves as a light source and a series of lenses and a beam splitter focus the light onto a test and reference silicon photodetector. A feedback circuit from the reference detector adjusts the lamp power (Fig. 21-2). Wavelength selection is accomplished by narrow band-pass interference filters with wavelength accuracy of ± 2 nm. The linear absorbance range is 0 to 2.0 OD at 340 nm. The contents of the flowcell is aspirated to waste when the next reaction vial is aspirated. Reaction vials in which a chemistry is not being performed contain deionized water, and this is aspirated in place of reactants. This ensures that the flowcell is always filled with liquid so that the introduction of air bubbles into the flowcell is minimized. One channel is devoted to a serum blank. Diluted specimen is aspirated into the spectrophotometer, which measures the absorbance of the sample at 500, 546, and 650 nm. Appropriate corrections for icterus, hemolysis, and turbidity that were developed by the company are then applied to each chemistry.

The flame photometer uses lithium as an internal reference. Two sets of fixed

Figure 21-2. Diagram of Parallel spectrophotometer. (Courtesy of American Monitor Corp, Indianapolis, IN)

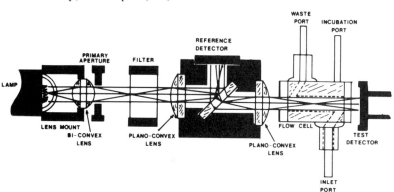

lenses and a beam splitter direct the light to the three photodetectors. Because sodium and potassium are determined simultaneously, they are counted as a single channel.

Reflex Reschedule Delta Detection and Encoded Test Selection

Reflex reschedule delta detection (R2D2) and encoded test selection (ETs) are two new additions to the Parallel instrument. Encoded test selection uses a bar-code printer (not supplied with the instrument) to print a bar code with patient demographic and test-selection information. This information is supplied via a terminal or can be downloaded from the laboratory computer through the bidi-rectional interface. Samples may then be loaded in the sample chain at any position and patient demographic and test-selection information is read by the bar-code reader and stored in the DEC computer.

The R2D2 system consists of a panel of light-emitting diodes (LEDs) and switches mounted on the front of the instrument and a small printer. Software for the system resides in the DEC computer. The R2D2 panel has three areas. One set of LEDs monitors each chemistry channel displaying the status of that channel. This warns the operator that a particular channel may need attention. The next section monitors the status of individual samples. For instance, if a particular sample has an enzyme value that exceeds the linear dynamic range of the instrument, this would be noted by a red LED on the panel. The operator may then dilute the sample and reschedule it. Because of the software associated with R2D2, the dilution ratio has been predetermined and the operator merely places the sample in an empty position and signals the instrument by pressing on LED. The instrument reads the bar code and automatically repeats the deter-mination that is necessary on the diluted sample and calculates the value. The dilution factors for each test are determined by the operator and are entered into the software. Other combinations of LEDs alert the operator to other problems and allow the operator to interact with the samples before observing a final print-out. This saves time and makes more efficient use of the instrument. The last area of the R2D2 panel is the stat pad. This combination of LEDs and switches allows the operator to schedule tests without interacting with a terminal. The printer is used to print an audit trail of the samples.

Standardization and Chemistries

A startup procedure is performed once a day and takes from 30 to 40 minutes. This includes powering up the computer and verifying spectrophotometer function and water regulation. Standardization, also done once every 24 hours, takes an additional 20 minutes. After these procedures, the instrument may be left in a standby status while not running samples. Shutdown is performed once per day as part of maintenance and requires about 25 minutes.

Twenty-eight chemistries are currently available on the instrument, with more under development. Sample volumes range from 3 to 80 μl with most tests re-quiring 30 μl or less. Tests may be ordered singly or in up to 99 user-defined profiles. Based on the 15-second cycle, the instrument is capable of processing 240 samples per hour for a theoretical test rate of 7200/hr if 30 tests per specimen are ordered. In practical terms, a throughput rate of 150 to 180 specimens per hour seems reasonable.

Interfacing

Almost every aspect of instrument operation is under some form of computer control or interaction. This is accomplished by a number of utility programs through which the operator can interact with the computer. These utilities control such options as choices of data acceptance, patient scheduling, quality control and standardization data review, selection of printout formats, and defining profiles.

The Parallel comes equipped with a bidirectional direct interface (RS232C) for communicating with a laboratory computer. An optional buffered interface is also available. Transmission lines in excess of 50 feet between the instrument and the laboratory computer require the use of a pair of modems. Because the interface is bidirectional, information concerning patient demographics and test ordering can be downloaded from the laboratory computer into the resident DEC computer in the Parallel. Data transmission from the Parallel to the laboratory computer usually consists of collated patient results.

SUMMARY

The American Monitor Parallel is a computerized, high-throughput instrument that is capable of performing multiple tests on a sample in a discrete test-selective manner. Microsampling and low reagent consumption make this an attractive instrument to the high-volume laboratory where speed of analysis, instrument availability, and minimal labor inputs are important.

Beckman ASTRA

The Beckman ASTRA* (Automated Stat/Routine Analyzer) was introduced in the late 1970s. It embodied several concepts that have become almost standard in subsequent instrumentation introduced for clinical chemistry analysis. The instrument was discrete and had random access (*i.e.,* only those tests ordered on a particular sample would be performed). It also allowed the operator to interact with the instrument via a keyboard and a video screen. The instrument originally came in two models. The ASTRA 4 is a bench-top model capable of containing four chemistry modules, and the ASTRA 8 can contain up to eight modules. A recently introduced ASTRA IDEAL System links two ASTRA 8s together with a data management system.

ASTRA OPERATING PRINCIPLES

The ASTRA has four main functional areas: (1) a sample turntable rotates under command of the instrument microcomputer and presents both specimens or calibrators to the sample pickup probes; (2) the chemistry modules receive and analyze specimens; (3) a disk-operating system contains operating programs; (4)

*Beckman Instruments, Brea, CA

a program keyboard allows the operator to enter instructions for specific speci-mens located on the sample turntable.

Sampling System

A 40-position sample turntable accepts various sizes of plastic sample cups. This turntable is under operator and computer control and automatically advances to present the next specimen or calibrator to the sample probes. A plastic sample tray hood is provided to lessen the evaporation of the specimens. Specimen sampling is accomplished by dual stainless steel probes controlled by the sample with the instrument via a keyboard and a video screen. The instrument originally came in two models. The ASTRA 4 is a bench-top model capable of containing four chemistry modules, and the ASTRA 8 can contain up to eight modules. A recently introduced ASTRA IDEAL System links two ASTRA 8s together with a data management system.

Each probe is under the control of a positive-displacement pump that is in-dividually driven by stepping motors controlled by the computer. The amount of specimen aspirated by the probes is determined by the tests ordered on a particular

Figure 21-3. Sample probe contents be-fore sample injection on ASTRA. (Cour-tesy of Beckman Instruments, Inc, Brea, CA)

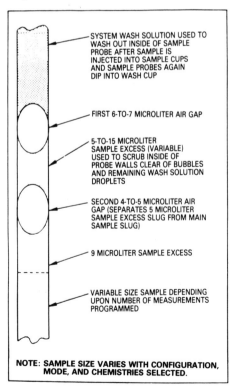

specimen. The probes dip twice into each specimen cup while the sample pumps are drawing up sample. This creates two 10-μl air slugs in each probe separated by a variable 5 to 15 μl of sample. This sample slug is to accumulate any drops of wash solution remaining along the wall of the probes and to scrub any accumulated bubbles. This excess sample slug used in cleaning the probe is not for testing. After the second air slug, a variable amount of specimen is drawn into the probes depending upon the tests ordered plus an 8-μl sample excess (Fig. 21-3). For example, 133 μl are required to perform blood urea nitrogen (BUN), creatinine, glucose, and the four electrolytes on the ASTRA 8. During sampling, a low-voltage ac signal is passed between the two sample probes. If this path is broken during aspiration of the sample, the instrument will abort the assays on that sample. With this method of short-sample detection, probes must be properly adjusted for the system to be functional.

After sampling from the turntable, the probes are dipped into the wash cup to clean the outside of the probes. The probes then separate and swing out over the reaction cups of the chemistry modules and then descend into the reaction cups where the appropriate amount of specimen is injected. If a particular analysis has not been ordered on a specimen, no sample is injected. The probes then move to the next set of reaction modules and the process is repeated. After the final injection of sample, the sample transport mechanism returns the probes to the wash cup where wash solution is rinsed through the probes and the outside of the probes is also cleaned.

Chemistry Modules

A unique feature of the ASTRA system is the chemistry module. This self-contained system contains the pumps necessary for transporting and removing reagents to the reaction cup as well as the analysis system (electrode or colorimetric) for each test (Fig. 21-4). Because of this modularity, the module can be quickly removed and replaced with another to resolve a problem with the analytic system. The module can also be removed to provide better access when performing maintenance. Reagents are mounted on a shelf above the analyzer and are not refrigerated during use. Several companies in addition to Beckman Instruments market reagents for the ASTRA system. As of this date, there are 24 chemistries available. Several of these chemistries can be performed on urine; glucose, chloride, and protein may be performed on cerebral spinal fluid. Representative chemistries will be discussed.

Sodium and potassium are measured simultaneously in a single module. Fifty microliters of specimen are injected into the reaction cup, which contains approximately 1.3 ml of high-ionic-strength buffer. The large dilution ensures that the amount of protein in the cup is negligible while the high ionic strength of the buffer swamps the activity contribution of ions other than sodium or potassium that may be present in the sample. The reaction cup is mixed by means of a Teflon-coated stirrer located in the bottom of the cup.

Sodium is measured by an ion-selective electrode in which sodium undergoes an ion exchange in the hydrated outer layer of the glass electrode. The voltage increases as the exchange takes place. This potential follows the Nernst equation

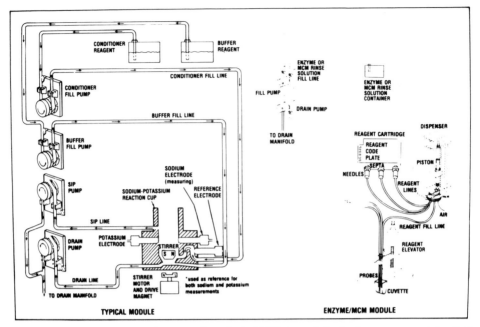

Figure 21-4. Schematic diagram of typical ASTRA module-dual reagent module (*left*), enzyme/multiple chemistry module (*right*). (Courtesy of Beckman Instruments, Inc, Brea, CA)

and allows calculation of the sodium concentration in the solution. The electrode has a selectivity of sodium over potassium of about 300 to 1. The sodium measurement on serum has a between-run standard deviation of 1.0 mEq/liter. The usable range for serum sodium is 100 to 300 mEq/liter and, for urine sodium, it is 10 to 300 mEq/liter.

The potassium electrode has a valinomycin membrane, which has a selectivity of potassium over sodium of about 1000 to 1. As the potassium ion complexes with the valinomycin membrane, a voltage develops that follows the Nernst equation. The valinomycin tips have a lifetime of about 2 months and then must be replaced. Between-run standard deviation for serum potassium is about 0.1 mEq/liter. Usable range for serum potassium is 1.0 to 10.0 mEq/liter and 2 to 300 mEq/liter for urine potassium. Sodiums and potassiums may be determined at a rate of 70 samples per hour. Both the sodium and potassium measurements have shown excellent agreement with flame photometer measurements.

Creatinine is determined in a single module using an alkaline picrate methodology. Thirty microliters of serum or 10 μl of urine are injected into the reaction cup containing approximately 2.6 ml of alkaline picrate reagent. A Teflon-coated stirring bar located in the bottom of the reaction cup ensures proper mixing; a heater maintains the temperature within the cup between 36° and 38°C with a variation of ± 0.1°C. The reagent is preheated before entering the cup. Light from a tungsten source lamp is directed through the reaction mixture and the transmitted light is detected by a photodiode fitted with a 520-nm narrow bandpass filter.

Instead of taking a single spectrophotometric measurement of the product at 520 nm, the ASTRA measures the rate of product formation at 25.6 seconds after sample injection. This time was chosen to eliminate interference from fast-reacting pseudocreatinine substances and before slow-reacting interferences have a chance to contribute. This method is not entirely successful because acetoacetate, a fast-reacting interference, causes a significant increase in the measured creatinine concentration in patients with diabetic ketoacidosis. This creatinine module displays a typical between-run precision of 0.1 mg/dl on serum. The usable range is 0 to 25 mg/dl for serum and 0 to 400 mg/dl for urine. Throughput is 70 specimens per hour.

Two modules recently introduced perform six enzymes. Each module performs three enzymes, two measured at 340 nm (aspartate transaminase [AST], alanine transaminase [ALT], lactate dehydrogenase [LD], or creatine kinase [CK]) and one measured at 405 nm (γ-glutamyl transferase [γGT] and alkaline phosphatase [AP]). Contained within each module is a carousel of 15 semidisposable cuvettes. Reagents, contained in cartridges of 50, 100, or 250 tests located on the module, are precisely dispensed into the cuvettes by dispensing syringes. Specimen is injected by the sample probes. Up to three injections for each patient sample per module can occur depending on what tests were ordered. Mixing is accomplished by a high-speed rotating rod that dips into each cuvette after the specimen has been injected. The carousel rotates completely every 400 seconds. A sample is injected every 80 seconds. The 80 seconds is divided into two phases— a rotational and a stationary phase. During the rotational phase, the specimen is injected, a sample blank is read, and the specimen and reagents are mixed. During the stationary phase, cuvettes are drained and washed, filled with new reagents, and absorbance measurements are taken. Ten absorbance measurements are taken over 30 seconds on each cuvette. A regression line is calculated on these points and the slope of the line is used to calculate enzyme activity. Substrate depletion is monitored and a system called Over-Range Detection and Correction (ORDAC) automatically samples a reduced amount of specimen and multiplies this answer by the appropriate dilution factor if the dynamic range is exceeded. Cuvettes are automatically checked for cleanliness and an enzyme multiplier factor can be used for correlation with other enzyme systems in the laboratory. Within-run precision is usually less than 4% and three enzymes can be run on 50 μl or less. Temperatures of either 30° or 37°C can be selected. After an initial delay of 2.5 minutes, the system can produce up to six enzyme results per patient every 80 seconds.

Calibration
Calibration is accomplished by two-level calibrating solutions. Calibrators can be aqueous or protein-based depending upon the tests desired. Aqueous calibrators may be used for electrolytes, BUN, creatinine, and glucose, whereas tests such as albumin require the protein-based calibrators. Bilirubin requires a special set of calibrators. Aqueous and protein-based calibrators may be used simultaneously (*i.e.,* calibrating some channels with aqueous and some with protein-based). The frequency of calibration varies with the test. Electrolytes, for instance, must be recalibrated every 8 hours whereas calcium calibration is stable for 4 hours and glucose is stable for 2 hours.

Each calibrator is sampled at least twice and up to four times. If calibration numbers are within preset precision limits, the first two replicates will be averaged. If outside these limits, the calibrator may be sampled up to two more times. If four replicates are outside the limits, a calibration error is printed for a particular channel. The channel may be bypassed or corrective action may be taken by the operator. Additional tests on the difference between the two calibration points is performed before calibration is accepted.

Keyboard

The operator interacts with the instrument through a system-program keyboard. The keyboard contains three functional areas: system command selections, measurement channel selections, and numerical data entry selections. The system command keys control major system tasks such as calibration, prime reagents, and stop. The measurement channel selection keys allow the operator to select the particular chemistries or panels desired on a particular specimen. The numerical data entry keys allow for the entry of patient identification numbers or items such as tray numbers and cup numbers. Three system-status indicator lamps (red, yellow, green) alert the operator to the various states of the instrument. An audible alarm sounds when there is an instrument malfunction or failure to calibrate. The keyboard is used in conjunction with a video display screen, which performs many functions such as aiding tray programming with patient samples or providing prompts for the operator when performing trouble-shooting options. Calibration and patient result data are printed on a thermal printer.

Disk Operating System

The operating system for the ASTRA is contained on 5¼-inch floppy disks. Two systems are available—Disk Operating System (DOS), which consists of two disk drives, and Disk Operating Reporting System (DORS), which consists of two additional disk drives and an off-line printer. This system is especially useful for those laboratories that do not have a laboratory computer to collate and generate patient reports. The operating system is contained on a set of two floppy disks that Beckman has routinely updated for maximum performance. To change operating systems, the operator merely loads a new set of disks. The operating system contains the programs for tray programming, calibration, instrument setup, and diagnostic programs. The diagnostic programs allow the operator to apply a number of tests to each chemistry module to help isolate a problem. The operating system can also perform calculations such as anion gap and certain ratios such as the BUN: creatinine ratio.

MAINTENANCE

Maintenance consists of tasks such as changing pump tubes, cleaning parts of modules, replacing electrode tips, and lubricating syringes. One unique feature of the instrument is the Rapid Kit. This option is a spare-parts bank that may include virtually all the parts of the instrument. A full complement of spare chemistry modules, circuit boards, printers, disk drives, and samplers is available.

This option allows the operator to switch out the faulty part once it has been discovered. A combination of the diagnostic program and a 24-hour hotline service is available to aid in trouble-shooting. This ensures that there will be little down-time on the instrument.

SUMMARY

The Beckman ASTRA is a discrete random-access analyzer that is capable of performing a wide range of analyses. Its several sizes and configurations make it useful in both large and small laboratories and its unique modular construction aids in maintenance and repair.

Kodak EKTACHEM

The Ektachem 400* and the Ektachem 700* are discrete chemistry analyzers capable of simultaneously performing a wide variety of analyses. The analyzers use slides composed of multiple layers of dry film to perform clinical chemistry tests. The construction of the slides is an extension of technology developed in the photographic industry. The multiple-layered slide technology offers significant advantages in both sensitivity and selectivity as compared with other commonly used chemistry analyzers.

Both the Ektachem 400 and Ektachem 700 require infrequent calibration and quality control procedures and require minimal operator maintenance. Sample throughput is approximately 500 tests per hour for each instrument. The Ektachem 400 is capable of performing colorimetric and potentiometric analyses. The Ektachem 700 has the additional capability of performing kinetic rate reactions as well as colorimetric and potentiometric tests.

COLORIMETRIC SLIDES

Colorimetric slides are composed of a spreading layer, one or more intermediate layers, and an indicator layer. The overall objective of the slide technology is to provide an accurate quantitation of the analyte with a minimum of interference from other materials present in the sample. A number of different techniques are employed to accomplish this desired result.[1,4] For example, interfering materials may be immobilized in one layer while the analyte is allowed to migrate to another place. In other cases, the interferent may be altered in one layer, making it nonreactive in the subsequent color reaction. Alternatively, the analyte itself may undergo a physical or chemical reaction in one layer, forming a product that then migrates to another layer where further reactions occur.

Spreading Layer

The spreading layer is composed of a highly porous polymer providing a capillary network designed to permit rapid and uniform sample spreading. Uniformity of the spreading layer is essential for good precision, especially should

*Eastman Kodak Company, Rochester, NY

there be a variation in sample volume. Uniform sample spreading is, in part, a result of the difference in time required for spreading to occur in the upper layer, compared with subsequent layers. The sample spreads quite rapidly in the porous spreading layer due to capillary action. Before the sample can penetrate the underlying gelatin layer, the gelatin must first become hydrated by moisture from the sample. The sample is, therefore, excluded momentarily from the underlying gelatin layers, allowing sufficient time for uniform sample spreading in the upper layer.

The spreading layer may be composed of cellulose acetate, microcrystalline cellulose, or plastic beads. Both the pore size and the thickness of the layer may vary depending upon the application. The spreading layer is usually designed to trap cellular material, crystals, and other particulate matter, as well as large protein molecules. This top layer may also be made reflective by the addition of TiO_2 or $BaSO_4$. These compounds may also serve to mask colored constituents within the sample. In some applications, additional chemical and physical reactions take place in the spreading layer.

Intermediate Layers

Just beneath the spreading layer are intermediate layers designed to screen out or alter interfering materials, and, if necessary, to convert the analyte into a substance suitable for quantitation. A wide variety of processes and reactions may be used in the construction of the intermediate layers. Filtration-type processes are commonly used (*e.g.*, dialysis and gel permeability). Selective absorbants such as ion-exchange resins and immunochemical reagents may be employed. Anchoring reagents and catalysts are used in some slides, including enzymes and beads containing scavengers. Reaction sequence and timing are controlled by such tools as competitive binding and controlled reagent diffusion.

Indicator Layer

The function of the indicator layer is to convert the analyte into its final color. This layer incorporates a mordant layered below a reflectant surface. As described earlier, the reflectant surface may be a part of the spreading layer or, alternatively, may be located in any position above the indicator layer.

Detection and Quantitation

Once the colorimetric slide is spotted, it is moved to a "precondition station" where the slide is brought to 37°C. This is accomplished in a 12-second period. The slide then moves into the colorimetric incubator where it remains for a period of approximately 5 minutes. Following incubation, the slide is moved to a read station. The major mechanical modules are shown in Figure 21-5. Within the read station, light from a tungsten-halogen lamp is passed through an appropriate filter, an optical system, and directed to the lower surface of the slide (indicator layer) at a 45° angle (Fig. 21-6). A photodetector is positioned at a 90° angle from the slide. Two additional readings are taken by this colorimetric reflectometer, one reading from a dark surface on the filter wheel before the slide enters the read station and a second reading on a white reference area. The reflection density

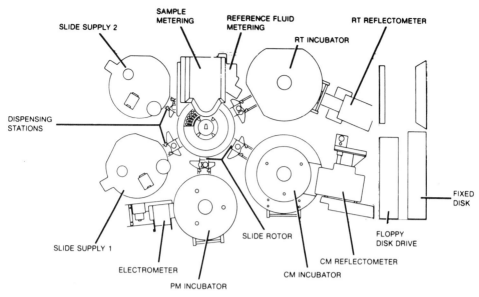

Figure 21-5. Major mechanical modules in Ektachem analyzer. (Courtesy of Eastman Kodak Company, Rochester, NY)

Figure 21-6. Optical system of Ektachem analyzer. (Courtesy of Eastman Kodak Company, Rochester, NY)

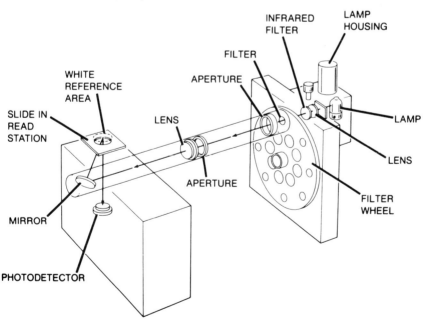

from the slide is related to the concentration of the analyte, by comparison with a series of calibrator samples. It should be pointed out that reflection density (unlike optical density in absorption spectroscopy) is related to concentration in a nonlinear fashion. The signal observed by the photodetector must be subjected to a linear data transformation before it can be properly interpreted.

POTENTIOMETRIC ANALYSES

Potentiometric slides used in the Ektachem consist of two identical ion-selective electrodes. The overall construction is illustrated in Figure 21-7. The electrodes consist of four layers.[3] The top layer is an ion-selective membrane that contains an appropriate ionophore. Next is an internal reference layer followed by a silver chloride layer and an underlying layer of silver. Sample fluid and reference fluid are simultaneously deposited on separate halves of the slide. The two half-cells are connected by a liquid junction provided by a paper bridge, forming a complete concentration cell. After the slides have been spotted, they are moved into an incubator where they remain for a 3-minute equilibration period and are then moved into an electrometer where the final reading is taken. The electrometer measures the potential difference in millivolts between the two electrodes of a potentiometric slide, one in contact with the sample and the other in contact with reference fluid. Because the concentration of the reference fluid is

Figure 21-7. Structure of an ion-specific electrode slide. (Courtesy of Eastman Kodak Company, Rochester, NY)

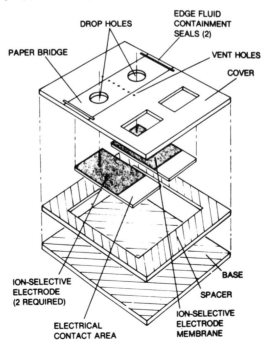

known, the ion concentration in the sample can be obtained by applying the Nernst equation.

This is a so-called "direct" potentiometric measurement and, as such, is not affected by severe hyperlipidemia, hyperproteinemia, or diabetic acidosis. "Indirect" potentiometric analysis (referring to measurements made after dilution with a diluent of fixed high ionic strength) and flame photometry are both subject to significant bias in these clinical conditions.[2]

RATE ANALYSIS

The Ektachem 700 is capable of performing multiple-rate tests. Slides used for rate analyses are constructed in a manner similar to those for colorimetric assays.[3] Once the slide has been spotted with a sample, it is moved to a precondition station where the temperature is brought to near 37°C. After a 12-second period in the precondition station, the slide is moved to the rate incubator where it remains for the required reaction time. The rate incubator is equipped with a reflectometer that operates on the same principle as the one used in the reflectance colorimeter. As the incubator disk rotates, a reading is taken of each slide as the slide passes over the "read station." A total of 54 readings are taken during the incubation period of approximately 5.5 minutes. Several steps are required in the calculation of enzyme activity. First, the reflectance of each reading is determined. Each data point is then transformed to density. The data is then systematically examined in order to provide optimum results. This includes the elimination of single-noise spikes, the discarding of early readings prior to steady-state conditions, and the discarding of late readings that fall beyond acceptable limits of constant slope. Final rate determinations are obtained by way of a linear "inside-out" regression technique, which limits slope determinations to the linear region. With some assays, data is fitted with a third-order polynomial in order to calculate maximum rate. The analyzer is capable of detecting several conditions that would produce adverse affects in determining enzyme activity. These include substrate depletion, too few data points in the linear region, the presence of multiple linear regions, and excessive curvature (high noise).

ENVIRONMENTAL CONTROL

Slide Supply

Depending upon the individual assay, slides may require fairly rigid environmental control. There are two slide supplies located within the instrument. One slide supply maintains a relative humidity between 25% and 45% using wet salt pads, and a second slide supply provides a dry environment with humidity being maintained at less than 20% using desiccant packs. Temperature is maintained in both slide supplies at 24°C or below using thermoelectric heat pumps.

Incubator Temperatures

The temperature within the colorimetric incubator is maintained at 37°C ± 1°C over an 8-hour period, by means of two resistance heaters—one above and one below the incubator disk. The potentiometric incubator is maintained at 25°C

± 0.1°C over an 8-hour period by means of a thermoelectric heat pump that provides both heating and cooling. Temperature in the rate incubator is maintained at 37°C ± 0.1°C by means of a heater and thermoelectric cooler located below the incubator disk.

COMPUTER SYSTEM

The entire operation of the Ektachem analyzer is controlled by a complex computer system. The Ektachem 700 is driven by two microcomputers communicating with one another over a high-speed data bus. The technologist enters sample identification and tests ordered, then signals when the sample is loaded and ready for processing through the computer system.

The master computer handles the operation of the analyzer as well as the data processing. The operator communicates with this unit through a keyboard and touch-sensitive monitor. Other communications, such as to printing devices, modems, or laboratory computers, are also controlled by this unit. Sample testing or calibration is initiated; test results, calibration, test reporting, and data transfer to fixed or floppy disks are all functions of this computer.

The purpose of the second computer, the mechanism computer, is to coordinate and direct all the mechanical and thermal components of the analyzer. Scheduling slides, synchronizing mechanical operation, maintaining temperature, and returning slide responses to the master computer for computation are all accomplished by 12 control software modules directed by the mechanism computer.

In conclusion, the Ektachem slide technology makes this analyzer unique; the ease of technologist interaction with the computer, the infrequent calibration and quality control required, and the speed of the analyzer make this instrumentation applicable to the modern clinical laboratory.

References

1. Curme HG, Columbus RL, Dappen Gm et al: Multilayer film elements for clinical analysis: General concepts. Clin Chem 24:1335, 1978
2. Maas AHJ, Siggaard-Andersen O, Weisburg HF, Zijlstra WG: Ion-selective electrodes for sodium and potassium: A new problem of what is measured and what should be reported. Clin Chem 31:482, 1985
3. Shirey TL: Development of a layered-coating technology for clinical chemistry. Clin Biochem 16:147, 1983
4. Spayd RW, Bruschi B, Burdick BA et al: Multilayer film elements for clinical analysis: Applications to representative chemical determinations. Clin Chem 24:1343, 1978

Suggested Reading

Finley PR, Williams RJ, Lichti DA, Thies AC: Evaluation of a new multi-channel analyzer, "Astra-8". Clin Chem 24:2125, 1978
Lloyd PH, Bicknell H, Broughton PMB: An evaluation of the Beckman Astra 8 analyzer. J Automated Chem 2:143, 1980

22

AUTOMATED MICROBIOLOGY SYSTEMS
Marietta M. Henry

Definitions

Abbott Cartridge: A plastic cuvette system with a linear arrangement of chambers, each containing a biochemical medium or an antibiotic for the performance of microbial identification or susceptibility analysis.

Aerobic: Microorganisms growing only in the presence of oxygen.

Autobac Cuvette: A plastic cuvette system with a linear arrangement of chambers, each containing biochemical test materials or antibiotic disks for the performance of microbial identification or susceptibility testing.

Facultatively Anaerobic: Microorganisms growing well under both aerobic and anaerobic conditions.

McFarland Standard: A barium chloride turbidity standard used to standardize bacterial inocula.

Microaerophilic: Microorganisms growing best in only a small amount of atmospheric oxygen (5%–10% CO_2).

Minimal Inhibitory Concentration (MIC): The lowest dilution of an antibiotic that inhibits visible growth. The basic MIC concept is based upon manual tube or microtube dilution procedures. Automation of MIC procedures involves the computer-assisted construction of a 2 or more point growth curve from which the MIC is mathematically determined.

Standard Microbiology Incubator: An incubator with temperature control and increased humidity.

Uniscept Strip: A disposable plastic carrier and strip of cupules containing biochemical and antimicrobial test materials.

Vitek Test Card: A thin rectangular plastic card containing biochemical media or dilutions of antimicrobial agents in test wells for the performance of microbial identification, enumeration, or susceptibility testing.

Introduction

Automated microbiology instruments have appeared in the past 10 years. The degree of automation varies considerably from essentially hands-off operations to manual manipulation of every step except growth assessment. An early partially automated microbiology instrument was the Bactec.* There have been three truly instrumental approaches to bacterial identification and susceptibility: the Vitek Automicrobic System (AMS),* the General Diagnostics Autobac IDX,* and the Abbott MS-2.* The latter instrument has been replaced by the Abbott Quantum II* and the Abbott Avantage.* Diagnostic testing in microbiology has relied upon tedious, repetitive manual techniques that took 18 hours to several days for completion. Automated instruments for bacterial identification and susceptibility testing allow a more rapid turnaround time for reporting to physicians, reduce the technologist's time, and reduce errors in identification and reporting. The time required for bacterial identification or susceptibility testing ranges from 4 to 13 hours. Most instruments are now also offering screening capabilities for urine cultures that utilize direct examination of the clinical specimens. Ranges of colony counts and identification of common urinary pathogens are produced in 4 to 13 hours as well.

Reduced technologist's time, accomplished by the automation of data acquisition, interpretations, and reporting, decreases labor costs and frees the technologist for other work. The potential for interfacing microbiology instruments to laboratory computers allows direct transfer of chartable information, diminishing the amount of the technologist's time required for information and communication. Many laboratory computer systems have not provided microbiology packages because of the complexity of the data required, the α-numeric format, and the long turnaround times for data acquisition. Therefore, most microbiology instrumentation companies had to enter the data processing field to provide chartable reports, susceptibility trend data, and hospital epidemiology packages.

Error reduction in identification, interpretation, and reporting have been accomplished by the automation of many operating steps. The potential for accuracy in the reporting steps has been increased by the use of a computer data base to reduce variability in terminology. The independent nature of microbiology procedures, with culture work spread out over several days and often performed by different technologists, is evened out by the use of instrumentation. This may be particularly important in smaller hospitals where technologists may work in more than one section of the laboratory and do not develop daily expertise with the unique demands of microbiology.

The Vitek Automicrobic System

The AMS is designed to detect, enumerate, identify, and establish the antimicrobic agent susceptibility of microorganisms. The AMS is the most automated of the presently marketed systems and is available in several configurations. The

*Products followed by an asterisk (*) when mentioned for the first time are listed with company name in the Appendix at the end of this chapter.

most common configuration consists of a filler-sealer module, a reader-incubator module, a computer-control module, a data terminal module, and a printer module. In addition to the modules, specially designed and manufactured test cards are an integral part of the system. The AMS provides multiple functions for the microbiology laboratory, including urine screening, enteric pathogen screens, antimicrobial susceptibility testing, and identification of gram-negative bacilli, gram-positive cocci, and yeasts.

TEST CARDS

The ability of the AMS to analyze clinical specimens is dependent upon the special media used both to support and inhibit the growth of microorganisms. The media particular to the type of test are contained in sealed plastic plates called test cards. The test cards contain 16, 20, or 30 wells into which micro-amounts of media are distributed and then dried. The cards are sealed with special tapes; the type of tape controls the level of aeration to the underlying wells. All wells of the card are connected to the injection port by distribution channels molded into the card, and to one or two smaller wells specifically designed to trap any air bubbles. The test cards are inoculated and the media are rehydrated by forcing the diluted specimen through the injection port and distribution channels, then into the wells. Biochemical media used in the identification test cards include both classic and novel test media. Highly selective media are contained in the urinary screen cards for identification of common urinary pathogens, even if the specimen is polymicrobic. Fortified broth media allow the enumeration of organisms in the specimens. Susceptibility cards contain dilutions of antimicrobials for the determination of minimum inhibitory concentration (MIC) values.

The test cards are inoculated with the diluted sample in the filling module. The test kit assembly (card, transfer tube, and sample) is placed into a chamber that is sealed and evacuated. As the pressure in the chamber drops, the air in the media wells and distribution channels is aspirated through the injector tube. When the vacuum reaches the required level, it is slowly released and the reduced air pressure aspirates the sample into the distribution channels and media wells. The bubble traps of each well capture any small air bubbles formed in the filling process. After the filling cycle, the cards are removed from the chamber and placed, one at a time, into the sealing apparatus to cut and seal the plastic transfer tube at the surface of the injector port of the card.

Each test card is precoded to identify the type of card. The operator must only mark the card to allow correct isolate identification when the card is being scanned by the reader head. Although the actual number assigned is left to the discretion of the laboratory, the number must be written in a squared-off style. Improperly marked cards are signified by a warning signal displayed on the data terminal module and the operator is notified by a single beeping sound and an error message.

Once coded and filled, the test cards are inserted into card trays in the reader-incubator module. The cards are designed so that they can be inserted only if they are properly aligned. Once started, the read cycle proceeds automatically and continuously until the system is shut down. Placing an isolate's identification card and susceptibility card in the same tray allows the computer to use the organism growth response data in the evaluation of susceptibility levels.

READER-INCUBATOR MODULE

The reader-incubator module consists of a temperature-controlled chamber containing the electromechanical devices necessary to process the inoculated test cards. The test card trays are then mounted on a revolving carousel within the chamber. Each tray of cards is processed by the AMS once each hour. Every 15 minutes, the carousel rotates 90° and places a different tray into the process position. In the process position, a particular tray is aligned with the reader head. The reader head consists of vertical and horizontal drive mechanisms and an electro-optical detection system. The drive mechanisms allow the reader head to slide down the tray in the processing position and to process any test cards present. Optical detectors align the reader head with the card. The reader head then extracts the card from the tray and sequentially indexes each set of wells into the optical reading position.

The processing of one tray (30 cards) requires 6 minutes. During tray processing, the system automatically secures the carousel access door to prevent aberrations of the reading process due to stray light or mechanical movement. Access for insertion or removal of cards is allowed at all other times. The optical system consists of a set of five light-emitting diodes (LEDs) and corresponding detectors. The LEDs emit light, at 660 nm, that is directed through the test card wells to phototransistor detectors to measure the attenuation of the light as it passes through the test card well. Each well detector is actually an array of four separate detectors to allow the system to obtain a correct reading even if a small air bubble or particulate matter is trapped in the well. The detector output will vary with the amount of bacterial growth or color change within a specific well; this data is computed and stored within the system computer.

There are 30 wells in the identification-type test cards which contain 29 biochemical broths and one growth control broth. Most of the tests are conventional biochemical tests with utilization of substrate causing a color change, either by *p*H change, chemical reaction, or growth in the presence of specific inhibitors (Table 22-1). The miniaturized concept of the test cards has uniquely reproduced aerobic and microaerophilic conditions suited for each test provided. The gram-negative identification (GNI) card (Fig. 22-1) utilizes the ability of an organism to utilize glucose fermentatively to determine into what group the AMS computer places the unknown organism for identification. The inoculum for identification and susceptibility testing is prepared by placing isolated, morphologically identical colonies into 1.8 ml of 0.45% to 0.5% sterile saline to make a suspension equivalent to the proper McFarland turbidity standard (Fig. 22-2).

The AMS-Vitek System is the only automated system currently providing identification of gram-positive organisms. The gram-positive identification card (GPI card) will identify clinically significant streptococci, staphylococci, and selected gram-positive bacilli. It is required that the isolate be screened for catalase

Table 22-1
Gram-Negative Identification Card

Aerobic	Microaerophilic
1. DP-3000	16. Raffinose
2. Glucose (oxidative)	17. Sorbitol
3. Growth control	18. Sucrose
4. Acetamide	19. Inositol
5. Esculin	20. Adonitol
6. Plant indican	21. *p*-Coumaric
7. Urea	22. H$_2$S
8. Citrate	23. ONPG
9. Malonate	24. Rhamnose
10. TDA	25. Arabinose
11. Polymyxin B	26. Glucose (fermentative)
12. Lactose/10%	27. Arginine
13. Maltose	28. Lysine
14. Mannitol	29. Base control
15. Xylose	30. Ornithine
	31. Code for oxidase reaction

Numbers correspond to numbered wells in Figure 22-1. A circular depression in the upper right of the card is for noting the oxidase reaction. No mark in the circular area indicates a negative oxidase reaction. A black mark in the area indicates a positive oxidase reaction.

reaction and the presence or absence of β-hemolysis on blood agar. If positive, these manual test results are entered on the GPI card by blackening small circles.

Enteric pathogen screen cards (EPS cards) allow automated screening of common oxidase negative enteric pathogens in 4 to 8 hours. The EPS card is similar in appearance to the urine screen card, with three sections, allowing

Figure 22-1. Vitek gram-negative identification card. (Courtesy of Vitek Systems)

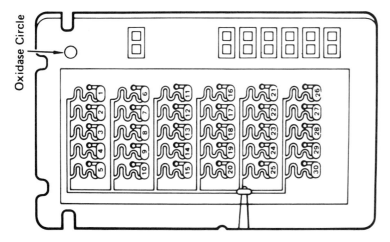

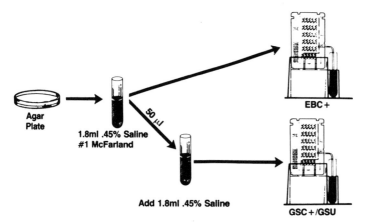

Figure 22-2. Gram-negative sample preparation for a Vitek instrument. (Courtesy of Vitek Systems)

simultaneous testing of three different isolates. Presumptive identification of the following organisms is made: possible *Edwardsiella tarda*, presumptive *Salmonella* species (*S. typhi*), presumptive *Shigella* species, presumptive *Shigella sonnei*, and possible *Yersinia enterocolitica*. If negative at 8 hours, a report is printed that states that the screening process is negative for *Salmonella, Shigella,* and *Yersinia*. This card reduces the use of multiple tube media and technologist time.

Susceptibility testing is performed by inoculating the proper susceptibility card. Eight standard and nine custom panels for gram-negative serum-level susceptibilities, one panel for gram-negative urine-level susceptibilities, and one panel for gram-positive serum-level susceptibilities are available. The multiple gram-negative serum-level panels allow tailoring of the panel to an individual institution's formulary. Each susceptibility card contains 29 wells with varying numbers of dilutions of specific antibiotics and a growth control well. Aminoglycoside wells are cation-supplemented with calcium and magnesium. Essentially, the cards are miniaturized and abbreviated versions of the doubling dilution technique for MIC determination. Once inoculated and placed in the reader-incubator, all wells of the cards are read hourly by the machine. When bacterial growth occurs at levels equal to or greater than a predetermined level, a regression approach is utilized (along with organism identification if available) to determine the appropriate MIC values for each antimicrobial agent. If during a 4- to 10-hour period, the organism reaches the growth threshold for an accurate call, a final status report is printed automatically for the card. If the growth threshold for an accurate call is not met in 4 to 10 hours, the final status is given as "insufficient growth in positive control well."

Urine screening is performed using a dilution of 200 μl of well-mixed clean-voided urine. Special transfer tubes and filling stands are provided. Three separate urine samples are tested simultaneously on one card. A final report is available at 1 to 13 hours. The urine screen card (Fig. 22-3) consists of 30 growth chambers, each containing dried growth media and sealed with oxygen-permeable tape. De-

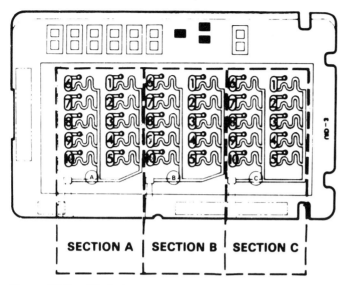

Figure 22-3. Vitek three-in-one urine screen card. (Courtesy of Vitek Systems)

tection, enumeration, and selective identification are performed for the following organisms: *Escherichia coli, Proteus species, Klebsiella/Enterobacter* species, *Citrobacter freundii, Pseudomonas aeruginosa, Serratia* species, Group D enterococci, *Staphylococcus* species, and yeast (Table 22-2). The media employed in the urine screen cards are nonclassical, rendered specific for a urinary organism's identification by the inclusion of both nutritionally selective components and unique metabolic inhibitors. The total enumeration is based upon the rate of growth of the organism in the growth wells. Enumeration is expressed as > 50,000 colony-forming units (CFU)/ml, 1,000 to 50,000 CFU/ml, or "no growth."

COMPUTER-CONTROL MODULE

The AMS is controlled by a minicomputer installed within the computer-control module. The computer contains memory for test card and data system instructions. The instructions (computer program) direct the instrument function and control important parameters of the system. Data storage for a particular test card begins after the first reading process. The program recognizes the new card and assigns the specimen identification to the corresponding tray position. The program then directs the processing of the card (once each hour) until the required number of readings has been achieved. The data is then processed and the final results are communicated to the operator.

Data analysis is performed by a variety of methods. Each method is chosen for the type of test card used. Biochemical reactions are compared to a probability table of known isolate reactions. The closest two patterns are compared and the identification probabilities for these two organisms are computed and reported. The susceptibility cards monitor the growth rate of the organism in the presence

Table 22-2
AMS-Vitek Urine Biochemical Reactions

Well No.	Organism	Active Component	Reaction
1	*Citrobacter freundii*	Rhamnose	Acid production and growth; indicator change
2	*Serratia* species	Esculin, ferric citrate	Enzymatic hydrolysis of esculin and precipitation of iron salt
3	*Klebsiella/Enterobacter* species	Cellobiose, *d*-biotin, Fildes enrichment	Acid production and growth; indicator change
4	*Proteus* species	Urea	Enzymatic degradation of urea; indicator change
5	*Escherichia coli*	Lactose, *l*-arabinose	Acid production and growth; indicator change
6	*Pseudomonas aeruginosa*	Cetrimide	Cetrimide tolerance
7	Yeast	Glucose	Acid production and indicator change
8	Group D enterococci	Esculin, ferric ammonium citrate	Enzymatic hydrolysis of esculin and precipitation of iron salts
9	*Staphylococcus* species	NaCl, DNA-methyl green	Enzyme hydrolysis; indicator change
10	Positive control	Peptones and carbohydrates	Acid production and growth; indicator change

of dilutions of antimicrobial agents and compare this data to the rate of growth in the positive control well. NCCLS (category) calls and MIC values are calculated from these differences. The urine screen card enumeration data are calculated by the most probable number theory and allow the estimation of the total colony-forming units per volume of sample.

Autobac IDX System

The Autobac system uses forward light scattering to optically monitor bacterial growth (Fig. 22-4). It is designed to perform antimicrobial susceptibility testing, gram-negative organism identification, and urine screening. The most common configuration of the Autobac consists of an incubator-shaker module, a photometer module, and a computer-data terminal-printer. Disposable plastic cuvettes are inoculated, incubated in the incubator-shaker module, and removed for reading in the photometer module. Extra information concerning an organism may be entered into the instrument's computer by the operator prior to reading for identification.

Identification and susceptibility testing are performed in 18-chamber disposable cuvettes. A standardized turbidity of inoculum is prepared and diluted with a low-thymidine eugonic broth for inoculation of a cuvette. Paper disks impregnated with identification compounds or antimicrobial agents are dispensed into

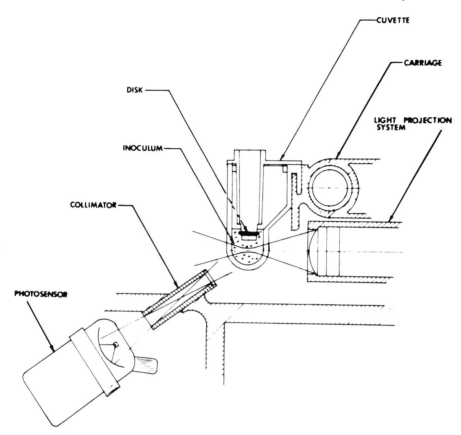

Figure 22-4. Optical arrangement of the cuvette in the Autobac photometer. (Prag-lin J, Curtis AC, Longhenry DK, McKie JE: Automation in Microbiology and Im-munology. New York, John Wiley & Sons, 1975)

the cuvette and the inoculum is added. The cuvette is then placed in the incubator-shaker and incubated for 3 hours. During incubation, the cuvettes are continuously shaken to ensure a homogeneous suspension of bacterial cells; this prevents bubble formation on the optical cell walls and permits rapid elution of antimicrobial agents or identification compounds from the paper disks.

Antimicrobial susceptibility testing yields category results (susceptible, in-termediate, or resistant) as well as statistically calculated MIC values. Those results are based upon comparisons of the amount of growth in the presence of the antimicrobial agents to the amount of growth after the same time in broth alone. The amount of growth is determined by forward light scattering, and a light scattering index (LSI) is derived by the computer. The LSI is a percent inhibition of growth parameter varying from 0 for resistant organisms to 1 for susceptible organisms.[2]

The Autobac data base for identification is nonclassical; it is based upon selective growth inhibition by dyes, antibiotics, and other compounds. Dyes used are acriflavine, brilliant green, malachite green, and methylene blue. Growth-inhibiting chemicals include cobalt chloride, 3,5-dibromosalicylic acid, dodecyl-amine hydrochloride, floxuridine, omadine disulfide, sodium azide, and thallous acetate. Selectively inhibiting antibiotics are carbenicillin, cephalothin, cycloser-ine, kanamycin, and novobiocin.[1] The Autobac data base also requires manual testing of the organism for additional information, including oxidase reaction, indole spot test, and swarming on blood agar. Manual testing is also required for documentation of growth, bile precipitation, and lactose fermentation on MacConkey's agar. If there is sufficient growth at the 3-hour reading, an identi-fication will be produced by the system. If growth is insufficient, the cuvette is reincubated and additional readings are required every 30 minutes for up to 6 hours.

Urine screening is performed by inoculating cuvette chambers with separate aliquots of urine. Once inoculated, the cuvette is placed in the photometer module for an initial reading. The cuvette is then placed in the incubator shaker and removed hourly for readings until positive or until 5 hours have elapsed. Significant bacterial growth is indicated by an appropriate change in LSI readings.

The Autobac System is only partially automated. An operator must dispense the disks, dilute the inoculum to a standard turbidity, and inoculate the cuvettes. After 3 hours, for identification or susceptibility determinations, the operator must manually transfer the cuvettes to the photometer module and, if sufficient growth has not occurred, repeat these transfers at 30-minute intervals for up to 6 hours elapsed time from inoculation. For urine screens, hourly transfer for readings are required.

Abbott MS-2 System

The Abbott MS-2 system is designed to perform urine screening, identification of both gram-negative bacteria and yeasts, and antimicrobial susceptibility testing. The MS-2 instrument consists of one or more analysis modules, which also func-tion as incubators for susceptibility testing and as a control module. Multiple analysis modules may be interfaced with one control module. Each analysis mod-ule has eight compartments for incubation that, for urine screens and susceptibility testing, allow automated optical monitoring of growth in plastic cuvettes. Iden-tification cuvettes are incubated off-line in a standard microbiologic incubator and are placed in the analysis module only for an initial reading and a reading at the end of 5 hours. Two new versions of the Abbott MS-2 have become available, the Abbott Quantum II and the Abbott Avantage. These systems use essentially the same plastic cuvettes as the MS-2, but the Quantum offers a coupled program of Abbott immunoassays and instrumentation for bacterial identification, and the Avantage offers increased automation of MS-2 functions and data management capabilities.

The Abbott bacterial identification system uses a disposable plastic cartridge with 20 lyophilized conventional biochemical substrates. A paper strip seals the top of the cartridge. Four or five well-isolated colonies are suspended in water and are adjusted to match a 0.5 McFarland standard. Then, 200 μl of inoculum per well is dispensed by puncturing the paper strip sealing each of the 20 cartridge chambers. A disposable inoculator is provided by the system. The cartridge is then inserted into the analysis module for an initial reading, incubated off-line for 4 hours, and reinserted into the analysis module for the final reading. Colorimetric analysis is completely automated to reduce the chance of error from interpretation or transcription. The same bacterial identification system, with off-line incubation, is used with the MS-2, Quantum II, and Avantage.

Susceptibility testing using the Abbott MS-2 and the Avantage instruments uses a separate 11-well cuvette cartridge into which antimicrobial disks are loaded and sealed. The remainder of the same standardized inoculum prepared for bacterial identification can be used for susceptibility testing. The upper growth chambers of the cuvette cartridge are filled with culture medium and inoculum. Specimen information is entered into the computer and the cuvette cartridge is inserted into the analysis module. When the proper cell density has been attained, indicating active log phase growth, the culture is automatically transferred from the upper to the lower cuvette chambers. Ten of the eleven chambers contain a specific antimicrobial disk; the eleventh chamber serves as a growth control. Once the culture is transferred, the growth within each chamber is photometrically monitored at 5-minute intervals. These readings are retained in the memory of the control module. A microcomputer utilizes an appropriate algorithm to compute each susceptibility result. Both qualitative and quantitative (MIC) results are printed out in 3 to 5 hours. Susceptibility testing is not available using the Quantum II.

A research cartridge is also available for the MS-2 and the Avantage. The open research cartridge permits the introduction of varying concentrations of test materials as well as organisms or media. Using multiple optical scanning systems to kinetically monitor turbidometric changes, the research cartridge performs special tests such as synergy studies, Schlichter testing, and minimum bactericidal (MBC) level testing.

Urine screening is performed using special test units, 100 μl of urine, and an adaptor for the analysis module. Eleven urine samples can be screened in one analysis module, which continuously monitors the presence or absence of growth for up to 5 hours. Detection of positives may occur as early as 40 minutes. Positive urines may then be plated in a conventional manner for later identification and susceptibility patterns.

Yeast identification by both the AMS-Vitek system and the Abbott automated systems involves the inoculation of a card or cartridge, off-line incubation at 30°C, and a final reading at 24 hours. Conventional biochemical reactions are used and germ tube reactions are part of the data base. Both systems print out the identification of the yeast with percentage probabilities.

Bactec System

The Bactec system is based upon a concept not previously applied to microbiology. It is an automated system for the detection of bacteremia and contains four components: (1) disposable culture vials that are inoculated with the patient's blood, (2) the Bactec instrument that automatically and sequentially tests the vials to determine microbial growth, (3) the culture gas and adaptors that regulate the flow of gas, and (4) a shaker that provides side-to-side agitation of aerobic vials.

The most commonly used Bactec system at this time is the Bactec 460, which has a reading capacity of 60 vials. The detection of microorganisms is based upon the microbial utilization of ^{14}C-labeled glucose and other substrates, with the subsequent production of $^{14}CO_2$, and upon measurement in a vial. Aerobic and anaerobic bacteria, fungi, and mycobacteria are detected.

CULTURE VIALS

Specific Bactec culture vials are designed for optimal growth of aerobic and anaerobic organisms, with or without resin for antimicrobial inactivation. A hypertonic (10% sucrose) medium is also available. Each vial contains culture medium with ^{14}C-labeled substrates in a sterile, ready-to-use form. After inoculation with 3 to 5 ml of blood, the vials are incubated off-line in a standard microbiology incubator at 35°C. The aerobic vials are placed on the Bactec shaker for the first 24 hours to achieve more rapid organism growth.

Culture vials are placed on the Bactec instrument in four-vial racks. Once the tops are cleansed with alcohol, the instrument automatically tests all 60 vials in 1 hour, without operator interaction. Testing is performed by aspirating the gas above the culture medium, measuring its radioactivity, and printing the result as a growth index (GI) number. A specific threshold is preset for aerobic and for anaerobic testing. If the measured radioactivity exceeds the threshold, a red indicator corresponding to the vial tested is lighted on the front panel and a positive (P) mark is made on the print-tape at that vial location.

Referring to Figure 22-5, the operation of the instrument begins with the pump producing a partial vacuum in the ion chamber. During this time, the twin 18-gauge needles are heated. The head valve then closes, lowering the moveable head and driving the testing needles through the rubber septum of the vial being tested. When the outlet valve closes, the inlet valve opens, drawing gas from a reserve cylinder through a filter and the culture vial. This flushes the atmosphere above the broth level into the ion chamber for measurement.

ELECTROMETER

The electrometer is a dipolar measurement system. Radioactive gas passing through the ion chamber changes the impedance between two poles. The impedance is converted to a GI number displayed on the front panel and printed on the tape.* If the GI value exceeds the preset threshold value, a red light will be seen. The head valve then opens and the head rises, after which the sample changer moves to bring the next vial into position. The pump draws room air through the dust filter, the flush valve, and the ion chamber, transferring all the $^{14}CO_2$ into the soda–lime CO_2 trap where it is retained. This cleanses the measuring system (electrometer) prior to the next reading cycle.

The major advantages of the Bactec system are the detection of positive blood

*From Geisler R, Johnston Laboratories, personal commmunication.

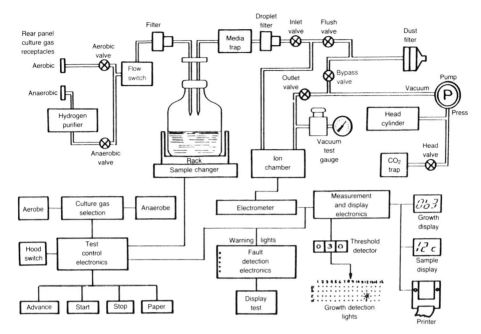

Figure 22-5. Flow diagram of the Bactec instrument. (Courtesy of Johnston Laboratories)

cultures earlier than conventional methods, the elimination of blind subcultures, and a significant decrease in the technologist's time. When combined with automated identification and susceptibility instruments, a report of a positive blood culture with the presumptive organism identification and susceptibilities can be made in 12 to 24 hours. This is possible with a high-grade bacteremia and a metabolically active organism.

The Bactec system is also capable of performing limited *Neisseria* identification and automated mycobacterial detection and susceptibilities. The *Neisseria* identification will separate *Neisseria gonorrhoeae, N. meningitidis,* and *N. lactamica* using ^{14}C-labeled sugars (glucose, maltose, or fructose) in specially formulated Bactec vials and a manually performed O-nitrophenyl-β-D-galactopyranoside (ONPG) test. The inoculated vials are incubated in a standard microbiology incubator for 3 hours at 35°C and then placed on the Bactec instrument for reading.

Radiometric detection of mycobacteria with the Bactec system employs a different detection hood (aerosol containment). The method relies upon the use of special Bactec vials, with 7H12 broth medium containing (1-^{14}C) palmitic acid. The detection of growth again uses the measurement of labeled CO_2 released by the metabolism of palmitic acid. Viable *Mycobacterium tuberculosis* can be detected from sputum specimens in 7 to 12 days, a great saving in detection time. Decontamination and concentration steps are still required. Use of a new growth medium containing an antibiotic supplement may further decrease time for detection of growth. Susceptibility testing of *M. tuberculosis,* using antibiotic dilutions in ^{14}C-labeled broth, has proved rapid and accurate. Atypical mycobacteria may be detected readily but their susceptibility testing is not yet standardized.

Bactec NR-660

Bactec Systems is now producing a new nonradioactive bacteremia-detection system, the Bactec NR-660.* The NR-660 detects bacterial growth by an infrared analysis of CO_2 content in the test vial. This system is significantly more automated because incubation and measurement take place in a single test module. When prompted by the system's computer, the operator loads the instrument with trays that hold up to 60 vials. The computer tracks the location of every vial in order to test it according to the correct schedule and sequence. Testing is completely automated; positive cultures are flagged and listed for each test, instrument status is monitored for quality assurance, and periodic maintenance is routinely monitored. To determine positive cultures, the instrument compares each vial's growth value (GV) reading with previously defined threshold and δ-GV criteria.

New Automated Systems

SENSITITRE MIC/ID

A new entry into the field of microbiologic automation is the Gibco Sensititre MIC/ID* system, which utilizes a unique fluorescent technology. A Sensititre automatic inoculator fills 96 wells of a microtiter plate with a precisely measured amount of organism suspension in less than 30 seconds. Prefilled test wells are available with a total of 22 different dehydrated antimicrobial agents arranged in twofold dilution steps. The inoculated plates are sealed, incubated in a standard microbiology incubator at 35°C, and read at 5 or 18 hours for same-day or overnight results.

Several substrates are used in the inoculum broth that are nonfluorescent in their native state. When hydrolyzed by bacterial enzymes, these substrates release chromophores that fluoresce upon excitation with ultraviolet light. The fluorescence produced is proportional to the increase in the number of cells. The addition of antimicrobial agents will, if inhibitory, prevent cell multiplication and decrease fluorescence. When placed in the new Sensititre Autoreader, each plate is read in less than 25 seconds. The Sensititre DEC Professional 350 computer compares fluorescence readings from the control well to fluorescence in wells containing dilutions of antimicrobial agents in order to construct a growth curve at the time of reading.

ALADIN

Another new concept in automation is the ALADIN,* a totally automated instrument designed to read all UniScept (API)* products.† After inoculation, the UniScept strips are placed in a labeled universal carrier, which is a disposable plastic frame responsible for standardizing the positioning of all UniScept tests with respect to the reagent dispenser and read stations. The universal carrier is then placed in the incubator module, which holds 60 carriers (as many as 180

†From Godsey JH, Analytab Products, personal communication.

individual tests). An electronic sensor enables ALADIN to continuously monitor the status and location of all in-progress tests. At the predetermined reading time, the universal carrier is transferred automatically to the reagent dispenser station where up to 20 different liquid reagents may be dispensed. The reagent dispenser station is preprogrammed to recognize the UniScept product and dispense reagents into the correct cupules. Each reagent reservoir is monitored, with an audible alarm sounding if the remaining reagent volume is insufficient.

The read station contains a video image processor that is used to interpret colored biochemical reactions or turbidometric growth patterns in susceptibility tests. Video image processing is a method of digitizing an image into a large matrix. Only those portions of the digital image that are of interest (microtiter wells and identification strip cupules) are maintained in the image processor's memory. The video image processor has the ability to look for signal changes from as many as 300 individual detectors located in a particular area of interest. Thus, various growth patterns in susceptibility wells are interpreted correctly, bubbles and particles are not read as positives, and biochemical reactions are thoroughly scanned.

After test interpretation, ALADIN has two options: (1) disposal of the universal carrier or (2) mechanical removal of the processed identification strip followed by return of the susceptibility test in the universal carrier to the incubator for continued incubation. The disposal station is located inside the ALADIN instrument and consists of an aluminum frame supporting a biohazard bag. As the universal carrier and its contents are dumped, the capacity of the bag is monitored. When the bag is full, a warning light is displayed.

Appendix

Trade Names	Company
1. Abbott Avantage	Abbott Laboratories Diagnostics Division Irving, TX
2. Abbott MS-2	Abbott Laboratories Diagnostics Division Irving, TX
3. Abbott Quantum II	Abbott Laboratories Diagnostics Division Irving, TX
4. ALADIN	Analytab Products Plainview, NY
5. Autobac IDX System	General Diagnostics Morris Plains, NJ
6. Automicrobic System	Vitek Systems, Inc. Hazelwood, MO
7. Bactec	Johnston Laboratories Cockeysville, MD
8. Sensititre MIC/ID	Gibco Laboratories Lawrence, MA
9. Uniscept	Analytab Products Plainview, NY

References

1. D'Amato RF, McLaughlin JC, Ferraro MJ: Rapid and mechanized/automated systems in microbiology. In Lennette EH (ed): Manual of Clinical Microbiology, 4th ed. Washington, DC, American Society for Microbiology, 1985
2. Heden CG, Illeni T: Automation in Microbiology and Immunology. New York, John Wiley & Sons, 1975

Suggested Reading

Auto Microbic System Operators Manual. Hazelwood, MO, Vitek Systems, Inc, 1982

Bactec NR-660 Operations and Maintenance Manual. Towson, MD, Johnston Laboratories, 1985

Heden CG, Illeni T: Automation in Microbiology and Immunology. New York, John Wiley & Sons, 1975

Kelly MT: Instruments for microbial identification. Clin Lab Med 5(1):91, 1985

Operation and Maintenance Manual for the Bactec 460. Cockeysville, MD, Johnston Laboratories, 1984

Staneck JL, Allen SD, Harris EE, Tilton RC: Automated reading of MIC microdilution trays containing fluorogenic enzyme substrates with the Sensititre Autoreader. JCM 22:187, 1985

Thornsberry C: Automated procedure for microbial susceptility tests. In Lennette E (ed): Manual of Clinical Microbiology, 4th ed. Washington, DC, American Society for Microbiology, 1985

INDEX

The letter *f* after a page number indicates a figure; *t* following a page number indicates tabular material.